The Children's Hospital at Westmead Handbook

GW00482891

the children's hospital at Westmead

The Children's Hospital at Westmead Handbook

Clinical practice guidelines
for paediatrics

HENRY KILHAM AND DAVID ISAACS, EDITORS

The McGraw-Hill Companies

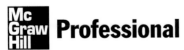

Professional

Text © 2004 Children's Hospital at Westmead
Illustrations and design © 2004 McGraw-Hill Australia Pty Ltd
Additional owners of copyright are acknowledged on the Acknowledgments page.

National Library of Australia Cataloguing-in-Publication data:

The Children's Hospital at Westmead handbook: clinical practice guidelines for Paediatrics.

Includes index.
ISBN 0 074 71161 X.

1.New Children's Hospital (Westmead, N.S.W.) – Handbooks, manuals etc. 2. Children – Hospital care – Handbooks, manuals etc. 3. Pediatrics – Handbooks, manuals, etc.
I. Kilham, Henry. II. Isaacs, David, MD.

618.92

Published in Australia by
McGraw-Hill Australia Pty Ltd
Level 2, 82 Waterloo Road, North Ryde NSW 2113
Acquisitions Editor: Meiling Voon
Associate Editor: Thu Nguyen
Production Editor: Kathryn Murphy
Editor: Joy Window
Proofreader: Tim Learner
Indexer: Glenda Browne
Designer (cover and interior): Jan Schmoeger
Illustrator: Alan Laver
Typeset in 9.5/11 pt Caslon by Midland Typesetters
Printed on 80 gsm matt art by Pantech Limited, Hong Kong.

The McGraw·Hill Companies

Contents

List of contributors   vii

Preface   ix

1   Practical paediatrics   1

2   Laboratory reference ranges   5

3   Emergencies   12

4   Nutrition and infant feeding   30

5   Haematology   42

6   Pain management   57

7   Fluid and electrolyte therapy   67

8   Neonatal medicine   80

9   Biochemical genetic emergencies   104

10   Anti-infective drugs and guidelines   112

11   Fever and severe infections   123

12   Infectious diseases and immunisation   139

13   Cardiology   154

14   Respiratory diseases   164

15   Endocrinology and diabetes   186

16   Gastroenterology   216

17   Neurology and neurosurgery   229

18	Renal medicine	248
19	Psychiatry	265
20	The adolescent patient	276
21	Oncological emergencies	292
22	Abuse of children	297
23	Important skin conditions	307
24	Ocular emergencies	318
25	Common ENT conditions	327
26	Dental and oro-facial emergencies	331
27	Acute poisoning and envenomation	337
28	Preanaesthetic preparation	343
29	Sedation for procedures	346
30	Management of burns	355
31	General surgery	363
32	Trauma and orthopaedics	374
33	Dying and death	383
34	Growth charts	389
35	Developmental assessment and screening	404
Appendix	Drug dosage guidelines	410
Index		487

List of contributors

The following members of the staff of the Children's Hospital at Westmead contributed material which was used by the editors in this handbook:

Stephen Alexander
Geoff Ambler
Jane Anthony
Peter Barr
Andrew Berry
Margaret Burgess
Danny Cass
Megan Chambers
Ray Chaseling
John Christodoulou
John Coakley
John Collins
Michael Cooper
Peter Cooper
Chris Cowell
Genevieve Cummins
Julie Curtin
Jonathan de Lima
Mark Dexter
David Dosseter
Carolyn Ellaway
Martin Glasson
Paddy Grattan-Smith
Robert Halliday
Victor Harrison
John Harvey
David Isaacs
Alyson Kakakios

Ramanand Kamath
Melissa Kang
Henry Kilham
Michael Kohn
Kasia Kozlowska
Robyn Lamb
Deborah Lewis
David Little
Peter McIntyre
Frank Martin
Hugh Martin
Ken Nunn
Tony O'Connell
Ted O'Loughlin
Kim Oates
Robert Ouvrier
Peter Procopis
Phil Renner
Maureen Rogers
David Schell
Hiran Selvadurai
Gary Sholler
Albert Shun
Michael Stevens
Jane Storman
Paul Tait
Sue Towns
Peter Van Asperen

Richard Widmer

Bridget Wilcken

Katrina Williams

Carola Wittekind

Julian Wojtulewicz

The exclusion of anyone from this list is purely accidental and in no way lessens the gratitude for contributions received.

Many other staff members have given much appreciated assistance via content evaluation and proofreading.

Preface

The *Royal Alexandra Hospital for Children (RAHC) Handbook* was first produced in 1964, for use by the hospital's resident medical staff. It has been progressively revised and rewritten, as the *Children's Hospital Handbook*, and (in 1999) as the *New Children's Hospital Handbook*, following the hospital's move to Westmead in 1995. This version carries the hospital's new name, the Children's Hospital at Westmead.

The handbook is intended to be a practical manual, and not a textbook. Emphasis is given to serious conditions, to common clinical situations where guidance is often needed and to frequently needed information such as laboratory reference ranges, drug doses, immunisation schedules and growth charts.

The handbook's new subtitling as 'clinical practice guidelines' is a reminder that such guidelines, evidence-based wherever possible, have been in use for decades. Guidelines are not intended to cover every possible clinical situation. They should be used as general guidance and as a check-list of actions to consider. Guidelines do not represent a 'standard of care' in medical, legal or other terms.

Great efforts have been made to make this handbook a useful and practical guide for good management of sick children. However, the handbook should not be used as a substitute for appropriate discussion and consultation. The responsibility for decisions made in management belong to the medical practitioner treating the patient. The final responsibility for hospital patients lies with the physician or surgeon in charge, whose clinical judgment and experience will ultimately determine the treatment used.

Many members of the hospital's staff have contributed to this and previous editions and their help is gratefully acknowledged. We particularly acknowledge the work of Mrs Kim Gillett in the completion of this edition.

HENRY KILHAM
Departments of General Medicine,
Respiratory Medicine, Clinical Toxicology
and Pain,
The Children's Hospital at Westmead
Associate Professor, Department of
Paediatrics and Child Health, The University
of Sydney

DAVID ISAACS
Departments of Education, and Immunology
and Infectious Diseases,
The Children's Hospital at Westmead
Clinical Professor, Department of Paediatrics
and Child Health, The University of Sydney

1

Practical paediatrics

This chapter includes:

- requirements of good paediatric practice
- making the diagnosis
- the child in hospital
- principles of good care.

Requirements of good paediatric practice

- A sound basic approach
- A working knowledge of child growth and development
- An appropriate history and physical examination
- Knowing where to find additional information
- Being ready to ask for advice if you don't know
- Recognising the family and social context
- Whenever possible, a sense of humour

More mistakes are made by not asking (that is, a poor history) and by not looking (that is, inadequate examination) than by not knowing.

Making the diagnosis

- Enquire about the presenting problem/s.
- Take whatever background history is relevant to the type of consultation. For a child requiring hospital admission, this will always include full past, family and social history. In any consultation ask about the child's immunisation status.
- Commence your examination with observation from 1–2 metres: does the child appear unwell, pale, afraid, short of breath, drowsy or abnormal in any other way? This part of the examination is often the most revealing.

- Continue the examination by going to the site of the presenting complaint, or to the system you think is most likely to be involved.
- Write down a differential diagnosis.
- Perform only simple investigations first.
- In an emergency situation, ask what has happened while assessing the urgent priorities—A (airway), B (breathing), C (circulation)—then direct the examination to the apparent problem. (See Chapter 3.)
- Explain to the parents and the child what you are doing at each stage.
- If unable to make a firm diagnosis, remember that you are more likely to be seeing an atypical or unusual presentation of a common illness, as opposed to a truly 'rare' condition.
- Where the diagnosis is unclear, tell the parents this and, also, your plan of action.
- Don't hesitate to consult if necessary.

The child in hospital

Effects of illness and being in hospital

- Children's thoughts and feelings about illness, injury, pain, operations and hospital can be difficult to discern.
- Some apparently 'good' children may in reality be depressed, withdrawn or in pain; many will 'overreact' to even comparatively harmless procedures.
- 'Needles' are universally feared and/or disliked by children.
- Regression to a less mature behaviour pattern is common, especially if the child is immobilised, is very unwell, or requires prolonged treatment.
- Separation from family is a most stressful aspect of hospital care. A very young child will often not understand why his or her mother has left, or that she will ever return.
- Children often misinterpret illness or treatment as punishment.

Some paediatric pitfalls

- Comments by hospital staff implying ineptitude of other doctors are common. In paediatrics such comments are often also made about parents and schoolteachers. Decry this unfair and useless

practice. If mistakes have indeed been made, learn from them yourself.
- Be wary of discounting parental anxiety. A mother's intuitive feeling that her young child is seriously unwell should be interpreted as a 'red flag', even if the child does not look especially unwell to you.
- Be wary of the quiet child: he/she may be the most emotionally disturbed one.
- Be wary of assuming what you say in the presence of any child will not be understood. This pitfall is especially relevant with a dysmorphic, physically impaired or apparently unconscious child.

Principles of good care

Active efforts are needed to minimise the separation, pain, unfamiliarity, loneliness and boredom that often accompany illness where hospital admission is required. Remember the importance of the family in the child's illness and the child's illness in the family.

Good medical care

- Minimise the number of procedures (injections, blood collection, catheterisations and so on) and perfect the skills in carrying out these procedures, to cause the least fear, suspense, pain, surprise or indignity.
- Carefully organise the investigation and treatment to minimise the length of admission.
- Use adequate analgesia for painful procedures, where necessary using injections or infusions of narcotic analgesics 'titrated against' the child's pain.
- Make hospital admissions as short as possible.

Appreciating the special vulnerability of some children:

- Very young children
- Those from broken or disturbed homes
- Those who have had previous illness or accidents
- Those suffering severe pain
- Those who react badly to change
- Those having eye, mouth, throat, genital and bowel operations
- Those who have suffered physical, sexual or emotional abuse

Avoiding separation from parents— especially the mother

This is a crucial countermeasure and it has the following benefits:

- It reduces distress in the child and parents.
- It promotes the relationship between mother and child.
- It promotes the parents' understanding of the child's illness and future needs.
- It helps medical and nursing staff to understand the child's unique characteristics and needs.
- It speeds convalescence.

Communicating

Parents must be kept appropriately informed about their child's progress and made to feel that their contribution is valued and taken into consideration. Try to talk directly with them each day. Family doctors must be kept informed of progress and the treatment plan at discharge.

Play and education

To a small child, 'play is work, thought, art and relaxation'. Providing opportunities for play serves many needs; possibly the most important is helping the child cope with the hospital experience. Older children should, whenever possible, continue schoolwork when in hospital.

2

Laboratory reference ranges

This chapter includes:

- haematology—reference ranges
- biochemistry—reference ranges.

Haematology

Correct collection of blood specimens is the cornerstone of accurate diagnosis in paediatric haematology.

Capillary collection techniques are essential for neonates and young children; free-flowing blood from the heel or a finger-prick is added to collection tubes with powdered EDTA (for blood counts and most other haematology tests) or sodium citrate (for coagulation studies) and mixed well. 'Direct' blood films (made at the time of collection from the skin-prick site or from the syringe) have the advantage of being free of the artefacts induced by anticoagulants and are better for the diagnosis of bacterial sepsis.

Always consider a problem with specimen collection if a result is inconsistent with the clinical findings. Common paediatric artefacts include:

- *a partially clotted sample.* This occurs because of 'slow' blood flow, inadequate mixing with the anticoagulant or adding too much blood for the amount of anticoagulant in the tube. This results in false thrombocytopenia, neutropenia or abnormal coagulation studies.
- *dilutional errors.* These can occur in samples collected on in-patients with intravenous lines if venous blood is collected proximal to the IV site or if blood is collected from an indwelling catheter without discarding the initial aliquot equivalent to 1.5 times the dead-space of the line. This results in falsely low blood counts or abnormal coagulation studies.
- *heparin contamination.* Minimal amounts of heparin in IV lines or

at three-way taps may give prolongation of the activated partial thromboplastin time (APTT).

Table 2.1 Normal haematological values

Coagulation studies	Normal range for children > 6 months
Plasma studies	
Prothrombin time (PT)	11–15 seconds
International normalised ratio (INR)	1.0–1.3
Activated partial thromboplastin time (APTT)	27–39 seconds
Fibrinogen	Above 1.5 g/L
D-dimer	< 0.2 mg/L
Lysate studies*	
Prothrombin index (PI)	80–100%
Kaolin clotting time (KCT)	Within 10–15 seconds of value recorded as calculated normal for packed cell volume

* Lysate studies are done when only capillary samples are obtainable.
For infants < 6 months of age, the normal ranges for some of these studies are prolonged. Any results that fall outside these normal ranges need to be discussed with a haematologist.

Miscellaneous haematological tests
Serum ferritin
- Age > 6 months: 10–150 mg/L
- Ferritin is an acute phase reactant and is raised in inflammation, liver disease and malignancy.

Haemoglobin electrophoresis
Haemoglobins A, F and A_2 are normally identified.

Test	Normal range (after 12 months of age)
HbA_2	2.1–3.7%
HbF	< 1.5% (alkali denaturation)
	< 1% acid resistant cells (Kleihauer)

Table 2.2 Haematological age-related reference ranges

Test	Units	Birth	1 week	1 month	3–12 months	5 years	10 years	Puberty
Haemoglobin	g/L	140–225	135–205	100–130	95–140	115–140	115–150	130–160 M 120–160 F
WBC (total)	× 10⁹/L	9–30	5–21	5–19	5–17	5–14.5	4.5–13.5	4.5–13
Platelets	× 10⁹/L	150–600	150–600	150–600	150–600	150–600	150–600	150–600
RBC indices								
Haematocrit	L/L	0.47–0.62	0.42–0.62	0.30–0.48	0.28–0.45	0.35–0.45	0.35–0.48	0.36–0.46 M 0.37–0.48 F
MCV	Fl	100–135	100–120	84–105	70–85	75–90	77–95	78–95
MCH	Pg	31–37	28–40	24–36	24–36	24–31	25–33	25–35
MCHC	%	32–36	32–36	32–36	32–36	32–36	32–36	32–36
White cells								
Neutrophils	× 10⁹/L	1.5–25	1.5–10	1–8	1–8	1–8	1.5–8	1.5–8
Lymphocytes	× 10⁹/L	2–11	2–17	2–13	2–13	1.5–10	1.5–7	1.0–6
Monocytes	× 10⁹/L	0.1–1.7	0.1–1.7	0.1–1.7	0.2–1.2	0.2–1.2	0.2–1.0	0.2–0.8
Eosinophils	× 10⁹/L	0.1–1.1	0.1–1.1	0.1–1.1	0.1–1.1	0.1–1.1	0.1–1.1	0.1–1.1
Other tests								
Reticulocytes	× 10⁹/L	110–450	<10–80	20–65	20–105	20–105	20–105	20–105
ESR*	mm/h		0–2	0–13	0–13	0–20	0–20	0–15 M 0–20 F

*The ESR may be artificially prolonged in anaemia unrelated to acute inflammation.

- Heterozygous β thalassaemia: Hb A_2 is raised and Hb F is slightly raised in 50% of cases.
- Homozygous β thalassaemia: Hb F > 50%; usually 90–100% of erythrocytes contain Hb F.

Heterophile antibody agglutination test ('monospot' or equivalent)

Antibodies of infectious mononucleosis are rarely present in the first week of the illness. They commonly appear towards the end of the second week or during the third week and may persist for 3 months. It is unusual to find them in children younger than 4 years of age. EBV IgM antibody testing is preferable in this age group.

Cold agglutinin titre

- This is a screening test done against adult group O cells.
- Normal range at 4°C: < 1:64

Biochemistry

Blood collection rounds

In-patient blood collection rounds occur each morning of the week except for Saturday and Sunday (when there are collections for urgent tests only). Another collection round occurs at 2 p.m. on weekdays, but this is only for tests which have missed the morning collection round and which require a result that day. Please contact the laboratory if you need an urgent blood collection or a collection on the 2 p.m. round.

Specimen requirements

As a general rule, 0.5 mL of blood is required for EUC, 0.5 mL for LFT and an extra 0.5 mL for every three of the common tests added on. Common tests are listed in Table 2.3. Most drug estimations require 0.5 mL of blood. Thyroid function tests require 3.0 mL of blood. For less common tests, contact the laboratory.

Special requirements

- Most tests can be done on plasma (lithium heparin tube). However, cyclosporin and tacrolimus require whole blood (0.5 mL EDTA for each drug).

Table 2.3 Common reference ranges

Test	Reference range	Age
Blood: electrolytes, urea, creatinine and total protein		
Sodium	135–145 mmol/L	All ages
Potassium	4.5–6.5 mmol/L	< 1 week
	3.8–6.0 mmol/L	1 week–1 month
	3.5–5.5 mmol/L	> 1 month
Chloride	95–110 mmol/L	All ages
Bicarbonate	18–24 mmol/L	< 2 years
	22–30 mmol/L	> 2 years
Urea	1.3–5.1 mmol/L	< 1 month
	2.0–6.7 mmol/L	1 month–4 years
	2.7–6.7 mmol/L	> 4 years
Creatinine	< 90 µmol/L	< 1 week
	20–50 µmol/L	1 week–1 month
	20–45 µmol/L	1 month–1 year
	25–50 µmol/L	1–4 years
	30–60 µmol/L	4–8 years
	40–70 µmol/L	8–12 years
	45–85 µmol/L	12–16 years
	45–100 µmol/L	> 16 years
Total protein	50–69 g/L	< 1 month
	52–74 g/L	1 month–1 year
	60–79 g/L	1–4 years
	62–83 g/L	> 4 years
Blood: liver function tests		
Albumin	26–38 g/L	< 1 month
	30–44 g/L	1 month–1 year
	30–45 g/L	1–5 years
	33–46 g/L	> 5 years
Total bilirubin	< 100 µmol/L	< 2 weeks
	< 30 µmol/L	2–4 weeks
	< 10 µmol/L	> 4 weeks
Direct bilirubin	< 10 µmol/L	All ages
ALT	20–60 U/L	< 1 month
(alanine transaminase)	10–50 U/L	> 1 month
GGT	25–200 U/L	< 1 month
(gamma glutamyl	17–150 U/L	1–3 months
transpeptidase)	4–33 U/L	> 3 months

continues . . .

Table 2.3 Common reference ranges *(continued)*

Test	Reference range	Age
ALP	160–400 U/L	< 6 months
(alkaline phosphatase)	140–360 U/L	6 months–2 years
	130–325 U/L	2–10 years
	80–355 U/L	> 10 years

Other common blood tests

Ammonia	20–100 µmol/L	< 1 month
	10–50 µmol/L	> 1 month
Amylase	5–45 U/L	< 1 year
	20–85 U/L	> 1 year
AST	20–90 U/L	< 1 month
(aspartate transaminase)	10–50 U/L	> 1 month
Calcium	1.80–2.65 mmol/L	< 2 weeks
	2.10–2.65 mmol/L	> 2 weeks
Cholesterol	2.9–5.3 mmol/L	
CK	24–215 U/L	> 1 month
(creatine kinase)		
Glucose	3.5–5.5 mmol/L	All ages
Lactate	< 2.0 mmol/L	All ages
Magnesium	0.71–0.96 mmol/L	All ages
Osmolality	265–295 mmol/kg	All ages
Phosphorus	1.5–2.7 mmol/L	< 2 weeks
	1.2–2.1 mmol/L	2 weeks–2 years
	1.0–1.8 mmol/L	2–16 years
	0.9–1.6 mmol/L	> 16 years
Triglyceride	0.5–1.4 mmol/L	< 5 years
(fasting)	0.6–1.7 mmol/L	> 5 years
Urate	0.10–0.30 mmol/L	1–3 years
	0.12–0.35 mmol/L	3–12 years

Serum drug levels

Carbamazepine	20–40 µmol/L
Cyclosporin	Dependent on transplant type
Digoxin	1.3–2.5 nmol/L
Phenobarbitone	40–130 µmol/L
Phenytoin	40–80 µmol/L
Theophylline	40–80 µmol/L neonatal apnoea
	55–110 µmol/L asthma
Valproate	300–700 µmol/L

Table 2.3 Common reference ranges *(continued)*

Test	Reference range	Age
Thyroid function tests		
Free T4	13–30 pmol/L	< 1 month
	10–20 pmol/L	> 1 month
TSH	< 40.0 mU/L	1–3 days
	< 25.0 mU/L	3–7 days
	< 10.0 mU/L	1–2 weeks
	0.4–5.0 mU/L	> 2 weeks
Cerebrospinal fluid		
Glucose	> 3.0 mmol/L	
Protein	< 1.20 g/L	Full-term newborn
	0.20–0.80 g/L	< 1 month
	0.15–0.42 g/L	> 1 month
Urine		
Protein/creatinine ratio	< 0.02 mg/µmol	

- Ammonia test—requires 0.5 mL of blood into a lithium heparin tube, placed immediately on ice and sent to the laboratory as soon as possible.
- Lactate test—requires exactly 0.5 mL of blood (fill to the mark) into a special tube available from Pathology, placed immediately on ice and sent to the laboratory as soon as possible.
- Tests for galactosaemia—contact the laboratory for special requirements.
- Sweat tests—must be pre-booked. Please contact the laboratory to arrange an appointment.

3

Emergencies

This chapter includes:

- cardiorespiratory arrest
- circulatory failure (shock)
- coma
- anaphylaxis
- guidelines for tracheal intubation
- emergency patient transport and medical retrieval.

Other emergencies included in other chapters are:

- neonatal (Chapter 8)
- burns resuscitation (Chapter 30)
- status epilepticus (Chapter 17)
- suspected bacterial meningitis (Chapter 11)
- suspected septicaemia (Chapter 11)
- acute upper airway obstruction (Chapter 14)
- acute severe asthma (Chapter 14)
- severe hypertension (Chapter 18)
- diabetic ketoacidosis (Chapter 15)
- acute poisoning (Chapter 27).

The Emergency Team is available by telephoning 444 (within the Children's Hospital at Westmead) and simply giving the location.

Cardiorespiratory arrest

- Most often, in children, this follows severe hypoxaemia or hypovolaemia (blood loss or dehydration).
- It occasionally follows arrhythmia, for example in drug overdose.
- Children often 'compensate', maintaining respiratory effort and circulation, but without anticipation and correction of the underlying problem, then deteriorate suddenly.

- Prevent cardiac arrest wherever possible by recognising and treating increasing respiratory distress, cardiovascular compromise, blood loss and so on.

Note: For successful cardiopulmonary resuscitation (CPR), adequate circulation and ventilation must be re-established before irreparable cerebral and cardiac damage have occurred.

Preparation for emergencies

- All medical and nursing staff must know how to perform external cardiac compression and assisted ventilation.
- Children at high risk must be cared for by appropriate personnel in well-equipped areas. Continuous pulse oximetry must be used in children at risk of hypoxia.
- All clinical areas of the hospital are equipped with resuscitation trolleys, with laryngoscopes, endotracheal tubes, ventilating circuits, airways suction devices, a cardiac arrest board and intravenous equipment.

Management of cardiac arrest

- *Immediate steps (ABC; E)*: Cardiopulmonary resuscitation (CPR) commences with the recognition that the child is unconscious. Consciousness in an infant or young child is judged by lack of a verbal response to a loud call or tapping the child. Yell for assistance while commencing basic life support:
  A Maintain AIRWAY (clear mouth and pharynx, lift chin up and forward, place a Guedel airway).
  B Determine if BREATHING is present: if not, give 2–5 slow breaths. Maintain breathing (bag and mask with oxygen; if unavailable, use 'Resuscitube' or mouth-to-mouth).
  C Maintain CIRCULATION (external cardiac compression—ECC; see below). Place the index finger of the lower hand on the sternum just under the intermammary line. The area of compression is at the location of the middle and ring fingers (the lower third of the sternum). A board is placed under the child's chest.
  E Summon the EMERGENCY TEAM (Ext. 444) whose first duties are to simultaneously:
    – secure the airway (usually by tracheal intubation);
    – achieve vascular access; and
    – diagnose the arrhythmia using ECG monitoring.

Endotracheal tube (ETT) sizes for different ages are listed in Table 3.4. The most senior member of the team will take charge.

- Ventilation must be adequate but not excessive. Duration of inspirations should be 1–1.5 seconds, at the rate 20/min. Ventilate with 100% oxygen, using bag-valve-mask/tube, at 15 L/min. Check the position of the tube with a stethoscope, and suction the tube as necessary. Place a nasogastric tube if abdominal distension appears.

- External cardiac compression is best done by a second person. Once the child is intubated, there is no longer a need to synchronise chest compression with ventilation. Compression should be a firm downwards movement, occupying 50% of each cycle. Commence ECC if the heart rate is < 80 bpm in an infant, < 60 bpm in a small child, or < 40 bpm in a large child.

- ECG monitoring: The initial rhythm is almost always asystole or bradycardia (over 95% of the time). See the cardiorespiratory arrest algorithm, Figure 3.1.

Supraventricular tachycardia (SVT) causing a pulseless state is uncommon in children. Beware the use of verapamil for this condition, since children have a higher incidence of profound hypotension and asystole with rapid boluses of this drug. Adenosine (see below) is now the preferred drug for SVT.

Vascular access

- Venous (IV):
  - Potential veins: external jugular, saphenous, superficial temporal, cubital and those on the back of the hand.
  - If no access is gained after 3 attempts or 90 seconds (whichever comes first) attempt intraosseous access.
- Intraosseous (IO):
  - Useful for both drugs and fluids in children aged up to 6 years.
  - Place the short intraosseous needle via the anteromedial surface of the upper tibia just below the tibial tuberosity.
  - Use a rotary movement through the bone cortex; a slight loss of resistance is felt.
- Endotracheal (ET):
  - Used if IV or IO access has not been achieved within 3–5 minutes.
  - Give adrenaline in 10 times the IV dose, diluted to 2 mL with normal saline.

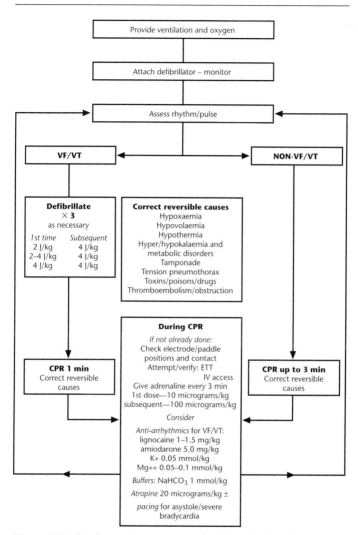

Figure 3.1 Cardiorespiratory arrest algorithm (adapted from Australian Resuscitation Council Guidelines)

- Use a syringe to squirt the drug into the ET tube, then 'bag' into the lungs.
- Use this route for atropine and lignocaine if needed.
- Intracardiac: ET use is now preferred to intracardiac for drugs, and IO route for fluids.

Drugs

Drug dosage is related to body mass (which may be unknown at the time of arrest). If necessary, use these equations to estimate body weight from age (which is usually known):

For children over 8 years of age: weight (kg) = 3 × age (years)

For children 1 to 8 years of age: weight (kg) = 8 + 2 × age (years)

- Adrenaline: The main drug for treating asystole and/or electro-mechanical dissociation (EMD). See Figure 3.1 for dosage.
- Sodium bicarbonate:
  - Recommended for hyperkalaemia, pre-existing bicarbonate-responsive metabolic acidosis, tricyclic antidepressant overdosage.
  - Now less strongly considered for acidosis after the return of circulation following prolonged arrest.
  - Initial dose is 1 mEq/kg (= 1 mL/kg of 8.4% solution).
  - Give further doses every 10 minutes while the arrest continues.
- Adenosine:
  - Now 'drug of choice' for SVT when the child is stable, or it can be given immediately in a child with IV access before cardioversion.
  - In the presence of circulatory instability use synchronised electrical cardioversion instead (0.5 J/kg).
  - Dose is 0.1 mg/kg; give as a rapid IV bolus.
- Atropine:
  - May be considered after adrenaline in bradycardia.
  - Use a minimum of 20 micrograms/kilogram to avoid paradox-ical bradycardia which occurs with lower doses.
- Bretylium: Not recommended.
- Calcium:
  - No longer recommended for asystole or EMD.
  - Indicated when hypocalcaemia has been proven; may be considered in treating hyperkalaemia, hypermagnesaemia and calcium channel blocker overdosage.

> – Dose is 0.2 mL/kg of 10% calcium chloride, repeated in 10 minutes if needed.

Fluids

- Blood volume must be returned to normal rapidly.
- In the short term, normal saline or Hartmann's solution will suffice regardless of the nature of the losses.
- Large losses must eventually be replaced with the appropriate solutions.
- Blood sugar levels should be monitored, especially in babies.
- Give 50% glucose (1 mL/kg) if blood sugar level is less than 3 mmol/L.
- Flushing solution during the arrest should be normal saline.
- After successful resuscitation, use dextrose-containing fluids to maintain blood sugar level in the range 3–10 mmol/L.

If CPR is successful

- Management of the post-arrest phase is as critical to recovery as that of the arrest.
- Secondary brain insults must be prevented—continue artificial ventilation, manage the child in the intensive care unit; monitor and manage post-arrest seizures, apnoea, myocardial failure, hypoglycaemia, electrolyte abnormalities and cerebral oedema (which may increase over 12 hours post-arrest).
- Reassess frequently; sedate for agitation; mildly hyperventilate.
- Where cardiac output remains low, and once euvolaemia has been achieved, consider inotrope infusion (for example, initially, adrenaline, 0.1 microgram/kg/min, or dopamine 5 micrograms/kg/min, or dobutamine 5 micrograms/kg/min).

When to stop

- The outcome in paediatric cardiac arrest is most often poor.
- In hypoxic arrest, failure to achieve the return of spontaneous circulation within 15 minutes is almost never followed by useful recovery.
- Exceptions include arrests associated with hyperkalaemia, hypothermia from immersion in water colder than 10°C, and cardiodepressant toxicity (for example, bupivicaine).
- The decision to terminate resuscitative efforts is difficult—consultation with a paediatric intensivist may help decision-making.

Documentation

Details of events and treatment are quickly forgotten unless promptly recorded. Where possible, one person is given this task.

Immediate investigations

- Obligatory: chest X-ray, pO_2, pH, pCO_2, haematocrit, blood sugar, serum electrolytes
- Other investigations, according to conditions present

Monitoring

- Obligatory: continuous ECG and pulse oximetry, blood gases, core body temperature, inspired oxygen concentration, urine output
- Other parameters, according to the conditions present

Circulatory failure (shock)

Physiologically, this can be defined as failure of the circulation to meet the metabolic needs of tissues. Clinically, it may be manifested as hypotension, usually tachycardia and pallor, and sometimes by cyanosis, sweating, oliguria, cold extremities, restlessness and an abnormal conscious state.

Progressive hypovolaemia is the primary problem in most children with shock; 'cardiogenic' shock is much less common; combinations of mechanisms may occur; for example in sepsis, decreased peripheral resistance, myocardial depression and hypovolaemia may coexist.

Remember that 'hidden' fluid losses (for example intraperitoneal in peritonitis, blood loss around major closed fractures) are usually underestimated. Abrupt changes in peripheral resistance or blood flow redistribution can lead to sudden shock with no external fluid losses (for example, in meningococcal septicaemia).

Immediate management

Simultaneously:

- Give 100% oxygen and respiratory support if necessary.
- Make an initial assessment on history and examination to determine aetiology.
- Place an intravenous cannula.
- Begin ECG monitoring.

Table 3.1 Causes and mechanisms of circulatory failure

Category	Subcategory	Examples
Hypovolaemic	Haemorrhagic	Trauma
	Other	Vomiting, diarrhoea, diuresis, increased skin and lung losses of water, heat exhaustion, hypoadrenal states
Cardiogenic	Intrinsic	Congenital heart disease, arrhythmia, myocarditis, drug-induced (arrhythmia or myocardial depression), severe outflow obstruction
	Extrinsic	Tension pneumothorax, severe asthma
Distributive or low resistance	Anaphylaxis	Anaphylaxis
	Sepsis	Meningococcaemia
	Neurogenic	Spinal cord injury

Unless immediate assessment indicates a cardiac cause, begin rapid infusion of crystalloid (for example, Hartmann's solution), 4% human albumin (Albumex), or blood (if cross-matched blood is immediately available) as appropriate, initially 20 mL/kg over 15–20 minutes.

Then:

- Arrange definitive investigations.
- If only partial or no improvement, establish central venous pressure (CVP) monitoring, and place urinary catheter.
- If CVP < 5 mmHg, continue rapid infusion of appropriate fluids with frequent reassessment, including validity of CVP readings.
- If CVP > 5 mmHg, proceed with further investigation (including chest X-ray, arterial blood gases, serum electrolytes, glucose, calcium). Consider correction of acidosis, electrolyte and other metabolic abnormalities; consider need for antibiotics if sepsis possible; consider need for cardiac output studies and the use of positive inotropic drugs.

At this stage an appropriate consultant should be involved, and the child should be in an intensive care location.

Inotropic drugs

A full account of these is beyond the scope of this book. The following brief details are provided as an introduction. Tachycardia, hypertension and tachyarrhythmias can occur with each of these, often as an indication of excessive dosage. These drugs must not be used in the presence of hypovolaemia.

- *Adrenaline* is a powerful sympathomimetic substance, reducing systemic vascular resistance in lower doses, and increasing systemic vascular resistance and cardiac output in higher doses. It is especially useful in anaphylaxis (see p. 23) and septic shock (if low peripheral resistance is a major factor). Initial dose: 0.2 microgram/kg/min—always given by constant infusion pump, the dosage increased in increments of 50% according to response.
- *Noradrenaline* is a naturally occurring inotrope which is a potent vasoconstrictor. It is useful for patients in whom inappropriately low systemic vascular resistance is a feature. The return of euvolaemia should always be attempted before vasoconstrictors are used in shock. Initial dose: 0.1 microgram/kg/min.
- *Dopamine* is a naturally occurring chemical precursor of adrenaline. In low doses (2–6 micrograms/kg/min) it increases renal, cardiac, coronary and cerebral blood flow. These doses sometimes help in cases of heart failure by decreasing peripheral vascular resistance. Intermediate doses (7–20 micrograms/kg/min) increase heart rate, myocardial contractility and hence cardiac output. High doses (20–30 micrograms/kg/min) may produce further inotropic effects, but can cause vasoconstriction and decreased renal blood flow. Dopamine is sometimes useful in increasing peripheral perfusion in sepsis and increasing cardiac output in shock after correction of hypovolaemia.

Coma

Any infant or child in coma should be evaluated and treated as a medical emergency.

Examination

- Carefully examine for signs of trauma.
- Examine the pupils:
  - The pupillary light reflex is *retained* until the terminal stages

Table 3.2 Causes of coma

Metabolic	E.g. electrolyte disturbance, pH disturbance, hypoglycaemia, hyperglycaemia, liver disease, uraemia, adrenal insufficiency, hypothyroidism, hypoxia, hypercapnia, inborn errors of metabolism, Reye's syndrome
Toxic	E.g. drugs, lead, ethanol, salicylates
Raised intracranial pressure with or without a space-occupying intracranial lesion	E.g. trauma (non-accidental injury, or other); tumour
Other	E.g. post-ictal, meningitis

of metabolic brain disease produce coma. Destructive lesions of the midbrain lead to abolition of the pupillary light reflex. Thus a comatose patient who has retained pupillary light reflexes most likely has a *toxic* or *metabolic disturbance*, or is post-ictal.

- A fixed and dilated pupil (or in the early stages an enlarged and/or poorly reactive pupil) indicates a third nerve lesion, most likely due to *raised intracranial pressure*. Horner's syndrome, midposition pupil, irregular pupils or bilateral small pupils indicate a brain stem lesion.
- Drugs may affect pupil size, for example small pupils with opiates, and large, unreactive pupils with atropine, glutethimide and severe barbiturate poisoning.
- Examine eye movements; oculocephalic reflex ('doll's eye manoeuvre'), ice water calorics. These reflexes are lost in structural lesions of the brainstem and drug overdoses. They are generally retained in metabolic causes of coma. Also note fixed deviation of eyes to one side.
- Examine fundi for papilloedema, haemorrhages, exudates and vessel changes.
- Do a full neurological examination: look for focal signs, signs of raised intracranial pressure (for example large head, full fontanelle, split sutures), decorticate or decerebrate posturing, and signs of chronic neurological disease.

- Do a general examination, especially of airway, ventilation and blood pressure. The patient's level of coma should be recorded using the Glasgow coma chart (see Table 3.3).

Investigation

Investigate at first to determine the cause as listed above, using clinical signs to suggest a toxic, metabolic or a structural cause.

Lumbar puncture is contraindicated in the presence of raised intracranial pressure. In a patient with a structural cause of coma, lumbar puncture should be deferred pending further investigation, to be determined by urgent consultation with a neurosurgeon and/or neurologist. If meningitis is suspected, take blood cultures, commence antibiotics immediately and consult.

A CT brain scan needs to be performed urgently in a coma not of toxic, infective or metabolic origin.

Treatment

- Maintain airway, oxygenation and ventilatory support.
- *Note*: CO_2 retention leads to increased intracranial pressure and worsening of the situation.
- Urgently treat raised intracranial pressure—hyperventilation (maintain arterial pCO_2 between 30 and 35 mmHg) and mannitol (0.5–1 g/kg as 10% or 20% solution).
- Treat the cause.

Glasgow Coma Scale (modified for use in children)

- Explanatory notes and references are printed on the back of the hospital's Coma Record Chart.
- The score is useful both for more accurate designation of the degree of coma, and for better recognition of changes in conscious level between observations.
- The coma scale shown (Table 3.3) is currently used at the Children's Hospital at Westmead.
- Note that there are other 'paediatric' versions of the original Glasgow Coma Scale, which was devised for use with adults.
- The hospital's Coma Record Chart also records:
  - pupil size in mm; pupillary reaction
  - pulse rate, BP, RR and temperature
  - arm and leg power.

Table 3.3 Children's modified Glasgow Coma Scale

Eyes open			
Any age			*Score*
Spontaneously			4
To speech			3
To pain			2
No response			1

Best verbal response			
> 5 years	*2–5 years*	*0–23 months*	*Score*
Orientated and converses	Appropriate words and phrases	Smiles, coos, cries appropriately	5
Confused	Inappropriate words	Cries but consolable	4
Inappropriate words	Cries and/or screams	Persistent cries and/or screams	3
Incomprehensible sounds	Grunts	Grunts	2
No response	No response	No response	1

Best motor response		
> 1 year	*< 1 year*	*Score*
Obeys command	Spontaneously moves	6
Localises pain	Localises pain	5
Flexion-withdrawal	Flexion-withdrawal	4
Flexion-abnormal (decorticate rigidity)	Flexion-abnormal (decorticate rigidity)	3
Extension (decerebrate)	Extension (decerebrate)	2
No response	No response	1

- Each component of the coma scale is given a score and then added, with 15 as the maximum, and 3 as the minimum.

Anaphylaxis

Anaphylaxis is an immediate hypersensitivity reaction usually mediated by IgE. Anaphylactoid reactions are not immunologically mediated but they are similar in clinical features and treatment.

Any symptoms of a systemic reaction following an injection or even ingestion of a possible antigen must be considered as potentially serious. *It cannot be overemphasised that for immediate therapy in the presence of a systemic reaction the drug of choice is adrenaline.*

Severe systemic reactions

Severe systemic reactions are identified by the presence of:

- upper respiratory tract obstruction including laryngospasm
- bronchospasm
- hypotension
- urticaria.

Treatment

- Give 100% oxygen; call the Emergency Team (ext. 444).
- Give adrenaline BP 1:1000—0.02 mL/kg IM (or lower dose IV). This may need to be repeated one or more times. It can be given via an endotracheal tube, if that is already in place.
- Secure intravenous access and give 4% albumin for hypotension; large amounts, over several hours, with CVP monitoring may be needed.
- Endotracheal intubation and respiratory support may be needed.
- If appropriate, apply venous tourniquet proximal to site of entry of the antigen.
- Antihistamines are not recommended in severe anaphylactic reactions in the emergency situation, but may be given after the appropriate use of adrenaline.

Mild systemic reactions

- Mild acute systemic anaphylactic reactions may be associated with the rapid development of urticaria and angioedema in the absence of severe upper or lower respiratory obstruction or hypotension.

Treatment

- Adrenaline BP 1:1000—0.01 mL/kg SC stat
- Antihistamine

Guidelines for tracheal intubation

The oral route is preferred for most anaesthetics and for resuscitation. The nasal route carries the risks of dislodgment of adenoid

Table 3.4 A guide to endotracheal tube size and length

| Age | Size (mm) | Insertion length (cm) | |
		Oral	Nasal
Premature	2.5	9	$1.5 \times kg + 6$
Newborn–4 months	3.0	10	10.5
4–9 months	3.5	11	12
9–18 months	4.0	12	14
18 months–3 years	4.5	13.5	15
3–5 years	5.0	14.5	17
5–7 years	5.5	16	19
7–9 years	6.0	18	21
9–10 years	6.5	19	23
11–12 years	7.0	20	24
12–13 years	7.5	21	25
14–15 years	8.0	22	26

tissue and epistaxis. Nevertheless, it has advantages in ease of fixation and is often preferable in children undergoing intensive care and requiring prolonged intubation.

The correct diameter tube is that which results in a small leak at a pressure of about 25 cm of water; the tip should be at mid-trachea (between the clavicles on an AP chest X-ray). The position of the tube must always be checked by auscultation (equal air entry each side) and, in long-term intubation, by chest X-ray.

Uncuffed tubes should be used in prepubescent children.

For intubation of 'croup' patients the next size smaller than usual for the patient's age should be initially tried. Ultimately the correct size is that associated with a small leak, though size 2.5 should not be used because of the likelihood of obstruction with thick secretions in this condition.

Emergency patient transport and medical retrieval

Different hospitals offer differing levels of care for sicker children. In Australia and New Zealand, critical care tends to be centralised in some tertiary hospitals. This principle is based on statistical comparisons which show that a 'centralised' approach produces better outcomes than having a larger number of hospitals in a region each doing a small amount of critical care:

- Most newborns requiring critical care are treated in neonatal intensive care units at obstetric units caring for women with high-risk pregnancies.
- Infants and children, and newborns with major surgical conditions or complex medical problems who require critical care, are treated in children's hospitals.

The primary principle of paediatric medical retrieval is to bring the required critical care skills to the patient from a centralised location and initiate that care prior to transport rather than to rush the patient in an unstable condition and risk en route deterioration.

This is contrary to the 'wrap and run' approach, which is sometimes seen when adult retrieval services become involved in emergency paediatric transport, especially of older children. It relies on the 'golden hour' concept, in which the outcome depends on the patient being on the operating table in less than an hour from injury. This evolved from management of penetrating trauma in military personnel during the Vietnam war, and is rarely relevant to critically ill children in Australia, except in some rescue situations (for instance, from the scene of an accident). It is tempting for adult or rescue retrieval services to take this approach with children and arrive with a patient who then needs resuscitation.

In recent years medical retrieval services for adults have developed and are now being based in both metropolitan and regional centres. It is important that paediatric clinicians have input into decisions made about any older children whom these services might plan to transport. Most often in these circumstances, a joint response to the primary hospital by a regional service and a specialist paediatric retrieval team may be more appropriate. Thereafter, the optimum destination (regional hospital or specialist children's hospital) for the patient can be determined.

Components of the process of emergency transport and medical retrieval

These components are:

1 the clinician treating the patient in the hospital and seeking his or her transfer (the *primary referring clinician*)

2 the clinical staff in the hospital to which the patient is being referred (the *tertiary receiving clinician*)

3 the medical retrieval process with its clinical staff (the *transport clinician* and the operational component, the *transport service*).

An organised and streamlined interaction between these components is required for the best results. Here is a summary of the expectations, roles and responsibilities for each.

The primary referring clinician

- Expects to make just one phone call to initiate the process.
- Focuses on the basic principles:
  - airway, breathing, circulation, for a child
  - 'warm, pink and sweet', for a newborn.
- Provides basic details of history, assessment, examination and interventions.
- Nominates a preferred destination based on clinical need, proximity, family and so on.

The tertiary receiving clinician

- Offers telephone advice about management.
- Elicits appropriate additional information from the referrer.
- Assumes some responsibility for the patient at this stage.
- Accepts the transfer or ensures an appropriate alternative is arranged.
- Ensures that others at the tertiary hospital are informed and involved.
- Is available to advise the referrer and/or transport team about further management.

The transport service

- Assesses the level of clinical care required to transport the patient.
- Selects the most appropriate (based on clinical skills) and best available (most timely) team to treat and escort the patient.
- Chooses the most appropriate transport vehicle (road or air, rotary or fixed wing), by liaising with ambulance and other vehicle providers.
- Offers a link between the referring clinician and the receiving physician. This is particularly relevant when there are several potential destination units.

The transport clinician

- Participates in or is informed about prior clinical discussions about the patient.
- Prepares for the obvious and considers the not-so-obvious possibilities while outbound to the patient.
- Assesses the patient at 'first look' and acts on clinical need.
- May re-triage to a different level of care and/or alternative transport.
- Chooses between rapid-sequence and full stabilisation retrieval.
- Stabilises the patient.
- Communicates with receiving clinicians.

Levels of urgency

1 *Immediate*: The patient is in extremis, or is deteriorating, or needs time-critical therapy.
2 *Urgent*: The patient has a serious condition and the treatment required is not possible in the referring hospital.
3 *Elective*: The timing of transfer is discretionary—hours or days.

Modes of transport

Available transport vehicles include road ambulances, planes and helicopters. The choice of vehicle depends on the nature of the illness, the distance and the total time involved in the outward and return journeys. Other considerations may include weather conditions and the availability of aircraft landing facilities.

It is not the vehicle per se which is important to the patient; it is the maximising of available treatment, in the least time reasonably possible, and movement to the tertiary centre in a careful, safe, controlled manner.

Availability of telephone advice

In remote areas, specialist paediatric retrieval is generally unavailable and general retrieval or transport services are used. Telephone advice is always available and is even more relevant when distance increases the overall process and the time taken to reach definitive care. The expertise of specialists in the areas of paediatric ICU, ED, surgery, burns, neonatology, other paediatric disciplines and poisons is available by telephone through regional, state and national networks.

Different systems operate in different states

The system of medical retrieval of children is managed differently across Australia. In some states there is a state-wide system and in others, tertiary hospitals operate separate medical retrieval services. The current contact numbers for all these services can be found at www.nets.org.au. Base hospitals provide an intermediate level of care and patients not sick enough to need critical care are transferred from hospitals within their region. These patients should not be sick enough to need medical retrieval and can be transferred by ambulance with or without nurse escort. If in doubt, consult.

Region	Newborn	Paediatric
NSW and ACT	1300 36 2500	
Your region		

4

Nutrition and infant feeding

This chapter includes:
- infant feeding guidelines
- recommended intakes of nutrients for healthy children
- infant formulae
- special formulae
- therapeutic diets.

Infant feeding guidelines

General

- Feeding should start in the first 6 hours of life.
- Breastfeeding is the best method of infant feeding. There are numerous advantages for mother and baby and the community at large.
- Health professionals should encourage the initiation of breast-feeding and support the mother to continue to breastfeed for at least the first year of life.
- There will always be some mothers who either choose not to start or cannot continue to breastfeed and hence need to use an infant formula.
- If an infant is not fed human milk, a standard commercial infant formula is recommended as the main drink until 12 months of age. At this age, solids are taken in reasonable amounts and a wide range of foods is being eaten.
- There are many brands of infant formula available and nutritional differences are negligible, supporting no clinical benefit between brands.
- Understanding formula preparation, feeding practices, parenting and normal infant development are important so as to avoid unnecessary formula changes.
- A follow-on or progress formula may be used after 6 months of

age (but not earlier). For healthy infants who commence solids around 6 months, these formulae offer no nutritional advantages over standard formulae, and standard formulae can be used for the whole of the first year of life.

- *Volume*: 60 mL/kg on the first day in a full-term baby increasing by 20–30 mL/kg/day to 150–180 mL/kg/day by 3–5 days. This amount will gradually be reduced to around 100 mL/kg/day by 12 months.
- *Feeding intervals*: 6–8 feeds per day will probably be necessary in the first week, decreasing to 5–6 per day by 6–8 weeks.

Introduction of solids

- Breastfeeding or infant formula is the only food required for the first 4–6 months of life. From 4–6 months infants are ready to start eating solids. Initially, the solids are educational in taste and texture and consist of rice cereal, pureed fruit and vegetables. Solids should be offered after a milk feed.
- From about 7 months other foods with a thicker texture (such as meat, chicken, egg yolk, other cereals and milk-based foods) can be introduced. These can be offered before breastfeeding or bottle.
- By age 9 months more solids can be eaten and the amount of human milk or formula will gradually decrease. By 12 months of age children can be eating the same foods as the rest of the family.
- From about 6 months, fluids other than milk can be offered from a cup. Infant formula is not necessary after the age of 12 months if the range of solids is varied.
- Salt, sugar or honey should not be added to the baby's food unless advised by a doctor/dietitian.
- Cow's milk and dairy products may be used in solids from the age of 6 months although it is not recommended that cow's milk be used as the major beverage until the age of 12 months because of its low iron content and high renal solute load.

Recommended intakes of nutrients for healthy children

Energy and protein

Daily protein and energy requirements vary with age and gender and tables containing specific information can be found in *The Feeding*

Guide by Jane Allen from the James Fairfax Institute of Paediatric Clinical Nutrition.

Vitamins and minerals

- The breastfed infant receives an adequate supply of all vitamins and minerals unless the mother's diet is very deficient. At risk are breastfed infants of mothers following a vegan diet (possible vitamin B12 deficiency).
- Commercial formulae meeting Australian standards contain adequate vitamins and minerals. No further supplements are needed.
- Cow's milk is deficient in both vitamins C and D and contains less vitamin A, when diluted for feeding, than required. Accordingly, supplements of these may be necessary in younger infants fed on cow's milk.
- Vitamin preparations should be given directly into the mouth rather than put into the bottle.
- Fresh goat's milk is deficient in folic acid as well as in vitamins A, C and D. A supplement of 50 micrograms per day of folic acid is necessary in addition to a standard vitamin supplement. Goat's milk should be pasteurised. Commercial infant formulae based on goat's milk are adequate until 6 months.
- Unsweetened diluted fruit juice (for example, orange juice) may be introduced in the later months of the first year as the vitamin C supplement. The use of vitamin C fortified syrups is not recommended because of the risk of dental caries.

Fluoride

Fluoride has been shown to reduce the incidence of dental caries. In fluoridated water areas such as Sydney, no supplements are recommended. In areas with a water supply containing less than 0.5 mg/L of fluoride, the dosage recommended is 0.25 mg per day up to 4 years of age, 0.5 mg per day from 4 to 8 years and 1 mg per day after 8 years (NHMRC). Overzealous use of supplements has been associated with fluorosis.

Infant formulae

Table 4.1 Approximate composition of milks per litre normal dilution

	Protein (g)	Fat (g)	Carbohydrate (lactose) (g)	Energy (kJ) (kcal)	Na (mmol)	K (mmol)
Human milk	10	42	74	2900 (693)	6	15
Infant formula	15–17	34–38	70–76	2729–2900 (653–693)	6–10	14–21
Follow-on formula	20–25	26–36	69–83	2710–2810 (648–672)	8–16	15–34
Cow's milk	34	39	48	2790 (670)	21	38
Goat's milk	34	47	48	3078 (735)	20	50

For current information on individual infant formulae and specialised feeds, *The Feeding Guide* by Jane Allen from the James Fairfax Institute of Paediatric Clinical Nutrition may be purchased from Kids Health, The Children's Hospital at Westmead, phone (02) 9845 3585.

Current infant formulae are listed in MIMS.

Special formulae

Descriptions of the major groups of formulae and additives most commonly used are given below. Detailed analysis of and information on other formulae are available from the Department of Nutrition and Dietetics or in Allen's *The Feeding Guide*. Patients being discharged on special formulae should be referred to the dietitian who will instruct on nutritional adequacy, formula preparation and/or any dietary restrictions.

Arrangements should be made for obtaining the formula on script or authority script where feasible and when long-term usage is necessary.

Table 4.2 Major groups of formulae and additives

Feed	Description and comments
Modified CHO feeds	
Delact (Sharpe Laboratories) S26 LF* (Wyeth)	95% lactose hydrolysed. For use in lactose intolerance up to 1 year of age, e.g. secondary to gastroenteritis. Easy to prepare and palatable.
Digestelact* (Sharpe Laboratories)	Suitable for children over 1 year for treatment of lactose intolerance.
Soy-based feeds	
Infasoy* (Wyeth) Karicare Soy (Nutricia)	Nutritionally adequate infant feeds free of lactose and cow's milk protein. The sucrose content differs between brands but this usually offers no clinical advantage. The use of soy formula is limited but is appropriate for vegan or vegetarian infants, for proven cow's milk allergy, and for infants with galactosaemia (consult the dietitian).
Pre-thickened formulae	
	Standard infant formulae with an added thickener agent such as rice starch, maltodextrin or cornstarch substituted for some of the lactose.
S26AR (Wyeth) KaricareAR (Nutricia)	The manufacturers claim 'designed for infants with reflux'. Contraindicated for infants with oesophagitis.

The formulae listed above are available from pharmacies and from some supermarkets. No prescription is required.

Elemental or partially elemental infant feeds	
Neocate Pepti-Junior (Nutricia)	Whey hydrolysate with 50% fat as MCT oil. CHO as glucose polymers. Suggested use: cow's milk and soy protein intolerance, severe enteropathy with disaccharidase deficiency, maldigestion and malabsorption disorders.

Table 4.2 Major groups of formulae and additives *(continued)*

Feed	Description and comments
Monogen (Nutricia)	93% of fat is present as MCT oil. Contains intact protein and carbohydrate as glucose. For those who cannot digest, absorb or transport long-chain fats, e.g. intestinal lymphangiectasia and abetalipoproteinaemia, chylothorax, long-chain fatty acid disorders.

Premature formulae

Pre-Nan (Nestlé) S26 Low Birth Weight* (Wyeth)	Increased protein, energy (340 kJ (81 kcal)/100 mL) and electrolyte content for low birth weight premature infants. Grade to standard formula at or before term.
FM85 (Nestlé)	Supplement for breast milk. Contains protein, carbohydrate, fat, vitamins and minerals.

Products to increase energy density of feeds
Carbohydrate

Polyjoule* (Sharpe Laboratories) Polycose (Abbott)	Glucose polymer of approximately 5 glucose units. 1/5th osmolality of glucose solution of same strength, and offers no taste. 16 kJ (4 kcal)/g

Fat

MCT oil* (Nutricia)	Primarily contains medium-chain triglycerides of C8 and C10 saturated fatty acids, which require little digestion by pancreatic enzymes and bile salts and are absorbed into the portal system rather than the lymphatics. 35 kJ (8.3 kcal)/mL Does *not* contain essential fatty acids.
Liquigen* (Sharpe Laboratories)	50:50 MCT oil and water emulsion. In most cases it is the preferred fat option to MCT oil as it mixes well with formulae. 18.5 KJ (4.5 Kcal)/mL. Does *not* contain essential fatty acids.

continues . . .

Table 4.2 Major groups of formulae and additives *(continued)*

Feed	Description and comments
Calogen* (Sharpe Laboratories)	50:50 long-chain fat and water emulsion. 18.5 KJ (4.5 Kcal)/mL

Products used to thicken feeds— refer to the fact sheet 'Thickened feeds'

Karicare Instant Food Thickener* (Nutricia)	Pregelatinised, unmodified corn starch. Used to thicken feeds for gastro-oesophageal reflux. For breastfed infants, make into gel. For bottlefed infants, use as a gel or mix into formula. See 'Thickened feeds' fact sheet or a dietitian for more information. Contributes energy.
Cornflour*	For infants > 6 weeks of age. Dilution = 1 tsp/100 mL of water. Water must be thickened and cooled prior to making up the formula. This is done by cooking the cornflour in the water. See 'Thickened feeds' fact sheet or a dietitian for more information. Contributes energy—approx. 18% energy increase.

Tube feeds

	For children < 1 year a standard infant formula can be used as the basis of tube feed. The feeds listed below are suitable for children > 1 year of age (if approx. 10 kg).
Osmolite (Abbott) Pediasure* (Abbott) Jevity* (Abbott)	Isotonic solution 4.4 kJ (1 kcal)/mL. Suitable for most tube feeding. Lactose free. Nutritionally complete. Pediasure is a standard enteral feed for 1–10-year-olds. Jevity contains fibre.
Ensure* (Abbott)	Non-isotonic tube feed. Contains lactose. Made up from a powder.
Ensure Plus (Abbott)	6.27 kJ (1.5 kcal)/mL
Nutrison Energy* (Nutricia)	Suitable for children with high nutrient needs and low fluid requirements.

Table 4.2 Major groups of formulae and additives *(continued)*

Feed	Description and comments
Vital* (Abbott)	Elemental feed. Nitrogen as peptides, and amino acids. 4.2 kJ (1 kcal)/mL. Strong taste and smell.

* Formulae currently available for patients at Children's Hospital at Westmead as per tender at time of printing. There are many other formulae and supplements available. Consult Allen's *The Feeding Guide* or a dietitian for more details.

Therapeutic diets

Special diets should be prescribed only after adequate clinical assessment, and in conjunction with a paediatric dietitian.

Carbohydrate malabsorption

Lactase deficiency

This may be congenital (rare) or primary, which can present between 3 and 20 years of age. It may be permanent (it is common in many racial groups, for example Australian Aborigines, Asians, Southern Mediterraneans) or temporary, secondary to gastroenteritis. Use a low-lactose formula (e.g. 'Delact' or 'S26LF') or a lactose-free milk such as 'Digestelact' or 'Lactaid' and have the child avoid foods high in lactose, e.g. milk, custard, ice-cream, yoghurt, cottage cheese and processed cheese.

Congenital sucrase-isomaltase deficiency

Avoid sucrose (cane sugar) and sucrose-containing foods.

Cow's milk protein intolerance (CMPI)

Use a cow's milk protein free diet for proven CMPI. Care is essential when eating processed foods which may contain milk, e.g. bread, margarine.

Initially, a formula containing cow's milk protein hydrolysate is used. Soy infant formula may be introduced later if it is tolerated, but intolerance to soy protein occurs in some infants with cow's milk protein intolerance.

Coeliac disease

This is a permanent intolerance to gliadin, a polypeptide of gluten, which is the protein component in wheat, malt, rye, barley and oats. A duodenal biopsy is essential to confirm the diagnosis. Dietary management is based on the strict avoidance of these cereals. Expert dietary advice is needed to avoid the small amounts of these grains which occur commonly in commercially prepared food and drugs. Once the diagnosis is established, avoidance is essential for life.

In the initial period of treatment, lactose intolerance secondary to intestinal mucosal damage may result in the diarrhoea continuing despite a gluten-free diet.

Cystic fibrosis

A high fat diet, along with appropriate enzyme, salt and vitamin supplementation, is recommended to meet the increased energy needs (120–150% normal).

Diabetes

(See also Chapter 15.) Diabetic diets routinely prescribed at this hospital are based on the control of the total amount of carbohydrate and its distribution through the day. The diet aims to provide 60% of the energy from carbohydrate, which effectively restricts fat intake to levels as recommended by the Australian Dietary Guidelines. The carbohydrate is measured in exchanges, each exchange containing approximately 15 g of carbohydrate. The carbohydrate distribution is based on obtaining a dietary history in order to estimate the total amount of carbohydrate normally eaten. If this is not available, the total energy requirement needs to be estimated accordingly and 60% of this provided by carbohydrate. This is achieved by calculating 60% of total energy requirements and dividing by 250 kJ (as 15 g of carbohydrate provides 250 kJ).

Exchanges are then increased according to appetite, as at initial diagnosis some weight loss may have occurred. The commencement of insulin also stimulates the appetite initially. The aim is to have a regular intake of carbohydrate over the day, every 2–3 hours. Nutrition education, where patients and their families are taught about the management of diabetes and food, is commenced after initial stabilisation.

Renal disease

Acute renal failure

A low potassium, low phosphate, low salt diet is often required and adjustments made according to biochemistry results. A high caloric intake is also recommended to stop catabolism and help control potassium and urea.

Chronic renal failure

Adequate nutrition is essential to maximise the growth of the child. A high caloric intake is also necessary to assist with stabilisation of urea and potassium. Protein restriction is not indicated as this may adversely affect the child's growth. Children with chronic renal failure are frequently anorexic and if dietary supplements are not tolerated nasogastric or gastrostomy feeding may be required.

Dietary phosphate restriction should be commenced once CRF is detected and phosphate binders used to maintain the serum phosphate in the low/normal range. A low potassium diet is instituted for medical control of hyperkalaemia. Sodium restriction is required if the children are hypertensive but children with salt wasting diseases (e.g. renal dysplasia) may require sodium supplementation.

Obesity

Dietary management of an obese child involves assessment of dietary habits and lifestyle habits (including activity) and education regarding appropriate changes. The aim of treatment is to allow for weight maintenance for an overweight child or a slow weight loss in the obese child. The principles of diet counselling follow the recommendations for the community for healthy eating and these are tailored to meet the needs of the individual child and the family. Foods to limit are those high in fat and sugar, and a reduction in total quantity of food eaten is usually necessary. The importance of altering the whole family eating style and increasing exercise is stressed, along with means of improving the child's self-esteem. Counselling parents of pre-adolescent children is more effective than individual counselling with the child. More extensive food restriction is not recommended as it may compromise growth and development, but may be necessary when the obesity is health-threatening. In conditions where energy needs are lower than normal, for example Prader-Willi or spina bifida, close monitoring is necessary to achieve adequate nutrient intake.

Community measures to prevent obesity are the key to preventing and controlling paediatric obesity.

Inherited metabolic disorders

Some of the most common inherited metabolic disorders requiring strict dietary manipulations for life are phenylketonuria (PKU) and galactosaemia. Others include hereditary fructose intolerance, maple syrup urine disease, ornithine transcarbamylase deficiency, tyrosinaemia and arginosuccinic aciduria.

Phenylketonuria (PKU)

The most commonly seen inborn error of amino acid metabolism is PKU. Dietary management involves a reduction in the intake of phenylalanine, which is an essential amino acid. The diet is very low in protein and is supplemented with an amino acid mixture containing all amino acids (except phenylalanine) and complete in all vitamins and minerals. All babies in NSW are screened in the newborn period and referred to the PKU clinic at RAHC with treatment commencing in the first or second week of life. Phenylalanine levels are monitored regularly and lifelong dietary management is recommended.

Galactosaemia

Galactosaemia is a condition in which the body is unable to metabolise galactose. Lactose is the major source of galactose in the diet. Dietary management is lifelong and entails complete avoidance of milk, milk products, processed foods and medications containing lactose as well as foods containing significant amounts of galactose. The infant cannot be breastfed as human milk contains lactose. A lactose-free infant formula such as soy infant formula is required. For children and adults a soy drink with added calcium is recommended. Calcium intake needs to be assessed regularly and calcium supplements may be necessary.

Ketogenic diet

The 'ketogenic diet' is sometimes prescribed in the treatment of seizure disorders that have failed to respond to drug medication. The aim of the diet is to achieve and maintain a state of ketosis. The diet provides 80% of the necessary energy intake for the child's weight from fat using a combination of half dietary fat and half MCT oil. The dietitian must be involved in the commencement and monitoring of the diet, and with parent education.

Food allergies and sensitivities

Many children have true food allergies to food proteins. The most common antigens are egg, peanuts and milk. Diagnosis is made on history and confirmed by skin-prick tests.

Some children with severe eczema, asthma or chronic urticaria benefit from a trial of an elimination diet for a couple of weeks, followed by food challenges to identify any provoking foods. The elimination diet is very restrictive and should not be used long term. Individual diets are based on challenge results and regular follow-up is essential to ensure adequate nutrition. The elimination diet is used when children exhibit symptoms similar to a food allergy, but the skin-prick tests are negative. The diet excludes all chemical additives—preservatives, antioxidants, colours, flavours—as well as naturally occurring chemicals such as amines, salicylates and glutamates.

Urinary collection for catecholamines

Restriction of foods which may give false elevated catecholamine levels in the urine is required one day prior to and during collection.

The foods to restrict include banana, tomato, nuts, fish, cheese, yoghurt, jam, chutneys, canned foods, highly coloured foods such as cordial, soft drink and sweets, foods containing vanilla, tea and coffee, and foods containing preservatives. A special diet should be ordered by the nursing staff via CBORD for hospital in-patients. Information regarding the diet is available from the Department of Nutrition and Dietetics.

Modified, supplementary and tube feeds

Diets of modified character and/or consistency, e.g. liquid, pureed and tube feeds, should be monitored by a dietitian to ensure adequate nutrient intake.

Tube feeding may be necessary for comatose children and children whose energy and protein needs are high and/or whose oral intake is poor, e.g. patients with burns, inflammatory bowel disease, cystic fibrosis, renal disease and cancer. Recommended tube feeds are outlined above.

5

Haematology

This chapter includes:
- blood transfusion
- blood products and their use
- treatment of congenital coagulation disorders (haemophilias)
- haematological emergencies.

Blood transfusion

- Medical staff must complete all questions on the request form for blood transfusion. They have a legal responsibility to ensure that the correct blood is transfused.
- Positive identification of the patient is essential, both when blood samples for cross-match are collected, and again before administering any blood unit.
- Identification details on the compatibility label must be checked with those on the patient's arm/leg band and transfusion sheet before commencing transfusion.
- Provided that blood of the appropriate group is 'in stock', a full cross-match will take 1 hour from the receipt of the patient's blood sample in the blood bank.
- When blood is required more quickly, medical staff should contact blood bank staff by telephone.
- In emergency situations of acute blood loss, blood may be issued after a shortened incubation time of the cross-match.
- In extreme emergencies before any cross-matching is possible, group O, Rh-negative, haemolysin-free blood should be used.

Transfusion in the newborn

For transfusion in newborn infants, the mother's blood sample should also be available for the cross-match. Any atypical antibodies will be present to a higher titre in her serum. Blood for transfusion should be selected within 7 days of collection. It is likely that whole blood will no longer be available for emergency exchange transfusion. (For exchange transfusion, see Chapter 8.)

Clinical transfusion practice

Acute blood loss

(See also Chapters 3 and 7.) Clinical signs of circulatory collapse may be minimal, even when substantial blood loss has occurred, particularly in a previously healthy child. Direct measurement of blood loss during surgical operations is an important guide to blood replacement, but requires experience when blood is mixed with body fluids.

Indications for transfusion in acute blood loss

If hypotensive shock is present, at least 10–20% of blood volume has been lost and red cell transfusion is indicated. Saline or a plasma expander, for example 4% human albumin (Albumex 4), may be used initially. When bleeding appears to be continuing, the rate of transfusion must be assessed by repeated careful observation of the child. Fresh blood should be used if the total volume or more is replaced within 24 hours.

Blood transfusion for massive and continuing blood loss is best managed in an intensive care ward.

Acute haemolytic anaemia

Anaemia may develop with such rapidity in children with G6PD deficiency and some autoimmune haemolytic anaemias that prompt transfusion is needed. Autoantibodies, especially high titre cold agglutinins, can lead to cross-matching difficulties. In acute haemolytic anaemia the planned transfusion management should be discussed fully with a haematologist.

Chronic anaemia

In chronic anaemia urgent transfusion is rarely required, and investigations to elucidate the cause of the anaemia should always be carried out prior to transfusion. Red cell concentrates are used in the correction of chronic anaemia in every instance.

Children who will need repeated transfusions (for example, for homozygous β thalassaemia) should receive phenotyped blood. The transfused blood should be leucocyte-poor to prevent febrile

43

transfusion reactions due to leucocyte antibodies. If filtered blood is not provided by the Australian Red Cross Blood Transfusion Service, leucodepletion is most easily achieved at the bedside through the use of a white cell filter in the infusion line. The alternative product is Triple Washed Packed Cells, provided by the Red Cross, which are both leucocyte-poor and plasma-poor (these are reserved for patients who have regular transfusions and who have repeated allergic reactions despite the use of filtered blood).

Administration of blood

Guide to transfusion volume

Red cell concentrates are as follows:

- in infants weighing less than 5 kg:
  volume to be given (mL) = $4.7 \times$ weight (kg) $\times D^*$
- in infants and children of 5 kg and over:
  volume to be given (mL) = $4 \times$ weight (kg) $\times D^*$
  $^*D$ = change in haemoglobin desired in g/dL

This formula is derived for red cell concentrates with a haematocrit of 50–60%. Caution must be exercised in the amount of blood given on any occasion, and the rate of its administration to any patient with anaemia, particularly acute anaemia, or with cardiac failure. In patients with chronic anaemia, it is often prudent to raise the haemoglobin to the desired level by two or three separate transfusions if the initial level is very low. As a rule of thumb the haemoglobin should not be increased by more than 50 g/L in any one transfusion.

Rate of administration

The following is a guide to maximum safe rates of administration of blood (either whole blood or packed cells) in most cases of chronic anaemia:

- up to 15 kg: weight in kg $\times$ 4 mL/h
- 15–30 kg: 60 mL/h
- over 30 kg: 80–100 mL/h

In severe chronic anaemia, cardiac failure or pulmonary disease, slower rates should be maintained.

Intravenous lines

To prevent osmotic lysis of red cells, glucose solutions or medications must not be added to blood bags or tubing containing blood.

Duration

Because of the risk of bacterial infection when blood products are maintained at room temperature, transfusion from any unit of blood (or plasma) must not be continued for longer than 6 hours after removal from monitored blood refrigerator. If the required volume has not been given within this time, blood from another unit of blood should be substituted.

Blood must be stored only in the monitored refrigerators of the blood bank or theatre.

Transfusion of blood or plasma of different groups

To avoid the risk of agglutination of red cells in the tubing it is recommended that the 'giving set' be changed when blood or plasma of a different group is given during a transfusion.

Irradiated blood

In order to prevent transfusion-associated graft-versus-host disease, all cellular blood products (including filtered products) should be irradiated in the following groups of patients at this hospital:

- congenital immunodeficiency syndromes
- all oncology patients
- all patients with aplastic anaemia
- bone marrow and solid organ transplant recipients
- low birth weight newborns (< 1.5 kg)
- HIV-1 positive patients
- transfusion from blood relatives
- cardiac patients with conotruncal problems (for example di George syndrome, Sprintzen syndrome, truncus arteriosus) where there may be thymic hypoplasia.

CMV negative blood

In order to prevent transfusion-acquired cytomegalovirus infection all cellular blood products should be negative for CMV antibodies in the following groups of patients who have not previously had CMV infection (that is, those who are CMV IgG and IgM negative) or if the patient's CMV status is unknown:

- congenital immunodeficiency syndromes
- oncology patients
- patients with aplastic anaemia
- bone marrow and solid organ transplant recipients (including patients being considered for transplant)
- low birth weight newborns (< 1.5 kg)
- HIV-1 positive patients
- cardiac patients with conotruncal problems (for example di George syndrome, Sprintzen syndrome, truncus arteriosus) where there may be thymic hypoplasia.

Transfusion reactions

The main types of transfusion reactions are:

- haemolytic (from incompatible, overheated or frozen blood)
- febrile reactions (due to white cell antibodies, infected blood or 'pyrogens')
- allergic reactions to plasma constituents
- circulatory overload.

The following symptoms and signs may indicate a transfusion reaction: back or loin pain, haemoglobinuria, rigors, fever (over 38°C in a previously afebrile patient), respiratory distress, rash, hypotension and tachycardia (not present before transfusion). Resident medical officers called to assess a patient suspected of having a transfusion reaction should check:

- the patient's identification data (verbally stated or wrist/leg band name) with that on the blood unit and transfusion sheet
- the blood group and expiry date on the unit being transfused.

Assess the patient clinically and determine the probable cause of the reaction. If an infected or incompatible blood transfusion is suspected, *stop the transfusion immediately*. All transfusion reactions or other untoward events must be notified to the hospital blood bank and the haematologist on call for immediate investigation.

Blood products and their use

The following products used in the treatment of bleeding disorders are issued from the hospital blood bank. As platelet packs may contain red cells, the group selected should be ABO- and rhesus-compatible with the recipient. Anti-A and Anti-B agglutinins are present in plasma products. The group of the plasma infused should be selected according to the recipient's blood group, especially if large volumes are to be given.

Patients with unexpected bleeding should be investigated prior to receiving blood or plasma products.

Platelet concentrates

Use: Severe thrombocytopenia associated with reduced marrow production. Platelets are almost never indicated in the treatment of immune thrombocytopenia.

Infusion: Infuse through standard (200 micron filter) 'giving set' with a white cell filter in the infusion line; rate is dependent on patient's weight and clinical indication.

Storage: Room temperature; maintained on 'platelet shaker' in hospital blood bank.

Three types of platelet concentrates are available:

1   Standard platelet concentrate
   Source: Centrifuged concentrate of platelets from a single blood donation in donor plasma.
   Pack volume: 30–60 mL
   Dosage: Depends on patient's weight (usually 2–6 bags are administered).

2   Pooled platelets
   Source: Four standard platelet concentrates are pooled and resuspended in platelet additive solution (Tsol) by the Red Cross blood bank.
   Pack volume: ~200 mL
   Dosage: One bag of pooled platelet concentrate is equivalent to four bags of standard platelet concentrate.

3   Single donor unit (SDU) platelet concentrates
   Source: Apheresis donation of platelets from a single donor.
   Pack volume: ~200 mL
   Dosage: 1 SDU is equivalent to about four bags of standard platelet concentrate.
   Indication: Patients in whom donor sensitisation is a problem (for example, aplastic anaemia); patients with

reduced platelet recovery secondary to HLA and platelet antibodies. (These patients often require cross-match-compatible platelets issued by the Red Cross.)

Fresh frozen plasma (FFP)

This is plasma from a single unit donation, frozen promptly after donation.

Pack volume: 150–250 mL approx. or pedipack of 50–60 mL
Storage: −20°C (blood bank freezer).
Use: Patients with multiple coagulation deficiencies (such as consumptive coagulopathy, after massive transfusion).
Dosage: To be discussed with the haematologist on call.
For infusion: Thaw quickly at 37°C; infuse the required volume within 6 hours.

Cryoprecipitate

This is prepared by thawing FFP between 1°C and 6°C and recovering the precipitate. The cold-insoluble fraction is refrozen. Cryoprecipitate contains fibrinogen, factor VIII, von Willebrand factor, factor XIII and fibronectin. On average, each bag of cryoprecipitate contains at least 15 mg of fibrinogen in less than 15 mL of plasma.

Pack volume: 20 mL approx.
Storage: −20°C (blood bank freezer).
Use: Source of concentrated fibrinogen. Used primarily as a supplement to FFP in patients with severe hypofibrinogenaemia. Should be given only after discussion with haematologists.
For infusion: Thaw quickly at 37°C. Infuse calculated dose as a 'bolus' intravenous injection.

Factor VIII concentrates

Recombinant factor VIII

This is prepared by recombinant DNA technology by several manufacturers. Note that human albumin is used as a stabiliser in many products currently available.

Bottle volume: 5–10 mL after reconstitution (depending on brand of product).

Storage: 4°C (blood bank refrigerator).
Use: Patients with haemophilia A (factor VIII deficiency).
For infusion: Reconstitute with water for injection, supplied in the pack. Factor VIII activity of bottle is stated on the label. Infuse calculated dose as a 'bolus' intravenous injection.

Anti-haemophilic factor (AHF)

This is prepared as a lyophilised powder from pooled donor plasma at Commonwealth Serum Laboratories.

Bottle volume: 10 mL after reconstitution.
Storage: 4°C (blood bank refrigerator).
Use: Patients with von Willebrand disease or haemophilia A (factor VIII deficiency).
For infusion: Reconstitute with 10 mL of water for injection. Factor VIII activity of bottle is stated on the label. Infuse calculated dose as a 'bolus' intravenous injection.

Factor IX concentrates

Recombinant factor IX

This is prepared by recombinant DNA technology by several manufacturers. Note that human albumin is used as a stabiliser in many products currently available.

Bottle volume: 5–10 mL after reconstitution (depending on brand of product).
Storage: 4°C (blood bank refrigerator).
Use: Patients with haemophilia B (factor IX deficiency).
For infusion: Reconstitute with water for injection, supplied in the pack. Factor IX activity of bottle is stated on the label. Infuse calculated dose as a 'bolus' intravenous injection.

Monofix

This is prepared as a lyophilised powder from pooled donor plasma at Commonwealth Serum Laboratories.

Bottle volume: 10 mL after reconstitution.
Storage: 4°C (blood bank refrigerator).
Use: Patients with haemophilia B (factor IX deficiency).
For Infusion: Reconstitute with 10 mL of water for injection. Factor IX activity of bottle is stated on the label. Infuse calculated dose as a 'bolus' intravenous injection.

Prothrombinex

This is prepared as a lyophilised powder from pooled donor plasma at Commonwealth Serum Laboratories. It contains concentrated coagulation factors II, IX and X.

Bottle volume: 20 mL after reconstitution.

Storage: 4°C (blood bank refrigerator).

Use: Patients with inhibitors to factor VIII.

For infusion: Reconstitute with 20 mL of water for injection. Factor IX activity of bottle is stated on the label. Infuse calculated dose as a 'bolus' intravenous injection.

FEIBA

This is prepared as a lyophilised powder from pooled donor plasma. It contains activated factor IX.

Bottle volume: 20 mL after reconstitution.

Storage: 4°C (blood bank refrigerator).

Use: Patients with inhibitors to factor VIII or factor IX.

For infusion: Reconstitute with 20 mL of water for injection. Factor Eight Bypassing Activity (FEIBA) is stated on label. Infuse calculated dose as a 'bolus' intravenous injection.

Note: To be administered only on the order of a consultant haematologist.

Novoseven (Activated Factor VIIa (Recombinant))

This is prepared by recombinant DNA technology.

Bottle volume: 1.2 mg, 2.4 mg or 4.8 mg per vial.

Storage: 4°C (blood bank or pharmacy refrigerator).

Use: Patients with inhibitors to factor VIII or factor IX. In exceptional circumstances, it may be used in circumstances of uncontrollable life-threatening haemorrhage.

For infusion: Reconstitute with water for injection as indicated on vial. After reconstitution with the specified volume of diluent each vial contains 0.6 mg/mL of factor VIIa. Infuse calculated dose as a 'bolus' intravenous injection.

Note: To be administered only on the order of a consultant haematologist.

Treatment of congenital coagulation disorders (haemophilias)

Planned treatment for patients with known congenital coagulation disorders must be discussed with the haematologist on call.

The following principles of management apply:
- A 'unit' of a particular coagulation factor is the activity of that factor present in 1 mL of fresh citrated pooled normal plasma.
- The following is a guide to the desired factor level for the treatment of bleeding in factor VIII and factor IX deficiency:

Site of bleed	Initial dose	Maintenance dose
Haemarthrosis	50%	30%
Haematoma	50%	40%
Surgical incisions	100%	> 50% until wound healing is complete
Head/neck injuries	100%—admit for observation	100%

- The dose of the coagulant product required can be calculated in 'units' by multiplying the patient's predicted plasma volume by the desired rise in coagulant factor activity:
  - Dose required = plasma volume (~45 mL/kg) × rise in factor desired (%)
  - Round the dose required up to the nearest whole bottle.

Example

The dose for a 20 kg patient with factor VIII deficiency of baseline activity 10% to increase to 50% would be:

$$20 \times 45 \times (50\% - 10\%) = 360 \text{ units}$$

As one bottle of factor VIII usually contains ~250 units, this patient should receive 2 bottles.

The *in vivo* half-life of factor VIII is 8–12 hours and of factor IX is 18–24 hours. In practice, factor VIII deficient patients require maintenance infusions twice daily, while factor IX deficient patients can be maintained with daily infusions.

Haematological emergencies

Acute anaemia

Life-threatening anaemia leading to cardiovascular collapse may occur in the following conditions.

Acute intravascular haemolysis

- *G6PD deficiency*: This is the commonest cause of intravascular haemolysis in childhood. The precipitating cause is almost always ingestion of fava beans or naphthalene exposure. The clinical clues for intravascular haemolysis are dark (or red) urine and/or jaundice ± abdominal pain and fever. Important clinical differential diagnoses include UTI and hepatitis. Examination of the blood film shows characteristic fragmented cells diagnostic of oxidant haemolysis. Rates of haemoglobin fall can be as high as 10 g/L (1 g/dL) hourly and therefore patients need close monitoring.

- *Autoimmune haemolytic anaemia (AIHA)*: This is seen as a rare sequel of viral or mycoplasma infection. Spherocytosis or auto-agglutination may be seen in the blood film. The direct Coombs test is positive with either IgG (warm AIHA) or complement (cold AIHA or paroxysmal cold haemoglobinuria [PCH]).

Urgent blood transfusion is often required in the treatment of children with acute intravascular haemolysis. In addition, those with cold AIHA or PCH should be kept warm to minimise further destruction of red cells.

Uncontrolled blood loss

This is seen in trauma victims, children with bleeding from GIT or occasionally postoperatively (for example, post-tonsillectomy). Children with bleeding disorders may swallow blood from lesions oozing continuously in the nose or oropharynx. Specific coagulation factor therapy as well as blood transfusion may be required.

Acute decompensation in a patient with known chronic anaemia

Children with chronic anaemia are often well compensated by increased levels of 2,3-DPG which allows a shift in the oxygen dissociation curve. Any condition which alters this compensated state, for example fever or development of acidosis, may result in acute deterioration in the child. In such circumstances transfusion is often indicated.

Bleeding disorders

The emergencies that may present in patients with congenital coagulation disorders or severe thrombocytopenia are intracerebral bleeding, intraocular bleeding, airway obstruction, and compartmental bleeding. These events may be the presenting manifestation of the disorder.

For patients with known coagulation factor deficiencies the appropriate factor concentrate should be given as soon as possible. Urgent factor supplement is required following trauma to the head, injuries about the neck, and muscle bleeds in the forearm and lower leg. If in doubt, treat and then investigate.

The approach to the thrombocytopenic patient

This depends on the aetiology of the condition. In conditions of poor platelet production (such as aplastic anaemia and marrow infiltration) or following chemotherapy, a platelet count of $< 20 \times 10^9/L$ could result in serious bleeding. Platelet transfusion is usually given to oncology patients at this hospital if the count is $< 10 \times 10^9/L$.

Immune thrombocytopenic purpura (ITP) in prepubertal children is usually of sudden onset. The numerous petechiae, widespread bruising and (often) mucosal bleeding are very worrying to family and medical staff. Although treatment is controversial, major complications (such as intracranial haemorrhage) are very rare. Perusal of the blood film often reveals large platelets not counted by the blood count analyser, so the platelet count may be higher than initially reported. Management of a bleeding child in ITP should be discussed with a consultant haematologist.

Neutropenia

Neutropenia is common in children with viral infections. Children with neutrophil counts $> 0.2 \times 10^9/L$ rarely have problems. With the exception of patients receiving chemotherapy, septicaemia due to neutropenia is rare.

Sickle cell disease

The most common presentation in children with sickle cell disease is painful vaso-occlusive crises. These can be managed with parenteral analgesia (morphine infusion is preferable) and hyper-hydration (fluids 1.5 × maintenance). Other very important presentations, however, are discussed below.

Acute splenic sequestration crisis

This presents with a rapid fall in haemoglobin and an enlarging spleen. This condition may proceed very rapidly to shock and death. These patients require:

- urgent blood transfusion (simple packed cell transfusion is often sufficient)
- supportive care and close monitoring.

Subsequently they may require a splenectomy because of the possibility of recurrence.

Chest crisis

This presents with chest pain, cough, fever and infiltrates on the CXR. It usually follows a veno-occlusive episode. It is very difficult to distinguish pulmonary infarction from infection, and often one leads to the other. These patients require:

- supplemental oxygen
- parenteral analgesia
- antibiotic cover (penicillin G or ampicillin).

If symptoms are worsening despite the above, transfusion may be indicated. Transfusion may take the form of a simple packed cell transfusion or an exchange transfusion. This decision should be made in consultation with the haematologist on call.

Cerebral infarction

This usually presents with the acute onset of focal neurological signs, altered level of consciousness or seizures. These patients require:

- supplemental oxygen
- exchange transfusion to reduce HbS < 30%.

Subsequently these patients require long-term transfusion because there is a 66% recurrence risk, the majority in the first 3 years after presentation.

Infection

Patients with sickle cell disease should all be considered hyposplenic because they autoinfarct their spleen. This puts them at risk of overwhelming bacterial infection, a leading cause of death in sickle-cell patients. Bacterial sepsis in these patients may follow a rapidly fulminant course leading to shock and even death within a few hours. Pneumococcus is by far the commonest organism, but sickle-cell patients are also susceptible to sepsis with meningococcus, Hib (if not immunised) and salmonella. Febrile patients with sickle cell disease require:

- careful assessment
- blood culture and FBC/film looking for toxic changes.

Keep a low threshold for admission and commencement of antibiotics while awaiting culture results.

Patients well enough not to require admission should be reassessed by a medical officer within 24 hours.

See Chapter 12, p. 150, on immunisation in hyposplenic children.

Thalassaemia

On the whole, patients with thalassaemia major or thalassaemia intermedia are generally well. However, there are a few important points to remember when assessing these patients with an acute illness. Firstly, quite a number of patients with thalassaemia major or thalassaemia intermedia have been splenectomised. This puts them at risk of overwhelming bacterial infection. Secondly, these patients are iron-overloaded and are therefore at increased risk of *Yersinia* septicaemia. This is particularly so for those patients on iron chelation. *Yersinia* septicaemia in these patients usually presents with fever and abdominal pain (often right iliac fossa pain), nausea and vomiting. Diarrhoea may be present. Distinguishing this presentation from acute appendicitis is difficult, and it is therefore important that *Yersinia* be considered in all iron-loaded patients before surgery for acute appendicitis. Febrile patients with thalassaemia major or intermedia require:

- careful assessment keeping bacterial sepsis and in particular *Yersinia* infection in mind
- blood culture and FBC/film looking for toxic changes
- stool culture for *Yersinia*.

Consider admission and broad spectrum antibiotic cover (especially if splenectomised).

If *Yersinia* infection is suspected, therapy with intravenous cefotaxime and gentamicin should be commenced empirically.

Withhold iron chelation during any febrile illness.

Patients well enough not to require admission should be reviewed by a medical officer within 24 hours.

6

Pain management

This chapter includes:

- types of pain in children
- general principles of analgesic prescription
- opioid analgesics
- patient-controlled analgesia (PCA)
- side-effects of opioids
- local anaesthetics
- nitrous oxide.

Types of pain in children

The amount of pain anyone experiences is a composite of physiological and psychological variables and is not determined solely by the extent of tissue damage. Context, biological variation, previous experience and a variety of psychological factors modify the experience of pain and must be considered in every assessment of a child in pain. Nociception refers to noxious sensation per se without regard to its emotional significance.

In the past, pain in children has been underestimated and undertreated, due to an exaggerated fear of respiratory depression and addiction to opioids, and to misconceptions such as:

- Children experience less pain than adults.
- Pain is character-building for children.
- Children have no memory of pain.

Simple measures for dealing with a child in pain are valuable but often forgotten. These include:

- explanation, reassurance, gentle handling, and a calm environment
- cold or hot packs, elevation of a painful limb, splinting of fractures
- cognitive-behavioural techniques of pain control (such as breathing exercises, guided imagery, hypnosis).

Acute pain is associated with a brief period of tissue injury or inflammation (such as postoperative pain, fractures, burns, medical procedures).

Chronic persistent pain describes conditions of persistent or near-constant pain over 3 months or longer. This is distinguished from recurrent pain for which repetitive painful episodes alternate with pain-free intervals (for example in headache, abdominal pain).

Assessment

The assessment of pain begins with a medical history and physical examination to determine the aetiology. Therapies should be directed then at both the primary cause and the resulting pain.

The assessment of pain includes measurement. Pain is measured as an estimate of pain severity and to gauge the efficacy of analgesia administered. There is a variety of pain measurement tools which include physiological (heart rate, respiratory rate, blood pressure), behavioural and self-report measures, such as the pain faces scale and the visual analogue scale (see Figure 6.1). These may be useful for older children.

- *Pain faces scale*: A number of versions exist: this version (Figure 6.1) is reproduced with permission.
- *Visual analogue scale*

  0 _____ 10

  no pain   worst imaginable pain

It can be difficult to assess pain in the preverbal or cognitively impaired child. Postoperative pain should always be measured at rest, not during movement or coughing.

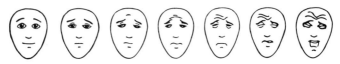

Figure 6.1 Pain faces scale
Source: Hicks CL, von Baeyer CL, Spafford P. et al. (2001) The faces pain scale—revised: toward a common metric in pediatric pain measurement, *Pain* **93**: 173–83.

General principles of analgesic prescription

The prescription of an analgesic is determined by the assessment of pain severity. *Mild* pain is treated with non-opioids, *moderate* pain is treated with opioids such as codeine, and *severe* pain is treated with opioids such as morphine, fentanyl or pethidine.

Oral analgesia is desirable in children whenever possible. Standard doses and dosage intervals will provide excellent analgesia for the majority of patients. The *intravenous* route of administration provides rapid onset of analgesia with the advantage of incremental intravenous titration with no discomfort to the child. Intramuscular injections should be avoided as children will often deny having pain rather than have repeated intramuscular injections.

The appropriate dose for the child (on a per kilogram basis), the route of administration and the dosage interval need to be individually determined. For severe and ongoing pain, the regular administration of an appropriate analgesic will provide better efficacy than 'p.r.n.' orders. Patient-controlled analgesia (PCA) and some opioid infusions need to be supervised by the Pain Service. Advanced regional anaesthetic techniques such as epidurals are the responsibility of the paediatric anaesthetist.

Non-opioid analgesics

The non-opioid analgesics are appropriately prescribed for mild pain or in combination with opioids for moderate to severe pain.

Paracetamol

This is an effective simple analgesic. The wide variety of different strengths of oral preparations demands additional care in prescribing. The major concern over toxicity (liver damage) from paracetamol arises when the drug is given repeatedly to sick, anorexic, febrile children over 48 hours or longer. In this situation the need for the drug and the dose should be frequently reassessed.

Dose: Oral or rectal—20 mg/kg for a single dose (up to 1 g), then 20 mg/kg if given regularly (4–6-hourly), to a maximum daily dose of 90 mg/kg/24 hours (up to 4 g/day); in a febrile, unwell child, give lower doses—60 mg/kg/24 hours (up to 2.4 g/day).

Paracetamol should be used with caution in children with liver or renal disease. Rectal suppositories are not appropriate in neutropenic patients.

Nonsteroidal anti-inflammatory drugs (NSAIDs)

NSAIDs are used for mild pain in children. Naproxen and ibuprofen are commonly used NSAIDs, and both are available as elixirs.

Contraindications to the use of NSAIDs

Contraindications include:

- gastrointestinal ulceration, ulcerative colitis or Crohn's disease
- liver dysfunction
- abnormal coagulation or potential for active bleeding
- asthma
- renal disease, diuretic therapy or decreased renal perfusion due to hypotension or hypovolaemia.

The non-opioid analgesics have a ceiling effect such that increasing doses do not provide increased analgesia. This is *not* the case for the opioids.

Aspirin is not widely used in children because of unproven concern that it may be a factor in causing Reye's syndrome. However, it continues to have specific indications, for instance in rheumatoid conditions.

Opioid analgesics

Oral opioids

Oral opioid analgesia is dependent upon oral bioavailability and dosage interval. The following are guidelines for starting doses of opioids.

Codeine

- 60–70% oral bioavailability
- Oral dose: 0.5–1 mg/kg 4-hourly

Morphine

- Poor oral bioavailability (30–40%)
- Oral dose (immediate release morphine): 0.3 mg/kg 4-hourly
- Sustained release preparations of morphine, such as MS

Contin™ (tablet, or powder for making up an oral liquid) and Kapanol™ (granules, which are not to be chewed), are available. These preparations are usually started after a total daily morphine dose has been determined by the prior use of immediate release oral morphine or intravenous morphine. The oral to IV morphine ratio is 3:1.

Methadone

- Available as tablets and oral liquid
- Good oral bioavailability and a long half-life
- Oral dose: 0.3 mg/kg/day, usually 8–12-hourly

Intermittent parenteral opioids

Intramuscular, intravenous

Opioid	Dose	Interval
Pethidine	1–2 mg/kg	3rd hourly
Morphine	0.1–0.15 mg/kg	3rd hourly

Intramuscular injections are not ideal due to the pain of injection. Following single injections (IM or IV) there is only a short duration of analgesic drug levels. An intravenous opioid infusion may be preferable if more than a few intermittent doses are required.

Subcutaneous

This can be administered through a subcutaneous 22-gauge cannula below the clavicle or over the deltoid muscle. The absorption characteristics are similar to IM injections. There is minimal discomfort if injected slowly.

Note:

- Only codeine and morphine should be given subcutaneously (pethidine stings). Doses are the same as for IM injections.
- This technique should not be used in a patient who is hypothermic, hypotensive or shocked, due to the risk of delayed absorption.

Intravenous opioid infusions

These are used for severe postoperative and other pain. Morphine is the drug of initial choice.

Note: Adequate intravenous loading should be used prior to the commencement of an infusion, for example morphine 0.1 mg/kg IV followed by 0.05 mg/kg boluses every 10 minutes until the patient is comfortable, then commence the infusion. Additional 'bolus' doses of morphine may be required after a morphine infusion has been started, to cover periods when pain may be greater, such as with bathing and during changing of dressings. Supplementary opioid doses are calculated as 5–10% of the total daily opioid dosage.

The continuous infusion dose/rate is:

morphine	10–50 micrograms/kg/h
fentanyl	1 microgram/kg/h

Codeine must not be given intravenously.

These doses are for children in a normal ward or high dependency unit. Methods of loading syringes and infusion rates are set out in *The Children's Hospital at Westmead Acute Pain Manual*. Pethidine infusions carry a risk of norpethidine toxicity—CNS irritability and convulsions.

Monitoring the child's condition during opioid infusion

Once analgesia has been achieved and an opioid infusion commenced, the child's oxygen saturation should be checked (via pulse oximetry) in room air, and oxygen commenced if necessary.

Respiratory rates and a sedation score should also be monitored hourly. Other parameters recorded hourly are pulse, pain score and complications.

Minimum respiratory rates		Sedation score
> 8 years	12 breaths/min	0 = unrousable
2–8 years	15 breaths/min	1 = asleep, rousable
3 months–2 years	20 breaths/min	2 = drowsy
< 3 months	25 breaths/min	3 = awake

Note: Immediate action must be taken to treat respiratory depression resulting from opiate therapy. See 'Side-effects of opioids' on p. 64.

Special considerations

The following groups may require special adjustments, observations and monitoring such as pulse oximetry with opioid infusions:

- *Infants < 6 months*: Use half the usual morphine infusion rate (that is, 5–15 micrograms/kg/h). These patients have a much longer half-life for opioids and should have constant pulse oximetry.
- *Children with renal failure*: Renal failure may cause delayed excretion of active morphine metabolites such as morphine 6-glucuronide, so lower infusion rates may be required.

Other high-risk children include those with:

- a difficult airway or airway pathology
- respiratory disease, such as pneumonia
- constrictive bandages around neck/chest/abdomen.

Patient-controlled analgesia (PCA)

PCA provides excellent analgesia. Preoperative education is valuable for children using PCA. Generally only the patient retains control of the button to self-administer a bolus. Before the use of PCA, adequate intravenous loading of the opioid must occur to achieve adequate blood levels (the same as for an opioid infusion).

There are two modes:

1 bolus only
2 bolus plus a small background continuous infusion (used for major surgery, for example scoliosis or thoracic surgery).

An hourly limit is set as an added safety mechanism.

Contraindications

- Children younger than 7 years old
- Cognitive impairment
- Inability to understand preoperative instruction on PCA (language barriers are a relative contraindication)
- Undiagnosed intra-abdominal or intracranial pathology
- Previous severe side-effects to opioids
- Patients with renal failure require bolus only

Drug	Bolus dose	Continuous infusion	Lock out interval	Hourly limit
Morphine	20 micrograms/ kg	10 micrograms/ kg/h	5 minutes	130 micrograms/ kg/h

Monitoring should be as for an opioid infusion. For further details on this technique see *The Children's Hospital at Westmead Acute Pain Manual.*

Side-effects of opioids

Respiratory depression

Respiratory depression is rare in the presence of acute pain and appropriate opioid dosing.

If sedation score = 0 (unrousable) and the respiratory rate less than the minimum for age then:

1 Stop infusion immediately.
2 Administer oxygen by mask.
3 Resuscitate as necessary.
4 Give naloxone 0.01 mg/kg stat, IV. Additional doses may be required.

> Extreme caution should be used in giving naloxone to patients who have been receiving chronic opioid therapy, since severe pain and symptoms of opioid withdrawal may ensue. Assisted ventilation may be a safer alternative.

Vomiting

Vomiting occurs commonly after surgery and is multifactorial in cause:

• Exclude non-opioid-related causes of vomiting.
• Adjust opioid dosing where possible or consider a switch to an alternative opioid.
• Ensure adequate hydration and normal serum electrolytes.

Drugs: Metoclopramide 0.15 mg/kg IV or IM 6-hourly, or ondansetron 0.15 mg/kg (usually maximum 8 mg) slowly over 15 minutes, if vomiting is refractory to metoclopramide.

Itch

• Exclude non-opioid-related causes (such as drug allergy, cholestasis).
• Consider antihistamines (for example, promethazine).
• Consider a switch to an alternative opioid.

Constipation

Patients receiving long-term opioids do not become tolerant to the constipating effects of opioids. Ensure the regular use of laxatives in these patients.

Local anaesthetics

- *EMLA™*: This is a topical anaesthetic cream mixture of lignocaine and prilocaine. It is useful for skin analgesia for procedures such as venous cannulation, long line insertion and lumbar puncture. It needs to be applied over the site (intact skin) thickly under an occlusive dressing for at least an hour prior to cannulation or other local anaesthetic infiltration. It is not normally used in children younger than 6 months of age due to the risk of methaemoglobinaemia. Increased absorption may occur if it is applied to mucous membranes.
- *Amethocaine (4% gel)*: This is a topical local anaesthetic that is useful prior to needle procedures, as an alternative to EMLA. It needs to be applied under an occlusive dressing at least 1 hour before a procedure. It may produce more skin reaction in comparison with EMLA.
- *Lignocaine (Xylocaine™)*: Usually used for local infiltration for cannulation and wound suturing. It has rapid onset of action and short duration (1–2 hours).
  - Maximum dose: lignocaine 4.5 mg/kg/dose
    lignocaine with adrenaline 7 mg/kg/dose
  - *Avoid using lignocaine with adrenaline in end-artery situations such as the digits or penis.*
- *Bupivacaine (Marcain™)*: Usually used as a specific nerve block or infiltration intraoperatively by the anaesthetist or surgeon as an adjunct to general anaesthesia and for postoperative analgesia, especially in day surgery, for example ilioinguinal/iliohypogastric nerve blocks for inguinal hernia repair. It has slower onset but longer duration of action (8–12 hours). Maximum dose: Bupivacaine 2.5 mg/kg (with or without adrenaline).

Nitrous oxide

Nitrous oxide (N_2O) is a short-acting analgesic gas used commonly in anaesthesia and for pain relief (for example lumbar puncture, bone marrow aspiration) or as Entonox (50% N_2O with 50% O_2) which is carried in ambulances. Patients should fast before its use.

Contraindications

- Difficult airway
- Impaired level of consciousness
- Undrained pneumothorax, recent middle ear surgery (nitrous oxide diffuses into gas-containing cavities)

The person administering the nitrous oxide must maintain verbal communication with the sedated child to ensure that analgesia is adequate but that the patient remains rousable.

7

Fluid and electrolyte therapy

This chapter includes:

- fundamental principles
- calculating fluids
- maintenance requirements
- deficit therapy
- fluid therapy in surgical conditions
- total parenteral nutrition.

Fundamental principles

- Blind guesses and unthinking application of 'rules-of-thumb' are recipes for disaster when calculating fluids and electrolytes.
- Calculations of *maintenance* needs versus *deficit* requirements are based on *different principles* and require *separate calculations*:
  - *Maintenance water requirements* relate directly to caloric expenditure. If metabolism is increased, water requirements are increased, and vice versa. Infants burn more energy to maintain their temperature and to grow. Fluid requirements gradually drop with increasing age and reach adult levels in adolescence.
  - *Deficit therapy* is based directly on the assessed degree of acute body weight loss, assuming this to be mostly water. Thus, a 5% dehydrated infant and a 5% dehydrated adult both need 5% of their weight replaced as water.
- A child with good cardiovascular and renal function can generally accommodate, without harm, considerable variations in both the volume and the electrolyte content of administered fluids.
- *Extreme caution* in fluid administration is required where there are pre-existing fluid overload, cerebral oedema, heart failure and/or renal impairment. Much smaller volumes will usually be required, and electrolyte content will require closer attention.

- Conversely, *severe dehydration* with circulatory impairment demands prompt fluid resuscitation to restore normal blood flow to vital organs and to prevent ischaemic damage to these.
- Giving dilute fluids (for example N/4 saline with 3.75% dextrose, N/5 saline with 4% dextrose, or dextrose 5% or 10%) to a child with low serum sodium is potentially dangerous. Even in moderate amounts, it risks acute brain swelling, raised intra-cranial pressure and death.
- Change in body weight is the best measure of change in hydration. An accurate bare weight on admission, then daily weighings, are essential in monitoring rehydration.

Calculating fluids

Table 7.1 Essential steps in calculating fluids

A	Is resuscitation required for circulatory failure? If yes, give resuscitation fluids at once; these are not to be included in subsequent calculations of fluid requirements.	Use Hartmann's solution or normal saline, 20 mL/kg over 10–20 minutes; repeat if necessary.	See p. 18.
B	Is there a fluid *deficit*— dehydration requiring correction? If yes, use calculation: weight × % dehydration (up to 5%) × 10	Deficit fluids are usually given as N/2 saline with 2.5% glucose (dextrose).	See p. 72.
C	What *maintenance volume* is required? (Table 7.2) Is correction needed for *modifying factors*? (Table 7.3)	Use N/4 saline with 3.75% glucose (dextrose), unless serum sodium is low.	See p. 69.
D	What allowance, if any, is needed for *continuing losses*?	Estimate a volume of a fluid with similar sodium content to that which is being lost, e.g. N/2 dextrose saline for diarrhoea.	

Table 7.1 Essential steps in calculating fluids (*continued*)

E   Write your calculations at the top of the IV Orders Sheet:
  • Add B + C + D, to calculate the estimated fluid volume for
    24 hours.
  • Generally, give the calculated volume at the same rate over
    24 hours, giving the chosen deficit replacement fluid first.
  • In any unstable or particularly unwell child, order fluids for
    4–8 hours only and then reassess the clinical state, urinary
    output and serum electrolytes to guide further therapy.

Maintenance requirements

Water

Maintenance requirements are *not* directly proportional to weight,
but to energy expenditure per unit mass. It is not convenient to have
to measure an individual's caloric expenditure to determine his or
her water requirements. Table 7.2 expresses the approximate water
requirements per kilogram according to age, taking varying energy
expenditure into account. The volumes shown are *not* 'basal'; they are
for normally active children, with good renal function, in usual
ranges of ambient temperature and humidity.

Table 7.2 Maintenance water requirements

Age	mL/kg/day
1st day of life	60
2nd day of life	90
Up to 9 months	120–140
12 months	90–100
2 years	80–90
4 years	70–80
8 years	60–70
12 years	50–60

The importance of modifying factors

The examples in Table 7.3, based on children of identical weight, show:

• how modifying factors can markedly increase or decrease fluids
• how allowing for correcting pre-existing dehydration, then also
  allowing for likely continuing losses (as in point 3 in Table 7.4)

69

may lead to an apparently alarmingly high calculated volume. Any calculated volume should be seen as a 'starting point'. Changes are then made according to frequent careful clinical observations, urine output and so on.

Table 7.3 Factors modifying water requirements

Extra required	Less required
Fever (add 10% for each °C above 37°C)	Hypothermia (subtract 10% for each °C below 37°C)
Hyperventilation	Very high humidity
High ambient temperature	Oliguria or anuria
Extreme activity	Extreme inactivity

Table 7.4 Examples of fluid calculation in clinical situations

1	10 kg child, nil-by-mouth following bowel surgery, is generally well, afebrile and reasonably active; serum electrolytes are normal.

A Resuscitation...nil
B Deficit therapy ....nil
C Maintenance 10 × 90 =...900 mL
D Continuing losses ....nil
B + C + D = 900 mL per day
Give as N/4 saline with 3.75% dextrose at 37 mL per hour.

2	10 kg child, 12 months, with head injury, unconscious and hypothermic (35°C), receiving artificial ventilation with humidified gases.

A Resuscitation...nil
B Deficit therapy ....nil
C Maintenance therapy 10 × 90 = 900 mL, reduced by
   modifying factors: less 200 mL (for hypothermia); 300 mL
   (allowance for pre-existing cerebral oedema, inactivity) ...400 mL
D Continuing losses ....nil
B + C + D = 400 mL per day
If serum sodium is normal, give as N/4 saline with 3.75% dextrose at 17 mL per hour and review often.

3	10 kg child, aged 12 months, with 5% dehydration, acidosis, protracted vomiting, continuing diarrhoea and persistent fever (38.5–40.5°C).

A Resuscitation...nil
B Deficit therapy 10 × 5 × 10 ....500 mL

Table 7.4 Examples of fluid calculation in clinical situations
(*continued*)

C Maintenance requirement (10 × 90 = 900 mL) plus
   400 mL for fever, hyperactivity..1300 mL
D For predicted ongoing losses via diarrhoea ....400 mL
B + C + D = 2200 mL per day
Review may demand an increase or decrease in this volume. Give as
N/2 saline with 2.5% dextrose (plus 10 mmol KCl per 500 mL
saline) at 92 mL per hour and review often.

Sodium

In the first week of life, normal babies require 1–1.5 mmol/kg/day
of sodium for maintenance, increasing to 3 mmol/kg/day by
age 2–3 months, then slowly decreasing to 2 mmol/kg/day by age
2 years.

In practice, giving 1/4 or 1/5 normal saline in maintenance
volumes will satisfy the maintenance sodium requirements in a child
with no abnormal sodium requirements or sodium losses. (Normal
saline contains 150 mmol sodium per litre, N/5 saline contains
30 mmol sodium per litre.) Deficit replacement is discussed below.

Potassium

Maintenance requirements are approximately 3 mmol/kg/day. It is
preferable to avoid a concentration of greater than 30 mmol/litre in
infusion fluid, and it is rarely wise or necessary to give potassium
before renal function has been established. Deficit replacement is
discussed below.

Vitamins

Except in severely ill or malnourished children, it is unnecessary
to add vitamins to intravenous fluids during the first 48 hours of
treatment.

Deficit therapy

Fluid and electrolyte deficits develop more rapidly in children than
in adults. Unlike maintenance volumes, deficit volumes are directly
related to body weight. Hence, a 7% acute loss of body weight
because of dehydration will be of similar seriousness in an individual

71

of any size, although it is likely to come about much more quickly in a smaller individual, even in just a few hours.

In treating a child with a water and electrolyte deficit, follow these steps:

- Assess the extent of deficit.
- Resuscitate where necessary—rapid fluid administration to improve circulation and renal function—when there is serious hypovolaemia.
- Otherwise, replace extracellular and intracellular fluid and electrolyte deficits slowly (over 24–72 hours).
- Even where the degree of dehydration is assessed as greater than 5%, the initial calculation of deficit replacement should be based upon 5%. Deficit therapy is usually given as N/2 saline with 2.5% dextrose.
- Include maintenance requirements, and allowances for continuing abnormal losses, in calculations of total water and electrolyte amounts to be given.
- Frequently reassess any child requiring replacement of water and electrolyte deficits.

Assessment of dehydration

Assessment of water deficit is based largely on symptoms and signs. Raised serum creatinine and blood urea may be an indication of dehydration. Otherwise, laboratory investigations are of most use in assessing coexisting electrolyte abnormalities. In the history, note the duration and severity of abnormal losses, recent fluid intake, thirst and urine output. On examination, note the pulse rate, blood pressure, circulatory state, skin tone, state of the fontanelle, ocular tension, degree of enophthalmos, mouth dryness, body temperature and mental state.

- *Mild dehydration* produces thirst and mild oliguria but *no detectable physical signs*; it equates with 5% acute weight loss.
- *Moderate dehydration* produces more thirst and oliguria, along with tachycardia, slightly sunken eyes, some alteration in skin tone, some loss of ocular tension and sunken fontanelle in infants; it equates with about 5–10% acute body weight loss.
- *Severe dehydration* produces marked tachycardia, obvious loss of skin tone and tissue turgor, sunken eyes, loss of ocular tension, severe oliguria or anuria, restlessness and apathy. It equates with

10% or greater acute weight loss. In addition, circulatory collapse, delirium, coma, hyperpyrexia and cyanosis may occur.

Physical examination can be misleading in the assessment of dehydration:

- Signs of dehydration, except tachycardia, are less apparent in obese infants.
- The degree of dehydration is often overestimated in marasmic infants.
- In hypernatraemic dehydration, the skin and circulatory changes may be deceptively inapparent, with neurological signs predominant.

Laboratory investigations

Children with mild water and electrolyte deficits can be treated adequately without laboratory investigations, but those dehydrated to the extent of needing intravenous therapy should have serum electrolytes measured initially and again at 6–8 hours. Serum electrolytes may reveal unexpected hyponatraemia, hypernatraemia or hypokalaemia, although serum potassium is of little use in indicating total body potassium. A raised blood urea may be an indication of dehydration more severe than it appears on physical signs, or may give a clue to underlying renal disease.

Resuscitation

Where severe dehydration has progressed to circulatory failure, rapid infusion of fluids is urgently needed to restore the circulation, to prevent hypoxaemic brain damage and renal failure.

- Either Hartmann's solution or normal saline, 20–40 mL/kg, is infused rapidly, for example over 10–20 minutes; the infusion is slowed when circulation improves and hypotension is relieved. Further deficit therapy then proceeds more slowly.
- Greater volumes are sometimes necessary when deficits are profound. If blood pressure remains low, continue rapid infusion, but look for other reasons for the poor response, such as myocardial dysfunction.
- Blood is used only if blood loss has occurred.
- In an emergency, if Hartmann's solution or normal saline are unavailable, use 4% albumin or N/2 dextrose saline.

Subsequent deficit therapy

- *Calculation of replacement therapy* following resuscitation:
  - Volume of rehydrating fluid (mL)
    = body weight (kg) × % estimated dehydration (up to 5%) × 10
  - *Note*: For oral rehydration in gastroenteritis, see Chapter 16.
- In gastroenteritis, the commonest condition in which deficit therapy is required, the sodium deficit is very variable. Even so, 1/2 normal saline with 2.5% dextrose has been found to be a satisfactory rehydrating fluid for most children with gastroenteritis, renal mechanisms ultimately adjusting total body sodium to normal. (See also Chapter 16.)
- Where sodium losses have been more severe, e.g. diabetic ketoacidosis, much larger amounts of sodium are required. (See Chapter 15.)
- In *hypernatraemic dehydration*, rehydrating fluid is still given as 1/2 normal saline, in order to prevent rapid movement of water across cellular membranes, and hence cerebral oedema. Oral correction of dehydration is often possible. The optimal management of hypernatraemia is controversial, but it appears that slow correction of dehydration (over 36–48 hours) is useful in reducing the risk of convulsions, cerebral damage and death associated with this condition.
- In *hyponatraemia*, rapid correction of the sodium deficit is required only in the rare circumstance of symptomatic hyponatraemia, in which the serum sodium will usually be below 115 mmol/L. Hypertonic (3%) saline is used only in exceptional circumstances; normal (0.9%) saline is usually more appropriate.
- The following formula gives an approximation of the amount required for sodium repletion in hyponatraemia; this amount is replaced over a 24–48 hour period:

  mmol Na required =
  (proposed serum Na − present serum Na) × 0.6 × weight in kg

Potassium

- Generally, have evidence of urinary output before the addition of the 'maintenance' potassium to the combined deficit and maintenance fluids.
- In any severely ill child, a serum potassium level should be available soon after admission. In some conditions (such as infantile

pyloric stenosis and diabetic ketoacidosis) the total body potassium deficit will be severe, regardless of the initial serum potassium; 5 mmol/kg/day of potassium (or more) may be necessary. Therapy must be guided by frequent serum potassium estimations.

Correction of acidosis

- Severe or moderate dehydration produces a metabolic acidosis which will usually resolve with rehydration, and without administration of alkali.
- In severe acidosis secondary to bicarbonate loss, particularly where circulatory impairment is present, use bicarbonate as follows:

$$\text{mmol of bicarbonate} = \text{base deficit} \times \text{weight (kg)} \times 0.3$$
(With 10% $NaHCO_3$, 1 mL = 1 mmol)

Fluid therapy in surgical conditions

General principles

Preoperative

- Children undergoing elective operations are generally healthy and can tolerate the necessary period without food or fluids before anaesthesia.
- This also applies to many children having urgent surgery, where abnormal fluid losses have not occurred.
- If shock, significant dehydration or serious electrolyte imbalance is present, preoperative correction with intravenous fluids will be needed to minimise the risks of anaesthesia and surgery.

Intraoperative

- Continue correcting existing dehydration and replace continuing losses during the operation.
- In most instances this can be achieved by the administration of Hartmann's solution or normal saline, 10 mL/kg, during the first hour of operation, and 5 mL/kg/h thereafter.
- Blood should be replaced when the measured blood loss exceeds 25–40% of the estimated blood volume. Where preoperative correction of anaemia is necessary, this should be carried out preferably 48 hours or more before the operation.

Postoperative

- Intravenous fluids are necessary until the child is able to tolerate oral fluids in adequate amounts. Following gastrointestinal surgery, this may take several days.
- Abnormal losses (for example, gastric or intestinal aspirate) are accurately measured and replacement volumes added to daily maintenance requirements. Some abnormal losses (such as evaporative and respiratory water loss in fever and hyperventilation) contain little or no electrolyte. These factors are taken into account in the electrolyte content of fluids given.

Surgery in the neonatal period

- Although healthy full-term newborn babies can usually tolerate low fluid intake during the first 1 or 2 days of life, unwell babies cannot. Intravenous fluids should be commenced immediately in babies with, for instance, intestinal obstruction or oesophageal atresia.
- Because babies do not tolerate hypothermia they should be kept warm and in a humid atmosphere during transport to the paediatric surgical unit and at all times thereafter.
- Because of the risk of hypoglycaemia in these neonates, intravenous fluids should be given as 10% dextrose in 1/4 normal saline, and the blood glucose level should be monitored regularly with Dextrostix.
- Gastric decompression with a nasogastric tube of adequate size is essential for those babies likely to vomit (such as those with intestinal obstruction) in order to prevent inhalation of vomitus.

Specific conditions

Intestinal obstruction

- Fluids must be given intravenously until the obstruction has been relieved and intestinal function has returned (bowel sounds are present, there is minimal or no gastric aspirate, flatus and/or stools are passed through the rectum).
- The surgeon decides when oral fluids may be recommenced.
- Intravenous fluids should be commenced on diagnosis and any existing dehydration corrected in the standard manner. Fluid and electrolyte resuscitation must be carried out before surgery.

- *Fluid regimen*: If serum sodium is normal, daily maintenance fluids are given as 1/4 normal saline with dextrose. Measured and/or expected abnormal losses are replaced with an appropriate fluid, such as 1/2 normal dextrose saline or Hartmann's solution for intestinal fluid losses. If renal function is adequate, potassium should be added; up to 5 mmol/kg per day may be required, because of abnormal losses due to the intestinal obstruction. Monitoring with daily serum electrolyte estimations and a record of urine output is essential.
- If the period of intravenous fluid therapy exceeds 4 days, total parenteral nutrition should be considered.

Pyloric stenosis

- Vomiting due to pyloric stenosis produces hypochloraemic metabolic alkalosis. If the diagnosis is delayed, the infant may develop gross dehydration and marasmus.
- Rehydration is carried out along standard lines with N/2 dextrose saline (or Hartmann's solution, then N/2 dextrose saline), maintenance requirements (as N/4 saline with dextrose) with added potassium (up to 5 mmol/kg). Although the initial serum potassium level may not be low, the total body potassium deficit is usually considerable.
- The operation for pyloric stenosis is not performed until the infant is well hydrated and has satisfactory serum electrolytes. In some instances, with late diagnosis, this state may not be achieved for 2 or 3 days. Conversely, operation must not be further delayed after a satisfactory clinical state is present.

Acute appendicitis

- Some children with acute appendicitis are not dehydrated at the time of admission and do not require preoperative intravenous fluids.
- In the presence of signs of dehydration, shock or peritonitis, normal saline or Hartmann's solution are required before the operation. The volumes required are very variable; usually a volume between 20 and 40 mL/kg is given in a 2–4 hour period.
- It is routine to administer intravenous fluids during appendicectomy and postoperatively until the child is able to tolerate oral fluids.

Intussusception

- Two-thirds of children with idiopathic intussusception are successfully treated with air or contrast enema reduction.
- An intravenous line should be secured before other treatment is commenced, but this should not unnecessarily delay the attempted non-surgical reduction.
- When air or contrast reduction fails, surgical treatment becomes necessary.
- When shock or dehydration is present, similar preoperative therapy to that described for acute appendicitis is necessary. The child must be resuscitated before any attempted reduction of the intussusception.
- Blood must always be cross-matched, and available before operation.

Total parenteral nutrition (TPN)

TPN aims to maintain a satisfactory nutritional state and growth with all nutrients given intravenously. This includes, then, all necessary amino acids, fat, glucose, electrolytes, vitamins, minerals, trace elements and water. TPN has been used in infants and children for more than 25 years, but remains an expensive, difficult and potentially dangerous therapy. It should not be considered in any child where enteral feeding remains possible.

When enteral feeds are contraindicated or are impossible, consider TPN:

- in malnourished and critically ill children when a metabolically stable situation has been achieved after initial resuscitation. In these patients usual intravenous fluids should not be continued for more than 24 hours.
- for children with adequate nutrition, if there is no oral intake beyond 4 days.
- for neonates if IV fluids are to be given beyond 48–72 hours.

Material and methods

TPN solutions

These are prepared under strict aseptic conditions in the hospital pharmacy.

Modes of administration

- By peripheral vein, if venous access is easy and if TPN is required for less than a week. Full caloric requirements are rarely supplied by this route.
- By *'peripheral-central' vein*: A silastic catheter is placed in a central vein or right atrium via a standard venipuncture needle in a scalp or limb vein. Full caloric requirements can be given.
- By *'central line'*: A silastic catheter is passed through a large vein into the right atrium. Use when long-term TPN is likely to be required.
- A constant infusion pump should always be used for TPN fluids.
- Protocols to be observed in using TPN are available in all wards.
- Never stop TPN abruptly (as this can lead to severe hypoglycaemia).

Patients receiving TPN have an increased risk of sepsis. Extravasation of fluid into the tissues may occur with central as well as peripheral lines and a chest X-ray may reveal fluid in the thoracic cavity. Under these circumstances, hypoglycaemia, as well as the local complications of leaking fluid, is likely unless an intravenous line is established quickly.

8

Neonatal medicine

This chapter includes:

- stabilisation and transport
- respiratory distress
- cyanosis and hypoxaemia
- neonatal sepsis
- neonatal jaundice
- hypoglycaemia
- intravenous fluid therapy
- examination of the newborn.

Stabilisation and transport

In about half of all cases, at-risk pregnancy or labour can be recognised early enough for the mother and foetus to be safely moved to a maternity hospital with a tertiary-level newborn intensive care nursery rather than moving the sick infant after birth.

Transport of the sick newborn infant is required where there is a diagnostic or therapeutic problem beyond the capacity of the local resources because of limitations in expertise, equipment or staff availability.

Initial stabilisation

- Initially, adept local staff should resuscitate the infant and maintain normal temperature, oxygenation, perfusion and blood sugar (TOPS).
- Communicate early with specialist staff to discuss management and seek advice. For very sick or small infants, this will be with a tertiary (Level 3) hospital or the Newborn and Paediatric Emergency Transport Service (NETS) (telephone: 1300 36 2500). For less sick infants, the duty paediatrician of a regional rural or suburban hospital would normally be contacted.

- Resist the commonplace urge to 'wrap and run' with the infant, as it regularly contributes to morbidity. Although referring hospitals may feel limited, the staff, their facilities and the environment of a hospital (with telephone support) are more able to support the infant than staff in the back of an ambulance.

Options for transport

The options for transport are to send an escort from the local hospital, arrange an ambulance escort or request retrieval. The local escort should have appropriate equipment, including an incubator with a thermal probe and an oximeter, and be familiar with their operation in an ambulance. The NSW Ambulance Service provides a skilled nurse escort for journeys by air ambulance.

For sicker infants, medical retrieval with Level 3 care is generally appropriate and NETS should be contacted.

Indications for transfer for Level 3 care include:

- $FiO_2 > 0.40$
- very low birth weight (< 1500 g)
- requirement for assisted ventilation
- oxygen saturation < 90% despite high ambient FiO_2
- Apgar score persistently < 7
- requirement for major operative surgery
- perinatal asphyxia
- meconium aspiration syndrome
- persistent pulmonary hypertension
- ductus-dependent congenital heart disease
- seizures
- apnoea.

All infants must be stabilised as far as possible before transfer, whoever might be escorting the infant. Except in rare circumstances, the infant should improve during the transfer rather than simply endure it.

Summary of stabilisation measures

Checks in ALL infants

- Oxygenation by pulse oximeter/blood gases
- Blood glucose by Dextrostix or formal laboratory measurement
- Temperature

- Respiratory status
- Circulation/fluid status

Requirements for MOST infants

- Intravenous fluids with 8% dextrose + N/5 or N/4 saline
- Gastric venting with size FG8 orogastric tube
- Monitoring of temperature and oxygenation

Pre-transport checklist

- TOPS? (Temperature, Oxygen, Perfusion, Sugar)
- IV line?
- Orogastric tube?
- Antibiotics?
- Vitamin K?
- Special considerations?
- Maternal blood sample? (10 mL clotted)

Documentation

- NETS Perinatal Transfer Form
- Referring letter
- Copies of relevant nursing and medical records
- Original X-rays, copies of laboratory results
- Consent for treatment (included in Perinatal Transfer Form)
- Ambulance form (air ambulance)

Communication

- Parents
- Local doctor(s)
- Destination hospital
- NETS Clinical Coordination

Drug treatment (first dose only)

- Suspected sepsis:
  - *Early onset* (< 48 hours): ampicillin 50–100 mg/kg + gentamicin 2.5 mg/kg
  - *Late onset* (≥ 48 hours): flucloxacillin 50–100 mg/kg or vancomycin 10 mg/kg + gentamicin 2.5 mg/kg
- Seizures: phenobarbitone 20 mg/kg
- Necrotising enterocolitis: clindamycin 10 mg/kg + gentamicin 2.5 mg/kg

Summary

These guidelines for newborn emergency transport should not be considered a substitute for timely discussions between the staff of the referring hospital, NETS and the accepting hospital.

NETS provides clinical advice, often drawing on its links with specialist staff in all perinatal referral centres and children's hospitals. Up to five medical retrieval teams are available from Sydney and another from Newcastle.

Bed availability information for possible *in utero* transfer and the bed status of all Newborn Intensive Care Units in NSW and the ACT is available. More detailed information is available from NETS on the NETSLine—1300 36 2500.

Respiratory distress

Although a structural lesion or disease process affecting the airway and/or the lung is the most likely cause for respiratory distress, it may be a nonspecific manifestation of many disorders.

Clinical evaluation

The cardinal signs are tachypnoea, intercostal recession, expiratory grunt and central cyanosis.

History

Pregnancy and intrapartum events, infant's gestation, birth weight, condition at birth and age at onset of the respiratory distress assist in diagnosis and management.

Chest radiograph

A chest X-ray is *essential* for evaluation. Auscultation of the newborn chest is unreliable.

Supportive treatment

Early and effective stabilisation and frequent reappraisal of the infant's condition are extremely important. Early consultation should be sought regarding the possible need for referral to a tertiary centre.

83

- The infant with *mild* respiratory distress requires:
  - continuous cardiorespiratory monitoring
  - blood gas monitoring
  - intravenous feeding.
- The infant with *severe* respiratory distress requires the above and provision for long-term mechanical ventilation.
- The infant should be observed in an incubator or on an open radiant heater bed and given sufficient head box or incubator oxygen to alleviate cyanosis. The inspired oxygen should be warmed and humidified and the concentration recorded continuously.
- A blood culture should be obtained and the infant treated with penicillin (or ampicillin) and gentamicin, unless there is immediate access to sensitive laboratory indices of neonatal sepsis.
- Keep nil by mouth and treat with intravenous dextrose saline and monitor the blood glucose regularly.
- Consider persistent pulmonary hypertension of the newborn (PPHN) in severe respiratory distress. Keep well oxygenated (oximeter saturation 95–98% and PaO_2 60–90 mmHg) until PPHN is excluded.

Indications for mechanical ventilation

Absolute indications for immediate endotracheal intubation and mechanical ventilation include:

- severe or persistent apnoea
- cardiocirculatory shock
- severe cyanosis and/or acidosis.

The need for assisted ventilation in the presence of respiratory failure may be apparent clinically (for example, birth weight < 1000 g or symptomatic congenital diaphragmatic hernia) but more often it is determined by the results of arterial blood gas and acid-base analysis (Table 8.1).

Initial mechanical ventilator settings

An infant must *never* be left to breathe spontaneously through an endotracheal tube without continuous positive airway pressure (CPAP).

- The infant should be given sufficient oxygen to relieve cyanosis and maintain normal oxygen saturation (92–96%) and/or normal PaO_2 (60–90 mmHg).

Table 8.1 Scoring system for grading severity of respiratory failure (RF)

	Score			
	0	**1**	**2**	**3**
Apnoea or shock	No	No	No	Yes
FiO_2	< 0.60	0.60–0.69	0.70–0.80	> 0.80
$PaCO_2$ (mmHg)	< 50	50–60	51–70	> 70
pH	> 7.30	7.25–7.30	7.00–7.24	< 7.00

Mild RF = 0; moderate RF = 1–2; severe RF = $\geq$ 3.
Total score (max = 12) $\geq$ 3 is an indication for mechanical ventilation.

- The peak inspiratory pressure (PIP) should be sufficient to produce discernible chest wall movement.
- Select a rate to produce a normal $PaCO_2$.
- The inspiratory time should be 0.4–0.7 seconds.
- The inspiratory:expiratory ratio should be 1:1.5–2.0 and never reversed.
- PEEP levels of 4–6 cm H_2O are appropriate.

Subsequent ventilator settings are determined by the infant's progress, the results of blood gas measurements and consultation with the Newborn Emergency Transport Service (NETS) or a tertiary-level neonatologist.

Cyanosis and hypoxaemia

- Hypoxaemia may be defined as an arterial oxygen tension (PaO_2) less than 50 mmHg or arterial oxygen saturation (SaO_2) less than 90%.
- Hypoxaemia may result in tissue hypoxia, anaerobic metabolism and metabolic (lactic) acidaemia (negative base excess), and/or hypoxic pulmonary vasoconstriction and persistent pulmonary hypertension.
- The presence of cyanosis is a guide to the presence of hypoxaemia but an infant may be cyanosed without being hypoxaemic (peripheral cyanosis and polycythaemia) or hypoxaemic without being cyanosed (anaemia and leftward shift of the oxygen dissociation curve by foetal haemoglobin, alkalosis and hypocapnoea).

- Methaemoglobinaemia should be considered in the infant with central cyanosis and norm- or hyperoxaemia.

Confirmation of hypoxaemia

- Pulse oximetry (SpO_2) and the PaO_2 should be measured.
- A capillary PO_2 is not accurate. Transcutaneous PO_2 ($tcPO_2$) is helpful in trend monitoring but it should not be the sole means by which oxygenation is monitored.
- The $tcPO_2$ and SpO_2 electrodes should be in the same position relative to the ductus arteriosus as the site of arterial blood sampling for PaO_2, thereby avoiding error from right-to-left shunting across the ductus.

Causes of hypoxaemia

The mechanisms and common causes of hypoxaemia include:
- alveolar hypoventilation:
  - central apnoea or hypopnoea—perinatal asphyxia and pre-maturity
  - airway obstruction—choanal atresia and Pierre-Robin sequence
  - pulmonary hypoplasia—oligohydramnios and diaphragmatic hernia
- ventilation/perfusion (V/Q) mismatch:
  - transient tachypnoea of the newborn
  - bronchopulmonary dysplasia
  - acyanotic congenital heart disease
- intrapulmonary or intracardiac right-to-left shunts:
  - severe parenchymal lung disease
  - hyaline membrane disease
  - massive aspiration syndrome
  - early-onset bacterial pneumonia
- persistent pulmonary hypertension
- cyanotic congenital heart disease.

Respiratory distress

- The presence or absence of respiratory distress may help define the cause of the cyanosis.
- Assure patency of the posterior nares (pass a narrow-bore feeding tube if necessary).
- *Cyanosis with intercostal retractions* indicates *decreased lung compli-*

ance, usually from parenchymal lung disease but perhaps due to congenital heart disease with pulmonary venous congestion or obstruction.

- *Cyanosis with tachypnoea* (rate > 60/min) *without intercostal retractions* is usually due to transient tachypnoea of the newborn (TTN) or cyanotic congenital heart disease. The cyanosis is relieved by oxygen in infants with TTN. The infant with hypoglycaemia or sepsis may present with cyanosis and an abnormal respiratory pattern without intercostal retractions.
- *Cyanosis with no respiratory distress* is usually due to cyanotic congenital heart disease, though idiopathic persistent pulmonary hypertension should also be considered.

Cardiovascular examination

- A cardiac murmur and a single second heart sound in a cyanosed infant usually indicate the presence of congenital heart disease (CHD). However, the absence of a murmur does not exclude CHD and the nature of the second heart sound may be difficult to appreciate.
- Examine the peripheral pulses carefully, especially the femoral pulses. A cardiac dysrhythmia, particularly a tachyarrhythmia, needs to be actively excluded. A non-sinus rhythm should be considered if the heart rate is < 80 bpm or > 280 bpm.

Investigations

Chest X-ray

- Look for evidence of parenchymal lung disease or an extra-pulmonary disorder such as a pneumothorax or pleural effusion. Look for pulmonary venous congestion or obstruction.
- Congenital heart disease is suggested by increased heart size, abnormal heart shape and/or increase or decrease in lung vascular markings, best assessed in the outer third of lung fields.

Electrocardiogram (ECG)

ECGs are less often done in 'modern' neonatology. This relates to a general lack of familiarity with the neonatal ECG, along with the ready availability of echocardiography.

Arterial blood gas analysis

- 'Normal' arterial blood gases:
  - PaO_2 60–90 mmHg
  - pHa 7.25–7.45
  - $PaCO_2$ 35–45 mmHg

Hyperoxia test (100% oxygen for 10 minutes)

- A true right-to-left intracardiac shunt (pulmonary atresia or isolated transposition of the great arteries) results in a PaO_2 < 100 mmHg in 100% ambient oxygen.
- Alveolar hypoventilation or V/Q mismatch results in a PaO_2 > 250 mmHg.
- Congenital heart disease and venous admixture (atrioventricular septal defect, double outlet right ventricle, complex transposition of the great arteries and persistent truncus arteriosus) and severe V/Q mismatching (massive aspiration syndromes) result in a PaO_2 of 100–250 mmHg in 100% ambient oxygen.
- Persistent pulmonary hypertension may be distinguished from cyanotic congenital heart disease by recording a PaO_2 > 100 mmHg during a period of hypocapnoea ($PaCO_2$ < 30 mmHg) induced by mechanical hyperventilation.

Arterial PCO$_2$

- Hypercapnoea ($PaCO_2$ > 45 mmHg) usually indicates parenchymal lung disease, but can be seen in congenital heart disease with pulmonary venous congestion or obstruction.
- Hypocapnoea ($PaCO_2$ < 30 mmHg) in the spontaneously breathing infant usually, but not invariably, indicates cyanotic congenital heart disease.
- Normocapnoea is not helpful in distinguishing cyanotic congenital heart disease from parenchymal lung disease.

Echocardiography

The infant with central cyanosis and hypoxaemia not demonstrably from intrapulmonary or extrapulmonary intrathoracic disease must have an urgent echocardiogram performed by a paediatric cardiologist to define the nature of an underlying congenital cardiac anomaly and to determine whether or not pulmonary blood flow is duct-dependent.

Oxygen therapy

- The fractional inspired oxygen (FiO_2) should be constantly monitored. The inspired gas should be humidified and heated to environmental thermal neutrality.
- Skin colour is not a reliable index of oxygenation; oxygen status should be monitored by SpO_2 or $tcPO_2$ or PaO_2 measurement.
- PaO_2 must be assessed when the SpO_2 is > 98%. Hyperoxia is one factor in the development of retinopathy of prematurity. The SpO_2 should be maintained in the range of 91–97% and the PaO_2 (or $tcPO_2$) should be measured in premature infants.
- The PaO_2 may be < 50 mmHg when the oxygen saturation is > 90% and the PaO_2 (or $tcPO_2$) should be measured if hypoxic pulmonary vasoconstriction and persistent pulmonary hypertension are present.
- If there is doubt about the cause of the cyanosis it is far better in the short term to give an infant too much oxygen rather than too little.

Neonatal sepsis

Neonatal sepsis is common, especially in neonatal intensive care units. Early signs are nonspecific and many infants will undergo diagnostic studies and initiation of treatment before the diagnosis has been confirmed. Neonatal sepsis is categorised as either 'early onset' (within 48–72 hours) or 'late onset' (after 72 hours). This classification is useful in guiding investigations and the choice of appropriate antibiotics.

- Early-onset sepsis syndrome is associated with infection in the peripartum period. Commoner micro-organisms implicated include group B streptococcus, *Escherichia coli*, *Haemophilus influenzae* and *Listeria monocytogenes*.
- Late-onset sepsis is usually acquired from the hospital environment. Commoner organisms implicated are *Staphylococcus epidermidis* and *Staphylococcus aureus*, *Escherichia coli*, *Klebsiella*, *Pseudomonas*, *Enterobacter* and *Candida*.

Risk factors

Early sepsis (48–72 hours old)

- Spontaneous premature onset of labour (< 37 weeks)

- Preterm premature rupture of membranes
- Prolonged rupture of membranes
- Maternal fever in labour
- Maternal group B streptococcal (GBS) colonisation
- Low Apgar scores

Late sepsis (> 72 hours old)

- Artificial ventilation with an endotracheal tube in place
- Intravascular catheters
- Extreme prematurity

Clinical picture

The signs of neonatal sepsis are often nonspecific and subtle. Early-onset sepsis is far more likely to be associated with respiratory distress and shock. The mortality is higher. Late-onset sepsis is often more insidious.

Important signs include:

- apnoea
- lethargy, irritability, seizures or unsettled behaviour
- tachycardia and peripheral circulatory failure
- feeding problems—reluctance to feed, abdominal distension and vomiting
- fever, though some may have hypothermia or temperature instability.

The differential diagnosis of suspected sepsis includes coarctation and other congenital cardiac disorders, intracranial haemorrhage and inborn errors of metabolism.

Investigations

Early-onset sepsis

- *Ear swab, gastric aspirate and surface swabs*: Gram stains are insufficiently sensitive and specific tests on which to base therapy, but the culture and sensitivity results of these swabs are often clinically useful.
- *Blood film*: The immature-to-total (I:T) neutrophil ratio is the most sensitive test for early sepsis, but may still be normal in severe sepsis.
- *Blood culture*: A blood culture should always be taken prior to

commencing antibiotics, if possible, although if there is great difficulty treatment should not be delayed.

- *Cerebrospinal fluid analysis*: Many clinicians perform a lumbar puncture only if the blood culture is positive or if there is a strong clinical suspicion that the baby has meningitis. We do not recommend routine lumbar puncture in possible early sepsis.
- *Chest X-ray*: Pneumonia due to GBS and other organisms may cause a diffuse reticulo-granular pattern indistinguishable from hyaline membrane disease.
- *Urine culture*: This does not constitute part of the routine screen for early-onset sepsis.

Late-onset sepsis

- *Blood film*: The I:T ratio may be helpful, but can be normal. Thrombocytopenia occurs in half of all babies with bacterial sepsis and almost all with fungal sepsis.
- *Blood cultures*: As above.
- *Lumbar puncture*: This should be performed when meningitis is suspected clinically and if blood cultures are growing an organism which may cause meningitis (this excludes coagulase negative staphylococci). A lumbar puncture is otherwise not routinely recommended in suspected late-onset sepsis.
- *Urine culture*: Mandatory.
- *Chest X-ray*: if there is respiratory distress. *Note*: Pneumonitis at 3–5 days of age may be due to HSV, and nasopharyngeal aspirate should be sent for immunofluorescence for HSV.
- *C-reactive protein*: This is sometimes used as a marker of sepsis but may be normal; it may be useful to monitor progress of treatment.

Treatment

- Empiric treatment with intravenous antibiotics is recommended and should be discontinued after 48–72 hours if blood cultures are negative and the infant appears well. The choice of antibiotics depends on the age of onset of infection, Gram stain results and the organisms prevalent in a particular nursery.
- Monitoring of vital signs, blood pressure, haematocrit, full blood count and platelets is also necessary.
- Infectious disease consultation is useful if an unusual clinical sign

such as an unknown rash is present, or if the infant is not responding to treatment.

Antibiotics therapy

- *Early-onset sepsis*: A combination of penicillin (or ampicillin) and gentamicin will provide coverage for Gram-positive organisms, especially GBS, as well as Gram-negative bacteria, such as *Escherichia coli*.
- *Late-onset sepsis*: Vancomycin and gentamicin are recommended as initial empirical therapy in this situation, unless there are other circumstances indicating a different regime.

Viral infections

- A picture of neonatal sepsis can also be caused by viral infection, for example with coxsackievirus, or herpes simplex virus (HSV).
- Babies with HSV infection may present with localised blistering infection of the skin, eye and/or mouth, which if untreated progresses to disseminated infection with hepatitis and DIC. Approximately one-third of neonates with HSV infection have isolated encephalitis and may present between 2 and 14 days with seizures, hypotonia and lethargy.

Investigations

- Swabs from mucocutaneous lesions for immunofluorescent (I/F) stains and culture for HSV
- Nasopharyngeal aspirate for I/F
- Lumbar puncture for virus isolation and PCR

Treatment

- Aciclovir should be started, after consultation with a senior colleague, if HSV infection is confirmed or strongly suspected.

Neonatal jaundice

- Jaundice in the newborn period is common.
- Jaundice may be a feature of a more serious yet potentially treatable disorder. If the level of bilirubin is sufficiently elevated, there is a risk of neurological damage.

Aetiology and investigation

- Jaundice present at birth or appearing in the first 24 hours is likely to be due to haemolysis or congenital infection whereas persistent jaundice beyond 7–10 days requires exclusion of bile duct obstruction.

- Jaundice is pathological if it:
  - appears too early (< 24 hours)
  - appears too late (after 3–4 days)
  - is too high (requires treatment)
  - lasts too long (> 2 weeks)
  - is associated with an elevated direct or conjugated fraction.
- Any infant with pathological jaundice should have the following investigations: total bilirubin, direct bilirubin, total protein, blood film to examine red cell morphology, blood group and direct Coombs test.
- Further investigation is usually required if there is evidence of haemolysis, prolonged jaundice (bilirubin > 170 μmol/L for > 10 days) or an elevated direct hyperbilirubinaemia.

Haemolysis

- Jaundice that appears during the first 24 hours suggests haemolysis, which can be immune or non-immune. The following investigations are required:
  - maternal and infant blood groups
  - direct Coombs test
  - total and direct serum bilirubin
  - full blood count and blood film.
- Non-immune causes of haemolysis include abnormalities of red cell shape (for example, hereditary spherocytosis), red cell enzyme defects (for example, glucose-6-phosphate dehydrogenase deficiency) and abnormal haemoglobins (for example, thalassaemia).
- Investigations required in the infant with non-immune haemolysis include autohaemolysis, glycerol lysis, red cell enzyme studies, haemoglobin electrophoresis and heat stability.

Prolonged unconjugated jaundice

- Prolonged jaundice for more than 2 weeks in a well infant is usually 'breast milk jaundice'.
- Differential diagnoses include congenital hypothyroidism or Crigler-Najjar syndrome.
- If the infant is unwell, consider urinary tract infection, galactosaemia and congenital hypopituitarism though infants with these conditions usually have an elevated direct reacting bilirubin as well.

- Investigations which may elucidate the cause are:
  - the newborn screening test
  - thyroid function tests
  - urine for non-glucose reducing substances
  - RBC galactose-1-phosphate uridyl transferase
  - urine culture
  - the plasma cortisol or short Synacthen test.

Neonatal cholestasis ('obstructive' or 'conjugated' or 'direct' jaundice)

- Neonatal cholestasis is present when the direct reacting (conjugated) serum bilirubin is > 25–35 μmol/L and generally more than 20% of the total serum bilirubin.
- Cholestasis may arise secondary to:
  - shock, parenteral nutrition or sepsis (bacterial or TORCH)
  - inborn errors of metabolism (such as galactosaemia)
  - biliary obstruction or hepatocellular disease
  - other rarer causes (Alagille's syndrome, cystic fibrosis, α-1-antitrypsin deficiency and congenital hypothyroidism).

Imaging

- Ultrasound can be useful in demonstrating extrahepatic biliary atresia and obstruction, such as choledochal cyst. It may provide information about the intrahepatic architecture.
- A DISIDA scan showing failure to excrete tracer into the bowel within 24 hours is strong evidence for extrahepatic biliary atresia, though tracer excretion in a 4–6-week-old infant does not exclude the diagnosis. Exclude α-1-antitrypsin deficiency (PiZZ phenotype), since the DISIDA scan and liver histopathology in this condition may be difficult to distinguish from those in biliary atresia.
- Occasionally, tracer does not appear in the bowel after 24 hours in infants with hepatocellular disease. Phenobarbitone (5 mg/kg/day) for 3 to 5 days prior to examination may encourage bile excretion and avoid confusion.

Treatment of hyperbilirubinaemia

The goal is to prevent unconjugated bilirubin reaching neurotoxic levels. This is achieved by combining phototherapy and exchange transfusion.

Phototherapy and exchange transfusion

The indications are determined by the cause, serum bilirubin, gestational age and birth weight (Table 8.2). Haemolysis, severe bruising, hypoproteinaemia, hypoalbuminaemia, hypoxaemia, acidaemia, hypercapnoea and sepsis may increase bilirubin toxicity.

- Phototherapy is conventionally delivered by a radiant light and may be assisted by the use of a fibre-optic blanket. Infants should be monitored and have their eyes covered.
- Check the SBR every 8 to 24 hours, depending on the rate of rise of bilirubin and the SBR level relative to that which would necessitate exchange transfusion. Cease phototherapy when the need for exchange transfusion has been averted.

Fluids

Additional fluids do not assist in decreasing bilirubin but may be required to compensate for increased insensible loss associated with phototherapy.

Rhesus isoimmunisation

- The infant with a cord haemoglobin less than 80–100 g/L should have an immediate simple packed RBC transfusion or, if hydrops

Table 8.2 Indications for phototherapy and exchange transfusion in infants with unconjugated jaundice after age 24 hours

Total bilirubin (µmol/L)*		
Birth weight	**Phototherapy**	**Exchange**
< 1000 g	100	200
1000–1499	150	250
1500–1999	200	300
2000–2499	250	350
> 2500 g†	350	450

* If haemolytic disease, severe bruising, hypoproteinaemia, hypoxaemia, acidaemia, hypercapnoea or proven sepsis are present then commence treatment at a level 50 µmol/L less than that shown.
† The normal birth weight infant with haemolytic disease of the newborn should commence phototherapy if the SBR > 250 µmol/L and an exchange transfusion should be performed when the SBR > 340–375 µmol/L.

is present, a packed red cell exchange transfusion, 30 mL/kg, and intensive double-light phototherapy should be commenced.

- During the first 24 hours, a double-volume exchange transfusion should be performed if the SBR increases by more than 10–12 μmol/L/h, despite intensive phototherapy. Thereafter, an exchange transfusion should be performed according to the modified recommendations in the table.

Breast milk jaundice

There is no need to discontinue breastfeeding in order to diagnose or treat breast milk jaundice, unless the SBR is within the range for exchange transfusion, despite intensive phototherapy.

Hypoglycaemia

Prolonged or recurrent hypoglycaemia in the newborn infant may cause brain damage.

Definition

- Neonatal hypoglycaemia is defined by a blood glucose < 2.2 mmol/L in term and preterm infants. Infants may have symptoms of hypoglycaemia at a blood glucose > 2.2 mmol/L, but this is quite unusual.
- Reagent strip measurement of blood glucose is unreliable and a formal laboratory measure should be used.

Aetiology

Transient hypoglycaemia

- Hypoglycaemia due to decreased production of glucose is usually mild and easily corrected with a glucose infusion rate of 6–7 mg/kg/min (approximately 10% dextrose at 90 mL/kg/day).
- Less commonly, hypoglycaemia may be due to increased glucose utilisation from hyperinsulinism (maternal diabetes, Beckwith-Wiedemann syndrome or transient idiopathic hyperinsulinism). It is usually short-lived and easy to control but may require high glucose infusion rates and treatment with glucagon.

Persistent hypoglycaemia

Hypoglycaemia lasting for longer than 2–3 days is usually due to hyperinsulinism (idiopathic hyperinsulinism, nesidioblastosis or pancreatic islet cell tumour), an inborn error of metabolism or a hormone deficiency.

Investigation

- If the cause is clinically apparent then the only laboratory investigations required are a haemoglobin to exclude polycythaemia and plasma insulin to document hyperinsulinism in the presence of hypoglycaemia.
- When the cause is not clinically apparent or if hypoglycaemia is severe, investigations to exclude persistent hyperinsulinism, inborn errors of metabolism and hormone deficiency should be performed and include:
  - plasma growth hormone
  - plasma cortisol or short Synacthen test
  - urine non-glucose reducing substances
  - pH and plasma lactate
  - plasma ammonia
  - liver function tests
  - RBC galactose-1-phosphate uridyl transferase
  - urine ketones
  - urine amino acids and organic acids.

Treatment of hypoglycaemia

Hypoglycaemic infants should be given enteral milk feeds, unless they are otherwise contraindicated.

Intravenous dextrose/saline solution

- Intravenous dextrose/saline therapy is required when hypoglycaemia is asymptomatic but not responding to enteral milk feeding or when symptomatic (extreme jitteriness or seizures).
- Increase the glucose infusion rate (GIR) if the blood glucose is < 2.2 mmol/L. This can be done by increasing the infusate glucose concentration or infusion rate. If symptomatic or the blood glucose is < 1.7 mmol/L, give a bolus dextrose 10%, 2 mL/kg (200 mg/kg), over 15 minutes prior to increasing the GIR.
- 10% dextrose/saline at 90–100 mL/kg/day (GIR of 6–7 mg/kg/min) should be sufficient to avert or correct hypoglycaemia secondary to decreased glucose production.
- Hyperinsulinism may require a GIR of approximately 12 mg/kg/min (15% dextrose saline at 120 mL/kg/day). This

should be given via a central venous catheter and used transiently while drug therapy is initiated.

Drug therapy

Transient hypoglycaemia

- Drug therapy is indicated if hypoglycaemia persists despite a GIR of approximately 8 mg/kg/min (10% dextrose saline at 120 mL/kg/day).
- If the infant is small for gestational age treatment with hydro-cortisone, 10 mg/kg/day, is likely to be effective.
- Infants with suspected hyperinsulinism should be treated with a glucagon infusion, 5–20 micrograms/kg/h.

Persistent hypoglycaemia

- Infants with persistent hyperinsulinism require treatment with diazoxide, 5–25 mg/kg/day, which inhibits insulin release from the pancreas.
- Subtotal pancreatectomy may sometimes be required if long-term diazoxide is ineffective or the side-effects are unacceptable.

Intravenous fluid therapy

Intravenous fluid therapy should be initiated in the following circumstances:

- birth weight < 1500 g or gestation < 32 weeks
- asymptomatic hypoglycaemia (plasma glucose < 2.2 mmol/L) despite enteral milk feeding; or symptomatic hypoglycaemia (plasma glucose < 2.6 mmol/L)
- moderate to severe respiratory distress (FiO_2 > 0.4)
- intestinal obstruction (functional or organic).

Water balance

- The goal of intravenous fluid therapy is to maintain zero water and sodium balance or the slightly positive balance necessary for growth.
- Urine flow rate should be 2.0–4.0 mL/kg/h.
- Zero water balance is achieved by matching water lost (notably skin and urine) with water gained (notably intravenous and oral fluids).

Water requirement

- The fluid infusion rate should commence at 60 mL/kg/day, except in infants with birth weight < 800 g in whom it should begin at 75–90 mL/kg/day.
- The water requirement changes with postnatal age, renal or cardiopulmonary function, exposure to radiant heat and phototherapy.
- The intravenous fluid requirement of an infant should be individualised.

Overhydration

- The newborn infant has a limited capacity to excrete a water load, particularly in the first 24 hours.
- To prevent overhydration the urine osmolality should be maintained at > 150–200 mosm/kg (urine specific gravity > 1.005) and the urine volume should be maintained at < 5.0 mL/kg/h.

Dehydration

- The newborn infant has a limited ability to concentrate the urine. The maximum urine osmolality achieved by the preterm infant is 400–500 mosm/kg, whereas the full-term infant can reach 700–800 mosm/kg.
- To avoid dehydration the urine osmolality should be kept at < 400–500 mosm/kg (urine specific gravity < 1.015) and urine volume should be kept at > 2.0 mL/kg/h.

Hyponatraemia (serum Na⁺ < 130 mmol/L)

- Hyponatraemia in the first 3 days is usually from iatrogenic overhydration. Other causes include salt wasting because of natriuresis (prematurity, diuretics, renal failure) or gastrointestinal losses (intestinal obstruction and stomal diarrhoea).
- The treatment of hyponatraemia depends on the cause but may include:
  - reduction of free water intake
  - replacement of sodium deficit over 24–48 hours according to the formula:

    sodium deficit = (desired serum Na − actual serum Na)
    $$\times 0.65 \times \text{weight (kg)}$$
  - increase in maintenance sodium.

Hypernatraemia (serum Na⁺ > 150 mmol/L)

- Hypernatraemia is usually the result of a free-water deficit, though it may be caused by an excessive intake of sodium, particularly in extremely preterm infants.
- Treatment depends on the cause, but usually requires an increase in free-water intake. Occasionally, the sodium intake needs to be decreased.

Sodium requirement

- The maintenance sodium requirement for full-term infants and preterm infants > 30–32 weeks gestation is 2–4 mmol/kg/day. Infants who are more premature, particularly those < 28 weeks gestation, may require > 5–12 mmol/kg/day to maintain positive sodium balance and prevent hyponatraemia.

Summary

- Intravenous fluid therapy should be initiated with 10% dextrose in 0.225% (N/4) saline at 60 mL/kg/day (75–90 mL/kg/day for infants with birth weight less than 800 g).
- The infant should be weighed daily. The preterm infant should lose 1.0–1.5% and the term infant 0.5–1.0% of birth weight daily for the first 7 to 10 days. Thereafter the body weight vis-à-vis water balance should remain relatively constant.
- The urine output and specific gravity should be measured. The urine flow rate and specific gravity should be 2.0–4.0 mL/kg/h after age 24 hours and 1.005–1.015, respectively.
- The plasma sodium should be measured every 12–48 hours and maintained at 135–145 mmol/L by adjusting the free-water intake.

Examination of the newborn

The examination should be done in a warm place with the infant in a quiet, alert state. The examination is unrewarding if the infant is highly aroused or asleep.

Neurobehaviour

- The head circumference should be measured.
- The cranial sutures should be separated or, if overriding, they should be mobile, thereby excluding craniostenosis.

- The infant's tone, power and movement should be symmetrical when the head is maintained in the midline.

Hearing and vision

- The infant should be able to establish visual contact with the examiner through the horizontal plane at a focal distance of 15–30 cm.
- The infant should attend to sound, particularly the human voice, as evidenced by a transient alteration in state such as the cessation of a previous activity like sucking, or purposeful eye movement, or a more generalised body movement.

Suck

The suck should be strong and rhythmical without biting or tongue thrusting.

Cry

The cry of an infant with possible neurological damage is mono-tonous, unremitting, unmodulated and vectorless compared with the purposeful pitch, loudness, modulation and direction of the cry of a normal infant.

Pull-to-sit manoeuvre

The pull-to-sit manoeuvre is the single most important procedure in the neurological examination. The manoeuvre allows an appreciation of the infant's grasp, limb and girdle tone, truncal tone and head control during the movement from supine to erect sitting.

Ventral suspension

When the infant is held supported in ventral suspension the back should form a gentle convexity with the head in line with the back and not extended, and the limbs should be slightly flexed against gravity.

Walking and stepping

The supported infant placed on a firm surface should make walking movements.

Moro test

A formal Moro test should not be performed because it intention-ally leaves the infant without apparent support and elicits fear.

Spine

- Inspect for abnormal curvature, midline birthmarks, pits and tufts of hair that may indicate an underlying abnormality such as diastematomyelia.
- Pits low in the natal cleft are not of clinical concern.

Heart

The examination should exclude two important conditions: coarctation of the aorta and pulmonary hypertension.

Coarctation of the aorta

- The femoral pulses *must* be felt to exclude coarctation of the aorta.
- An equivalent blood pressure in the upper and lower limbs by Doppler measurement does not rule out coarctation of the aorta.

Pulmonary hypertension

- Pulmonary hypertension beyond the first 3 days may be because of transient persistence of the foetal state but may signal a large systemic-to-pulmonary communication or obstructed left heart lesion.
- Pulmonary hypertension may not be associated with an impressive cardiac murmur but the right ventricle will be overactive and the second heart sound will be loud and closely split or single.

Respiratory

- Auscultation of the newborn chest is unreliable.
- Examine for signs of respiratory distress (tachypnoea, intercostal recession, expiratory grunt and cyanosis).

Eyes

- The eye examination can be facilitated by having the infant suck on the examiner's finger.
- Fundi are not examined routinely but the eyes should be examined for colobomata, glaucoma (hazy cornea) and a full range of external ocular movements.

Palate

- The infant will open the mouth if gentle downward traction is applied to the chin.

- Carefully examine for a cleft, including a submucous cleft. Feeling the palate with the finger is unreliable.

Abdomen

- The abdomen should be examined for prominent vascular patterns, inguinal hernias, masses and organ enlargement.
- The anus should be examined for patency and normal position.

Genitalia

- Confirm that both testes have descended completely into the scrotum. Do not retract the foreskin but if possible observe the urinary stream.
- Inspect the genitalia for hyperpigmentation that would raise concern about congenital adrenal hyperplasia.
- If the genitalia are ambiguous the assignment of sex of rearing should be deferred until genetic, endocrine and genitourinary investigations have been performed.

Feet

Postural talipes is not uncommon and does not require treatment if the foot is fully mobile. Full inversion means the foot can be positioned so the sole is vertically aligned. Full eversion means the foot can be turned out beyond the horizontal.

Hips

- Ligamentous or muscular 'clicks' or 'snaps' are not significant, providing the hip is stable. The stability of the hip is tested by grasping the thigh between the examiner's thumb placed anteriorly over the femoral neck with fingers positioned posteriorly over the greater trochanter and then adducting, internally rotating, and displacing the thigh backwards—a 'clunk' from posterior displacement of the femoral head out of the acetabulum indicates that the hip is dislocatable. The thigh is then abducted and externally rotated—a 'clunk' owing to anterior replacement of the femoral head within the acetabulum indicates the hip is dislocated or dislocatable.
- An ultrasound examination of the hips should be performed if clinical examination indicates they are unstable.

9

Biochemical genetic emergencies

This chapter includes:
- inborn errors of metabolism
- emergency treatment of inborn errors
- perimortem evaluation.

Inborn errors of metabolism

- Over 500 inborn errors have been described to date, many of them associated with episodes of acute metabolic decompensation.
- Despite the vast array of potential biochemical defects, most disorders can be categorised into a handful of clinical presentations.
- The judicious use of simple screening measures can often yield a specific diagnosis quickly.

Many inborn errors of metabolism may have their first presentation in the newborn period, but as the newborn has a relatively limited repertoire of rather nonspecific responses to severe illness (including lethargy, vomiting, poor sucking reflex, hypotonia, diarrhoea, dehydration, respiratory distress, and seizures), the clinical features in the neonate do not provide particularly specific clues to a precise diagnosis. Moreover, in up to one-third of children with so-called 'small molecule' disorders, the initial presentation may not be till late infancy or even beyond.

The importance of rapid identification and treatment of metabolic defects

- Emergency treatment is often available, particularly for disorders presenting very early and can significantly reduce or even prevent the development of permanent physical or neurological damage. Because of the nonspecific nature of symptoms of metabolic disorders, rapid and accurate diagnosis will be made only if screening tests, and often consultation with the metabolic team, are considered at the outset in an undiagnosed, sick child.

- These disorders by definition are genetic, making genetic counselling of crucial importance, in terms of both prognosis and the various aspects of inheritance of these disorders, which need to be addressed.
- Infants and children with known metabolic disorders presenting to the Emergency Department always need rapid triage and implementation of emergency metabolic treatment, as serious decompensation can occur rapidly.

When should a genetic metabolic disorder be considered?

Any of the following should prompt consideration of the possibility of an inborn error of metabolism in any neonate, infant or child:

- unexplained cardio-respiratory collapse
- acute encephalopathy
- acute liver failure
- hypoglycaemia
- metabolic acidosis ($\pm$ ketosis)
- lactic acidaemia
- hyperammonaemia.

History

As well as taking a routine history, ask specifically about:

- family history (similar illnesses in siblings, unexplained deaths, stillbirths and so on)
- consanguinity (most inborn errors of metabolism are autosomal recessive)
- intercurrent illnesses
- dietary history (especially any recent changes to the diet, or periods of fasting).

Physical examination

Physical examination is rarely helpful in determining the precise diagnosis; however, always take note of:

- level of consciousness (Glasgow Coma Scale)

- hepatomegaly
- focal neurological signs
- unusual odour (urine should be kept in a sealed, sterile container for at least 5 minutes at room temperature before testing).

Types of genetic metabolic diseases to consider

- Amino acidopathies, for example maple syrup urine disease
- Organic acidopathies, for example methylmalonic acidaemia
- Fatty acid oxidation defects, for example medium chain acyl-CoA dehydrogenase deficiency (MCAD)
- Urea cycle defects, for example ornithine transcarbamylase (OTC) deficiency
- Primary lactic acidosis disorders including defects of:
  - gluconeogenesis
  - the Krebs cycle
  - pyruvate metabolism, for example pyruvate dehydrogenase deficiency
  - mitochondrial respiratory chain
- Disorders causing acute liver failure (including galactosaemia, tyrosinaemia type I and hereditary fructose intolerance).

Those disorders presenting with acute metabolic decompensation by and large fit into the category of 'small molecule' disorders. Small molecules can be defined as small, water-soluble chemicals that are found in virtually all body fluids. In some of these disorders, the small-molecule level in body fluids may be several orders of magnitude greater than that normally seen; small molecules may exert their harmful effects by virtue of their toxic nature. Examples of this type of disorder include the amino acidopathies, the organic acidopathies and the urea cycle defects. In other small-molecule disorders, while there is an accumulation of some metabolites, a primary problem is that there is a defect of energy production. Examples include the fatty acid oxidation defects and the primary lactic acidosis disorders.

Screening tests

Where a particular genetic metabolic disorder is being considered, there is no substitute for performing the specific investigations. However, as the clinical presentations for many of these disorders overlap, the following set of investigations will screen for most genetic metabolic disorders:

- urine:
  - dipstick tests for ketones
  - reducing substances (both Clinitest and Clinistix)
  - amino and organic acid screens (urine metabolic screen)
- blood:
  - full blood count/film
  - urea, electrolytes, creatinine
  - glucose
  - calcium
  - blood gases
  - liver enzymes
  - ammonium
  - lactate and pyruvate
  - amino acids*
  - carnitine*
- cerebrospinal fluid:
  - lactate and pyruvate
  - amino acids*

Tests marked * should be ordered only after consultation.

- In the case of hypoglycaemia collect blood for the following when the child is hypoglycaemic (see the 'Hypoglycaemia Kit' in the Emergency Department):
  - growth hormone
  - cortisol
  - insulin
  - free fatty acids
  - β-hydroxybutyrate
  - acyl carnitine profile.

Urine should always be collected at the time of hypoglycaemia.

To obtain meaningful results, many of these samples require special handling (particularly for lactate, pyruvate, ammonium and amino acids) and, if in doubt, discussions should be held with either the metabolic physician or the biochemical geneticist on call before the samples are collected.

Table 9.1 summarises the biochemical clues to some of the inborn errors of metabolism that can present as acute metabolic emergencies.

Table 9.1 Clues to certain classes of inborn errors of metabolism

	FBC and coags	Ketosis	Metabolic acidosis	Anion gap	Blood lactate	Blood glucose	Blood NH_4^+	Other clinical and biochemical clues
Amino acidopathies	Normal	No→+++	No→++	Normal	Normal	N→↓	Normal	Relationship to dietary protein intake and catabolic episodes
Organic acidopathies	↓Platelets ↓WCC	++	+++	↑	N or ↑	N→↓	↑→↑↑	Relationship to dietary protein intake and catabolic episodes
Fatty acid oxidation or ketogenesis defects	Normal	No→+	No→+	N or ↑	N or ↑	↓↓	↑→↑↑	Often precipitated by fasting or catabolic illness, liver/cardiac symptoms
Urea cycle defects	Normal	No	No	Normal	N	Normal	↑→↑↑↑	Respiratory alkalosis, tachypnoea
Primary lactic acidosis								
• PDH deficiency	Normal	No	No→+++	N or ↑	↑	N→↓	N→↑	'Cerebral' lactic acidosis
• PC deficiency	Normal	++	++	N→↑↑	↑	N→↓	N→↑	
• Gluconeogenesis defects	Normal	No→+++	++	N or ↑	↑↑	N→↓↓	N→↑	Hepatomegaly
• TCA defects	Normal	+	++	N or ↑	↑	Normal	Normal	
• ETC defects	Normal	No→+	No→+++	N or ↑	N→↑↑	N→↓	Normal	Multi-system disorder
Acute hepatic failure (incl. galactosaemia, tyrosinaemia type 1, HFI)	Hlysis, consumption	No→+	No→+	Normal	↑	N→↓	N→↑	Cataracts (gal.) raised AFP (tyr.) Hx of fructose intake (HFI)

Legend: N = normal
PDH = pyruvate dehydrogenase deficiency
TCA = tricarboxylic acid (Krebs) cycle
ETC = electron transport chain
PC = pyruvate carboxylase deficiency
Hlysis = haemolysis

Emergency treatment of inborn errors

Acute resuscitative measures

Initial resuscitation must be undertaken in parallel with the diagnostic work-up, may be life-saving, and can be initiated at any hospital. Important components include the following.

Correction of dehydration, electrolyte imbalance and hypoglycaemia

A recommended initial fluid mixture to use is N/2 saline, made up to 5% dextrose, run at maintenance, and supplemented with the daily requirement of potassium. In addition, other sources of non-protein calories, such as intravenous intralipid, are likely to be needed to reduce catabolism, but should be used only in consultation with the metabolic team. Fluid restriction may be necessary if cerebral oedema is suspected, and a high glucose intake is contraindicated where pyruvate dehydrogenase deficiency is suspected. Because of the risk of hyponatraemia, electrolytes should be monitored carefully.

Correction of metabolic acidosis

Intravenous sodium bicarbonate administration is recommended if the serum bicarbonate is < 15 mEq/L. Overcorrection should be avoided; stop once the bicarbonate level has reached 15 mEq/L. Beware also of iatrogenic hypernatraemia, although sometimes this may be unavoidable and may necessitate dialysis.

Haemofiltration, haemodialysis, or peritoneal dialysis

This may prove necessary if there is a rapid clinical and/or biochemical deterioration despite appropriate initial resuscitative therapy.

Specific therapies according to the disease

Such modalities include:

- nutritional modifications (such as intralipid, specific amino acid supplements)
- cofactor administration (such as specific vitamins)
- specific therapeutic agents (such as sodium benzoate and arginine for hyperammonaemia).

109

Long-term (dietary) therapy

With successful acute resuscitation, long-term management goals need to be developed, and for many of these disorders are centred on modifications to the diet. The aim is to provide nutrients in sufficient amounts to allow normal growth, but to prevent the accumulation of potentially toxic metabolites. Thus, it is necessary to impose restriction of protein in amino acidopathies, long-chain fat in long-chain fatty acid oxidation defects, and specific carbohydrates for carbohydrate disorders. Supplements of specific amino acid mixtures, fatty acids or other food supplements may be needed. Cofactors in pharmacological doses are necessary for certain disorders and agents enhancing certain pathways, or the excretion of particular classes of compounds, can be used.

The principles outlined above can be applied to a range of many other metabolic disorders. Regular consultation with expert biochemical and clinical geneticists and metabolic dietitians is required.

Whenever there is any uncertainty as to appropriate investigation and management of children suspected of having a genetic metabolic disorder, it is highly recommended that urgent consultation take place with one of the members of the New South Wales Biochemical Genetic Service, which is located at the Children's Hospital at Westmead. The metabolic physician on call can be contacted through the hospital's switchboard 24 hours a day.

Perimortem evaluation

The unexpected death of a child, including one with multiple congenital anomalies or suspected bony dysplasia, warrants careful consideration of the possibility of a genetic disorder. While this period is possibly the most distressing time parents of a dying child will ever have to face, without timely and sensitive discussion of the need for perimortem sample collection the precise diagnosis may not be made. This has important implications for the parents in terms of future genetic risks.

Guidelines have been developed by the New South Wales Genetics Advisory Committee regarding the genetic autopsy. Only certain components of these guidelines may need to be followed in certain circumstances. Most important of all is the need to consult with a clinical or biochemical geneticist as soon as possible, so that direction on appropriate additional investigations can be made.

Details of the protocol can be found at the Children's Hospital at Westmead Internet site at:

http://www.chw.edu.au/prof/services/biogen/biogen07.htm

10

Anti-infective drugs and guidelines

This chapter includes:
- notes on antibiotic therapy
- guidelines on empiric antibiotic therapy
- indications for the use of aciclovir.

Notes on antibiotic therapy

Choice of agent

- Before antibiotic treatment is started, it is important to obtain appropriate specimens (for example blood, urine, CSF, pus, pleural fluid).
- Immediate results to guide therapy may be available from Gram stains on urine, CSF or pus.
- When the organism has been isolated and its sensitivities determined, any initial antibiotic regimen may need revision.
- In general, use drugs with the narrowest spectrum for the organisms most likely to be responsible for the infection.

Dosage

- It is important to check the manufacturer's recommendations when unfamiliar with any drug.
- When a drug is prescribed for older children on a dose per weight basis, there is a risk of overdosage. The maximum dosage usually should not exceed that calculated for a 40 kg individual.
- Neonatal doses are often higher or lower than those for older children, more usually lower because of decreased renal clearance.
- Doses calculated on body surface area are often much higher than those calculated on the basis of weight; the latter option is preferred.
- Doses should be adjusted in children with impaired renal

function. Consult Pharmacy or read *Therapeutic Guidelines: Antibiotic* (Therapeutic Guidelines Ltd, Melbourne).

Route

- The oral route is preferred when possible. Because food often interferes with the absorption of oral antibiotics, administration within an hour of mealtimes should be avoided (except with amoxycillin).
- When parenteral therapy is necessary, the intravenous route is preferable when possible; the intramuscular injection of antibiotics is painful and may give unpredictable blood levels with some antibiotics.
- Neonates absorb antibiotics erratically and antibiotics should generally be given to them parenterally for the entire course.

Toxic effects

- During treatment, the child should be examined daily for the appearance of toxic effects.
- The prescriber should be familiar with the toxicity of antibiotics in use, as prompt cessation of treatment may be essential if toxicity appears.

Dissolving antibiotics for injection

- The manufacturer's recommendations on solvent dilution and storage of prepared solutions must be observed strictly.
- With rare exceptions, intravenous antibiotics are given by separate injection, and not added to the intravenous fluids in the drip chamber.

Antibiotic assay

- Antibiotic assay should be used to monitor blood levels of potentially toxic drugs, such as aminoglycosides and vancomycin unless these are stopped within 2–3 days.
- Monitoring during continued administration of an aminoglycoside will vary depending upon which dosing regimen is adopted—once-daily or 8- to 12-hourly.
  For twice- or thrice-daily dosing monitor on day 2 or 3, then every 3–5 days:
  - Trough levels are collected during the hour before the next dose is given.

- Peak levels are collected as follows:
  1 hour after IM or IV bolus
  30 minutes after an infusion.

For once-daily dosing:

- A single blood level is used to monitor once daily aminoglycoside therapy (gentamicin or tobramycin). This is taken 6–14 hours after the daily dose, to measure the area under the curve (see standard nomogram in Figure 10.1).
- Each assay requires 1 mL of blood.
- Failure to collect specimens at the appropriate times makes the results uninterpretable.

For once-daily dosing of gentamicin, netilmicin or tobramycin, up to 7 mg/kg/day, a single measurement of plasma concentration should be made between 6 and 14 hours after the end of the infusion. This plasma concentration is then compared to the graph. The aim is to keep this plasma concentration between the two lines on the graph. Therefore, if the plotted plasma concentration is between the two lines on the graph, no dosage adjustment is required. If the plasma concentration is above the top line or below the bottom line, a proportional decrease or increase in dose is recommended.

For example:

Dose of aminoglycoside = 7 mg/kg

Actual concentration at 9 hours = 6 mg/L

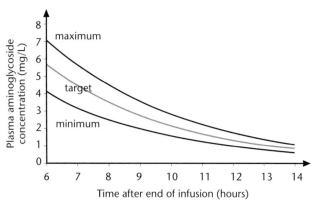

Figure 10.1 Time after end of infusion

Target concentration, calculated from the midpoint of the two lines = 3 mg/L

Next dose = (target concentration/actual concentration)
$\times$ initial dose
= (3/6) $\times$ 7 mg/kg
= 3.5 mg/kg

This method of dose adjustment applies to gentamicin, netilmicin and tobramycin. For once-daily amikacin dosing, up to 30 mg/kg/day, divide the measured concentration by four and use the same graph.

Dosage adjustment should be applied after the first dose. It should be repeated daily if the clinical state, especially renal function, is unstable and otherwise every 3 to 5 days.

Electrolyte content of antibiotics

* Some antibiotics, particularly the penicillins, have a very high sodium or potassium content, depending on the preparation used.
* Whenever high doses are being used, this must be taken into account, and the content of sodium or potassium in feedings or intravenous fluids lowered accordingly.

Guidelines on empiric antibiotic therapy

Antibiotic therapy should be directed by the results of Gram stains and cultures. However, when these are not yet available, empiric therapy is often needed. The following regimens are recommended, but should be reviewed in the light of culture results. See the Appendix for dosage information.

Table 10.1 Empiric antibiotic therapy guidelines

Condition	Age	Antibiotics
Fever		
Fever with no focus: (normal CSF and urine microscopy) if antibiotics indicated. See Chapter 11.	0–3 months	IV ampicillin plus gentamicin
	4 months–4 years	IV benzylpenicillin
	Over 4 years	IV benzylpenicillin plus flucloxacillin

continues . . .

Table 10.1 Empiric antibiotic therapy guidelines *(continued)*

Condition	Age	Antibiotics
Upper respiratory tract		
Acute otitis media		PO amoxycillin (if allergic use cotrimoxazole)
Acute OM with poor response to amoxycillin	Any age	PO amoxycillin/ clavulanate
Acute tonsillitis if antibiotics indicated	Any age (most children with streptococcal sore throat are > 4 years)	PO phenoxymethyl-penicillin (erythromycin or roxithromycin if penicillin allergic)
Epiglottitis	Any age	IV cefotaxime
Lower respiratory tract		
Pneumonia (community acquired)	Neonatal (birth to 1 week)	IV penicillin and gentamicin (consider HSV pneumonitis if onset between days 3 and 7)
Mild, afebrile pneumonitis	1 week–3 months	PO erythromycin
Mild-to-moderate	Over 3 months	PO amoxycillin or (over 5 years) erythromycin or roxithromycin
Moderate (needs hospitalisation)	Under 5 years	IV benzylpenicillin
	5 years and over	IV benzylpenicillin and PO roxithromycin
Severe (= systemic toxicity or effusion or pneumatocoeles)	Any age	IV cefotaxime plus flucloxacillin
Pneumonia (hospital-acquired)		
Mild postoperative	Any age	PO amoxycillin/ clavulanate
Moderate postoperative	Any age	IV benzylpenicillin plus gentamicin
Probable aspiration	Any age	IV benzylpenicillin plus IV metronidazole plus IV gentamicin *or* IV clindamycin plus IV gentamicin *or* IV ticarcillin/clavulanate alone

Table 10.1 Empiric antibiotic therapy guidelines *(continued)*

Condition	Age	Antibiotics
Diabetes/coma/renal failure	Any age	IV flucloxacillin plus gentamicin
Severe, hospital-acquired	Any age	IV gentamicin plus either ticarcillin/clavulanate or ceftazidime (or use IV imipenem or IV ciprofloxacin), and add vancomycin if MRSA likely
Pneumocystis carinii pneumonia (PCP)		
Proven or strongly suspected PCP; mild to moderate (pO$_2$ > 70, O$_2$ sat. > 94%, A–a gradient < 30)	Any age	PO cotrimoxazole
Severe	Any age	IV cotrimoxazole
Central nervous system		
Meningitis	Any age	See Chapter 11.
CSF shunt infections Base therapy on Gram-stain result.	Any age	IV and often intraventricular vancomycin
Brain abscess		
Neonatal	< 4 weeks	Seek specialist advice
Post-neonatal	> 4 weeks	IV benzylpenicillin plus cefotaxime plus metronidazole
Subdural empyema		
Neonatal	< 4 weeks	Seek specialist advice
Post-neonatal	> 4 weeks	IV benzylpenicillin plus cefotaxime plus metronidazole
Epidural abscess	Any age	IV flucloxacillin plus cefotaxime
Skin		
Cellulitis—orbital/ periorbital	Under 5 years	PO amoxicillin-clavulanate or (if ill) IV cefotaxime
Preseptal cellulitis (mild lid infection)	Over 5 years	PO or (if ill) IV flucloxacillin

continues . . .

117

Table 10.1 Empiric antibiotic therapy guidelines *(continued)*

Condition	Age	Antibiotics
Orbital cellulitis (proptosis, chemosis, toxic)	Any age	IV cefotaxime plus flucloxacillin
Cellulitis		
Facial	Any age	IV cefotaxime plus flucloxacillin
Not facial or periorbital	Any age	IV flucloxacillin (if due to *Streptococcus pyogenes* use IV benzylpenicillin)
Impetigo		
Streptococcal	Any age	PO phenoxymethyl-penicillin
Staphylococcal	Any age	PO flucloxacillin
Furunculosis/boils	Any age	PO flucloxacillin or cephalexin
Urinary tract infection		
Neonatal	Under 4 weeks	IV ampicillin plus gentamicin
Mild infection	Any age except neonate	PO cephalexin or PO amoxycillin/clavulanate or PO trimethoprim
Severe infection (acute pyelonephitis)	Any age	IV ampicillin plus gentamicin
Prophylaxis	Any age	PO cephalexin or trimethoprim or nitrofurantoin
Gastrointestinal		
Gastroenteritis		
Antibiotics not usually indicated, unless septicaemia suspected, e.g. high swinging fever in an infant		
Campylobacter	Any age	None usually PO or IV erythromycin for severe disease/septicaemia
Shigella	Any age	PO ampicillin or PO cotrimoxazole

Table 10.1 Empiric antibiotic therapy guidelines *(continued)*

Condition	Age	Antibiotics
Salmonella (non-typhoid)	Any age	None usually IV ciprofloxacin or IV cefotaxime or IV ceftriaxone for septicaemia
Enteric fever (typhoid or paratyphoid)	Any age	PO or IV ciprofloxacin or IV cefotaxime or IV ceftriaxone
Giardiasis		
Acute	Any age	PO metronidazole for 3 days or tinidazole single dose
Chronic	Any age	PO metronidazole for 7 days
Ascending cholangitis	Any age	IV ampicillin plus gentamicin plus metronidazole
Acute peritonitis Perforated viscus	Any age	IV ampicillin plus gentamicin plus metronidazole or cefotaxime plus metronidazole *or* ticarcillin/clavulanate alone
Peritoneal Dialysis-associated	Any age	Intraperitoneal (IP) cephalothin plus IP gentamicin (IP vancomycin only if proven methicillin-resistant organism)
Cardiac		
Bacterial endocarditis		
Community-acquired	Any age	IV benzylpenicillin plus flucloxacillin plus gentamicin
Hospital-acquired (or penicillin allergic)	Any age	IV vancomycin plus gentamicin

continues . . .

Table 10.1 Empiric antibiotic therapy guidelines *(continued)*

Condition	Age	Antibiotics
Osteomyelitis and/or septic arthritis		
Neonatal	Under 4 weeks	IV cefotaxime plus flucloxacillin for full course (oral antibiotics poorly absorbed)
Children	Under 5 years	IV cefotaxime plus flucloxacillin until fever and pain settled (usually 3–6 days) followed by PO flucloxacillin and/or PO amoxycillin/ clavulanate for at least 3 weeks
	Over 5 years	IV flucloxacillin until settled (usually 3–6 days) followed by PO flucloxacillin for at least 3 weeks

Indications for the use of aciclovir

Neonatal HSV infection

- Localised to skin, eye or mouth
- Encephalitis (presents at age 3–28 days)
- Pneumonitis (presents at age 2–7 days)
- Aciclovir *must* be given IV, not orally, at dose of 20 mg/kg/dose 8-hourly for 14 days, but for 21 days for encephalitis

Encephalitis

IV aciclovir is indicated in acute encephalitis, particularly when there are focal features or intractable seizures, pending results of tests.

Dermatological

IV aciclovir is indicated in HSV infection in patients with eczema, when it is severe, spreading rapidly and/or threatening the eyes (consult a dermatologist first).

Gingivostomatitis

IV aciclovir is indicated when a child with primary herpetic gingivo-stomatitis is ill enough to require hospital admission and IV fluids.

Immunocompromised patients

- *Proven* herpetic stomatitis
- *Stomatitis* in which results of HSV immunofluorescence are not yet back, *but* aciclovir should be stopped if HSV negative

Varicella zoster infection

- Any child with immune deficiency who develops chickenpox or zoster (IV aciclovir 10 mg/kg/dose to maximum 800 mg 8-hourly)
- Severe varicella infection in a normal child (same dose)
- Neonatal varicella infection under special circumstances (consult!)

For any other indications the approval of a consultant in micro-biology or infectious diseases is required.

Table 10.2 Summary of indications for the use of aciclovir

Absolute indications	
HSV encephalitis (proven or suspected)	Parenteral
Neonatal HSV infection (proven or suspected)	Parenteral (60 mg/kg/day)
Eczema herpeticum	Parenteral
Primary ocular HSV infection	Parenteral and topical
Varicella or zoster in immunocompromised child	Parenteral (30 mg/kg/day)
Severe varicella in normal child, e.g. pneumonitis	Parenteral (30 mg/kg/day)
Relative indications	
Severe primary HSV gingivostomatitis	Parenteral
HSV infections in immunocompromised patients	Parenteral
HSV infections in burns patients	Parenteral
Recurrent whitlow	Parenteral
Recurrent severe skin lesions	Oral*
Recurrent erythema multiforme	Oral*
Primary or recurrent genital HSV	Parenteral or Oral*

continued . . .

Table 10.2 Summary of indications for the use of aciclovir *(continued)*

Recurrent skin infections following neonatal HSV infection	Oral*
Painful herpes zoster	Oral
Neonatal varicella	Consult

Aciclovir *not* indicated
Mild to moderate HSV primary gingivostomatitis
Recurrent cold sores (unless exceptional circumstances)

* Oral aciclovir suspension is not available in Australia. Aciclovir is supplied as 200 mg tablets.

11

Fever and severe infections

This chapter includes:

- management of the febrile child
- bacterial meningitis
- septicaemia
- acute osteomyelitis
- septic arthritis
- toxic shock syndrome
- Kawasaki syndrome.

Management of the febrile child

Definitions

- Fever = temperature: rectal > 38°C or oral/axillary > 38.5°C
- Serious bacterial infection = meningitis, septicaemia, bone or joint infection, UTI, pneumonia, bacterial enteritis.
- Occult bacteraemia = blood-stream bacterial infection in child without focus of infection.
- Toxic appearance = lethargy (reduced consciousness with poor or absent eye contact), poor perfusion, hypoventilation, hyperventilation, cyanosis.

Early recognition and effective treatment of serious sepsis is of the highest priority.

History and examination

The history of the febrile illness may suggest a likely cause:

- Respiratory symptoms such as cough or tachypnoea suggest pneumonia (although young children with meningitis are often tachypnoeic and young children with pneumonia may have little or no cough).
- Abdominal pain may suggest UTI or enteritis.

- History of foreign travel should be sought.
- History of animal contact, for example cat-scratch, should be sought.

Apart from a careful clinical examination, an assessment should be made of whether or not the child is 'toxic'.

Toxicity

The following signs and symptoms can help distinguish the infant with serious illness:

- **A** for poor **a**rousal, reduced **a**lertness and reduced **a**ctivity
- **B** for **b**reathing difficulty (grunting, tachypnoea, increased respiratory effort)
- **C** for **c**irculatory impairment (mottling, tachycardia, decreased capillary return, hypotension) and **c**olour (pale)
- **D** for **d**ecreased **d**rinking, **d**ecreased output (drinking less than half the usual amounts in the past 24 hours; having fewer than four wet nappies in 24 hours).

Sinister signs include apnoea, convulsions, cyanosis and petechial rash.

- The more features present, the greater the likelihood of severe illness.
- The younger the infant, the more likely are the signs of serious illness to be subtle and/or atypical.
- The absence of any of the factors listed above does not exclude a serious illness.
- Recent antibiotic therapy may obscure clinical signs of sepsis.

Febrile child without a focus

If after a careful history and examination, a non-toxic, febrile child under 3 years old has no obviously detectable focus of infection, the most likely diagnosis is a viral infection.

The child may nevertheless have a serious bacterial infection, such as meningitis, UTI or pneumonia.

- Up to 10% of febrile children with no focus will have occult bacteraemia—positive blood cultures but normal urine and CSF cultures, and normal chest X-ray.
- *Streptococcus pneumoniae* (pneumococcus) is by far the commonest organism causing occult bacteraemia but others are *Haemophilus influenzae* type b (Hib) (rare since Hib immunisation was intro-

duced); *Neisseria meningitidis* (meningococcus); and *Salmonella* species.

- Most children with occult bacteraemia due to pneumococcus will recover spontaneously without antibiotic therapy.
- Without parenteral antibiotics, 1–2% of children with occult pneumococcal bacteraemia will develop meningitis.
- Children with occult Hib or meningococcal bacteraemia are highly likely to develop meningitis if untreated.
- Factors known to increase the risk of serious bacterial infection are:
  - neonate
  - high fever
  - raised blood total white cell count
  - the toxic appearance of the child.
- Clinical acumen is important in deciding which febrile children need any investigations and which need admission and empirical antibiotics.
- The investigation of the febrile child may include FBC, blood culture, MSU, LP and chest X-ray. Strategies are suggested below.

Management of the febrile child without focus

1 Immediate admission, investigation and empirical antibiotics:
   - all febrile neonates < 28 days old and infants < 3 months old
   - all toxic-appearing febrile children < 36 months old
2 No investigations, review in emergency department:
   - well-looking febrile child, aged 3–36 months, who will reliably be returned for follow-up
3 Make investigations and decide accordingly:
   - moderately unwell children, 3–36 months old.

Algorithm for child < 3 years old with fever

Figure 11.1 shows a general management guideline for this situation.

Bacterial meningitis

Diagnostic principles

- Meningitis should be considered in any child with unexplained fever.

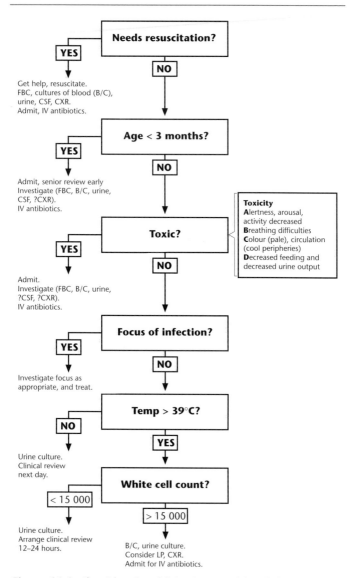

Figure 11.1 Algorithm for child < 3 years old with fever > 38°C axillary

- Headache, photophobia, neck stiffness and drowsiness are more likely to occur in older infants and children; any of these may be absent.
- Very young infants may have only nonspecific signs of sepsis, such as lethargy, reluctance to feed, weak cry, apnoea, hypothermia and shock.
- The presence of an apparent explanation for fever, such as pharyngitis or otitis media, should not divert from the possibility of meningitis.
- Meningitis needs to be considered in a child presenting with a first febrile seizure.
- Using oral antibiotics for unexplained fever often delays diagnosis.
- A common error is to consider a child 'too well' to have meningitis.

Differential diagnosis of bacterial meningitis

This includes:

- viral, fungal and protozoal intracranial infections, including malaria
- intracranial abscess or haemorrhage
- tuberculous meningitis.

Raised intracranial pressure

This is the most serious complication of bacterial meningitis and may appear at the outset (due to severe cerebral oedema) or later (due to subdural collection or acute hydrocephalus).

It should be suspected when there are:

- focal neurological signs
- rapidly deteriorating consciousness or deep coma (Glasgow Coma Scale < 8; see Chapter 3)
- signs of transtentorial herniation, such as one or both pupils dilated and poorly reacting, decorticate or decerebrate posture, abnormal fluctuations in pulse, BP or RR, and episodic apnoea
- fundoscopic changes consistent with papilloedema
- continuous uncontrolled seizures.

Under these circumstances lumbar puncture may be fatal and should not be performed. In the presence of a strong presumptive diagnosis of meningitis:

- Commence appropriate antibiotics.
- Lower intracranial pressure (if necessary, by use of mannitol or hyperventilation in intensive care—see Chapter 3).
- Exclude space-occupying pathology (CT head scan) only once the child's condition is stable.
- Attempt bacteriological diagnosis via blood and urine cultures and urinary antigen studies.
- Reconsider lumbar puncture later when it can be done more safely.

Lumbar puncture (LP)

This is indicated when meningitis is suspected: see the diagnostic principles above.

Contraindications

- Evidence of raised intracranial pressure (see above)
- Immediately overlying skin infection
- Bleeding disorder (prior to clotting factor replacement)

Distance to dura

An approximate guide is:
- 1.5 mm/kg (< 10 kg)
- 1 mm/kg (10–40 kg).

Procedure

- Give an appropriate explanation to the child.
- Use local anaesthetic cream (if LP can be safely deferred for an hour); arrange nitrous oxide analgesia (if possible); use 1% xylocaine under the skin and 2/3 the estimated distance to the dura.
- Use sterile technique, gloves and an alcohol-based skin preparation.
- Restrain the child in the lateral position with the thoraco-lumbar spine well flexed. The back should be perpendicular; avoid neck flexion.
- Carry out lumbar puncture between the posterior superior iliac crests, in the midline, using a 22-gauge cannula with trochar (the short version for children less than 8 years).
- Attempt pressure measurement, then collect 2–4 mL CSF in two tubes; contact the laboratory for the total volume needed if virology or other tests are requested.

- If CSF is blood-stained, collect small amounts in successive tubes to assess if clearing is occurring (indicating a traumatic tap).
- Send CSF to the laboratory immediately, requesting cell count, glucose, protein, direct smear for organisms and culture.

Initial assessment

This is the same as for any acutely unwell child, but with special attention to antibiotic allergy, developmental history and neurological signs including head circumference, circulation and hydration.

Do 'Dextrostix' on admission and formal blood sugar if Dextrostix is low. Arrange full blood count, blood culture and serum electrolytes. If serum sodium is less than 130 mmol/L, suspect the syndrome of inappropriate ADH secretion and assess further with serum osmolality and urine osmolality (see Chapter 15).

CT brain scan is not routinely required. It should be requested urgently if there are signs of raised intracranial pressure (see above) or where the diagnosis of meningitis is in doubt. CT brain scan is useful in demonstrating space-occupying lesions including hydrocephalus. It is not a method for demonstrating raised intracranial pressure.

Initial management

- *Fluids*: Correct shock with a bolus of normal saline or Hartmann's solution; for subsequent deficit and maintenance therapy, see Chapter 7.
- *Fluid restriction*: This is necessary for the syndrome of inappropriate ADH secretion but not otherwise; it should never be considered prior to correction of shock and dehydration.
- *Steroids*: Some authorities advocate the use of dexamethasone (0.4 mg/kg/dose 12-hourly × 2 days) which reduces complications in Hib and pneumococcal meningitis. This should ideally be given about 10 minutes before the first dose of antibiotics.
- Give antibiotics promptly. Do not delay for CT scan, etc.
- Treat seizures.
- Consider artificial ventilation for severe disease.
- Use rifampicin prophylaxis for the family and child with Hib or with suspected or proven meningococcal infection.

Antibiotic therapy

Intravenous antibiotic therapy should start as soon as possible. Whenever possible, the choice of antibiotic therapy will be based on expert microbiological assessment of the CSF—both Gram stain and subsequent culture. As pneumococci are increasingly insensitive to both penicillin and cefotaxime, it is now considered appropriate to include vancomycin in the initial therapy where there is a strong possibility of pneumococcal meningitis. Antibiotic therapy must be reviewed once reliable culture and sensitivity results are available. See the Appendix for antibiotic dosage guidelines; choose high dosage levels. A minimum of 7 days IV therapy is used for meningococcal meningitis and 10 days for most other types of meningitis. A longer duration may be chosen for severe or compli-cated meningitis.

Table 11.1 Summary of initial antibiotic therapy for suspected or proven bacterial meningitis

Age	Situation	Antibiotics
0–6 months	Presumed bacterial meningitis without bacteriological confirmation	Ampicillin and cefotaxime*
> 6 months	Presumed bacterial meningitis without bacteriological confirmation	Cefotaxime*
Any age	Meningitis due to *Haemophilus influenzae* type b, culture-proven, or urinary antigen positive	Cefotaxime
Any age	Meningitis where pneumococcus is considered to be a strong possibility, e.g. Gram-positive cocci on microscopy, severe meningitis when LP contraindicated	Cefotaxime and vancomycin
Any age	Suspected meningococcal meningitis	Cefotaxime
Any age	Culture-proven meningococcal meningitis	Penicillin

*Add vancomycin where *Streptococcus pneumoniae* (pneumococcus) is considered to be a strong possibility.

Septicaemia

- Septicaemia (bacterial invasion of the bloodstream) precedes bacterial meningitis.
- If septicaemia is fulminant, as in some cases of meningococcal infection, then meningitis may not have had time to develop.
- The clinical signs of septicaemia are very variable, and may

include toxic appearance, pallor, fever or hypothermia, shock, respiratory distress, altered consciousness, seizures and bleeding.

- Blood cultures should *always* be taken if there is any suspicion of septicaemia.
  - *Rash*: The rash of meningococcal infection (septicaemia with or without meningitis) is usually purpuric, but may be maculopapular with purpuric elements, or purely maculopapular. When purpuric rash is present, a rapid diagnosis of meningococcaemia may be made by performing a Gram stain on a smear of the fluid obtained by pricking a spot with an orange needle, squeezing the spot and dabbing a microscope slide onto the fluid thus expressed.

    Treatment: Penicillin G or ampicillin or cefotaxime
  - *Line-associated*: If suspected septicaemia occurs in association with a peripheral or central venous line, then there is a high risk of staphylococcal infection (*S. aureus* or *S. epidermidis*).

    Treatment: Flucloxacillin or vancomycin should be included in the regimen.
  - *Immunosuppressed*: Immunocompromised children, such as children on chemotherapy for malignancy or neutropenic children, are at risk for Gram-negative bacillary sepsis.

    Treatment: Usually according to a protocol and will vary according to the nature of the immune compromise, but will usually include Gram-negative cover (for example ticarcillin-clavulanate and/or gentamicin) and staphylococcal cover. Specialist advice is essential.
  - *Urinary tract*: The presence of organisms, white cell casts or > 100×10^6/L white cells in the urine suggests a UTI. The likelihood of this diagnosis is increased by the presence of urinary symptoms in an older child and of abdominal pain and/or rigors in an infant.

    Treatment: See Chapters 10 and 18.
  - *Pneumonia*: A chest radiograph should be obtained, as the signs of pneumonia are not always evident, and as the empiric management of pneumonia differs from that of septicaemia.

    Treatment: See Chapters 10 and 14.
  - *Gastrointestinal tract*: Children with severe chronic gastrointestinal disease are at risk for Gram-negative enteric bacillary sepsis.

    Treatment: Seek specialist advice.

General principles in management of suspected septicaemia

- Take history and examine for underlying predisposing conditions and important clinical signs.
- Take blood cultures.
- Establishment of vascular abscess is a priority.
- Correct shock if present (see Chapters 3 and 7).
- *Antibiotic selection*: Consider if any of the above conditions apply. If not, use empiric treatment based on the *Antibiotic Guidelines* described for fever without focus in Chapter 10.

Acute osteomyelitis

The treatment of acute osteomyelitis is based on early commencement of effective antibiotic therapy. This requires that a presumptive diagnosis be made on clinical features and treatment instituted promptly. Investigations and subsequent progress may require changes in treatment, sometimes including consideration of another diagnosis.

Diagnosis

Acute osteomyelitis should be suggested by pain of recent onset, usually in a limb and near a joint; the pain is usually, though not always, associated with fever and toxaemia. Limitation of movement and localised bony tenderness are found, with or without swelling and redness. The differential diagnosis includes septic arthritis, rheumatoid arthritis, trauma, early poliomyelitis, scurvy, cellulitis, leukaemia and bony tumours.

Investigations

- Collection of blood for culture, and swabs from any infective skin lesions for culture
- Examination of blood film, white cell count, ESR and serum C-reactive protein (CRP); useful as a 'baseline' for later comparison
- X-ray of the affected part (knowing that this will be normal in early osteomyelitis). The X-ray is useful for excluding other diseases, and as a 'baseline' for subsequent X-ray examinations
- Bone scan, which is more useful than X-ray in the early stages of osteomyelitis

Bacteriology

In over 80% of children with acute osteomyelitis the infecting organism is *Staphylococcus aureus*; *S. pyogenes*, *S. pneumoniae*, Hib and *Salmonella* account for most of the remainder.

Management

- *Antibiotic therapy*: Flucloxacillin (plus cefotaxime for children under 5 years not immunised against Hib) should be given intravenously, in the upper limits of dosage as set out in the Appendix.
- This choice may need to be modified when the results of cultures and sensitivities become available.
- If there is a history of penicillin allergy, cefotaxime is the initial antibiotic of choice.
- Antibiotics are given intravenously until the patient becomes afebrile, local swelling and tenderness have diminished and the CRP is decreasing. This may take several days.
- Oral antibiotics should then be commenced on an in-patient basis in older children to assess tolerance and continued on an out-patient basis for a total of at least 3–4 weeks.
- Antibiotic therapy should be intravenous for the entire course for newborns and young infants, who absorb oral antibiotics poorly.
- *General care*: Adequate analgesia, sedation and splinting should be instituted.
- *Surgery* is indicated when a collection of pus develops. This may be intraosseous, subperiosteal, intra-articular or in the soft tissues. This is most likely to occur when the diagnosis has been delayed.
- Antibiotics are not effective in the presence of pus and failure to drain may lead to chronic osteomyelitis.

Septic arthritis

Acute septic arthritis may be of haematogenous origin or due to spread from a neighbouring bone lesion.

Diagnosis

The onset is acute and the symptoms are at first those of acute osteomyelitis, with malaise, pyrexia and pain. Joint involvement may be indicated by effusion. Spasm and severe pain on the slightest movement of the joint are present.

Investigations

- Blood culture and culture of any skin lesions, white cell count, ESR, CRP and blood film are carried out, for the same reasons as stated for acute osteomyelitis.
- An X-ray of the joint may initially show soft tissue swelling and later porosis of the bone ends.
- An ultrasound scan will demonstrate the presence of a joint effusion, but is usually not necessary.
- Joint aspiration may be useful for therapeutic as well as diagnostic reasons. It should be performed under sterile conditions, preferably in the operating room under a general anaesthetic. The presence of organisms in the fluid on Gram stain or culture will confirm the diagnosis.
- Bone scan is sometimes required to exclude osteomyelitis.

Bacteriology

Infection is due to *Staphylococcus aureus*, *S. pyogenes* (group A streptococcus), Hib, *N. meningitidis* or *S. pneumoniae*. Hib should be considered in unimmunised children under 5 years old.

Management

- *Antibiotic therapy*: Following blood cultures and joint aspiration, treatment is commenced with flucloxacillin (and cefotaxime in children under 5 years not immunised against Hib), in the upper limits of dosage as set out in the Appendix. Appropriate changes are later made according to the results of bacteriological investigations. When a response to treatment is evident, antibiotics may be given orally, though not to neonates or young infants. If treatment is commenced early, a total of 3 weeks is sufficient.
- *General care*: Adequate sedation and analgesia.
- *Surgery*: In the weight-bearing joints, particularly the hip, early surgical drainage and lavage by arthroscopy or arthrotomy will decrease the risk of late degenerative arthritis.

Toxic shock syndrome

Toxic shock syndrome (TSS) is caused by strains of toxin-secreting *Staphylococcus aureus*. Staphylococcal TSS can occur following focal *S. aureus* infection, or even colonisation, in children of any age, including neonates.

- TSS may occur with no preceding predisposing cause.
- Recognised associations with TSS are:
  - tampon-associated (now rare)
  - abrasions
  - scalds or burns
  - osteomyelitis
  - abscess
  - wound infections
  - nasal surgery
  - sinusitis
  - empyema
  - peritonsillar abscess
  - tracheitis
  - preceding influenza-like illness.

Most children with staphylococcal TSS do not have positive blood cultures for *S. aureus*.

Other organisms such as streptococcus and (rarely) Gram-negative organisms can cause a clinical picture indistinguishable from staphylococcal TSS. The re-emergence of severe invasive streptococcal disease in the 1980s has coincided with the appearance of a streptococcal toxic shock syndrome which is similar to the descriptions of toxic scarlet fever in the 19th and 20th centuries.

- Most cases (around 70%) of streptococcal TSS are bacteraemic, in contrast to staphylococcal TSS.
- In many cases there is cutaneous evidence of pyogenic exotoxin activity in the form of bullae, erythema or focal swelling (necrotising fasciitis).
- Chickenpox predisposes to group A streptococcal infections, including streptococcal TSS.

The clinical characteristics of TSS are of a multi-system disease, of which the generally accepted criteria are shown in Table 11.2.

- The rash looks like diffuse sunburn and blanches on pressure.
- There may be a strawberry tongue and non-exudative conjunctivitis which can show limbal sparing, like Kawasaki syndrome.
- Shock can be profound, and the patient may develop adult respiratory distress syndrome, DIC, anaemia and/or cardiomyopathy.

TSS is a toxin-mediated disease. Exotoxins produced by bacteria initiate widespread inflammation, with the synthesis of cytokines such

Table 11.2 Clinical criteria for diagnosis of toxic shock syndrome

Fever	39°C or higher
Rash	Diffuse erythroderma
Desquamation	Particularly palms and soles after 1–2 weeks
Shock	Hypotension
and 3 or more of the following:	
Gastrointestinal	Vomiting or diarrhoea
Muscular	Severe myalgia or CPK at least twice normal
Mucous membranes	Conjunctival or oropharyngeal hyperaemia
Renal	Urea or creatinine at least twice normal, or sterile pyuria
Hepatic	Serum transaminases at least twice normal
CNS	Encephalopathy or alteration of consciousness
Blood	Thrombocytopenia (platelets < 100)

as tumour necrosis factor-alpha, interleukin-1 and interleukin-6. *S. aureus* strains causing TSS usually produce toxic shock syndrome toxin-1 (TSST-1) as described by Todd, although other staphylococcal enterotoxins have been implicated. Group A streptococci produce exotoxins A or C. Staphylococcal and streptococcal toxins are thought to act as so-called 'superantigens', capable of activating many different T-cells without prior sensitisation.

Treatment is in an intensive care ward and is supportive, with antibiotics (for example high-dose flucloxacillin) and the urgent correction of shock as priorities. Infected tampons should be removed and any abscesses identified and drained. Intravenous immunoglobulin may be beneficial in refractory cases.

Kawasaki syndrome

- Kawasaki syndrome (KS) is a multi-system vasculitis of unknown aetiology.
- It affects primarily preschool children, with the peak incidence in the first year of life.
- If untreated, approximately 25% of affected children will develop coronary artery vasculitis with a mortality of 2–3%.
- Treatment within 10 days of onset with intravenous

immunoglobulin (IVIG) reduces the risk of coronary involvement to about 8%.

Diagnosis

There are no absolute diagnostic criteria for KS and other diseases must be excluded. The diagnosis is largely a clinical one, based on the epidemiological criteria set out in Table 11.3.

- Other common clinical features are irritability, diarrhoea, cough and arthralgia or arthritis.
- Blood tests are nonspecific, but usually show neutrophil leucocytosis with toxic changes and raised ESR or CRP. Thrombocythaemia develops after 1–2 weeks but the platelet count may initially be normal. Transaminases may be raised. Sterile pyuria is common and aseptic meningitis may occur.
- Abdominal ultrasound scan may show hydrops of the gall-bladder, a nonspecific but suggestive finding.
- Echocardiography is indicated in all children with suspected KS, but does not need to be abnormal to make the diagnosis of KS. It can be delayed for a day or two for convenience, such as in country areas.
- Not all children with KS meet the epidemiological criteria. Some children develop coronary artery aneurysms, but have only three of the criteria.

Table 11.3 Epidemiological criteria for diagnosis of Kawasaki syndrome

Fever for 5 or more days, and 4 or 5 out of:	
Eyes	Non-exudative conjunctivitis with limbal sparing (giving a white halo around the iris)
Mucosa	Dry, cracked, red lips (the 'lipstick sign') and/or strawberry tongue and/or pharyngitis
Peripheral	Non-pitting oedema of the hands and feet or red palms and soles (desquamation is usually delayed for a week or two)
Rash	Variable, may be transient, maculopapular, urticarial, follicular. Peeling in the napkin area of the groin is very suggestive of KS.
Cervical adenopathy	There may be a unilateral mass resembling an abscess or discrete bilateral enlargement of nodes > 1.5 cm diameter.

- The differential diagnosis of KS includes group A streptococcal infection, measles and toxic shock syndrome (TSS). If a child with suspected KS is hypotensive either they are in severe heart failure due to cardiomyopathy or they actually have TSS (see above).
- The current treatment of KS is with a single infusion of IVIG 2 g/kg given over 8–12 hours. IVIG is obtained from the Red Cross blood bank. Low dose salicylate (2–5 mg/kg once daily) is started and continued until a convalescent echocardiogram (usually at 4–6 weeks) is normal.
- Failure of the fever to defervesce with IVIG casts doubt on the diagnosis of KS.
- Recurrence of fever after initial defervescence is usually treated with a second infusion of 2 g/kg a day or two after the first dose.

12

Infectious diseases and immunisation

This chapter includes:

- universal precautions against transmission of blood-borne viruses
- needlestick injury
- incubation periods, school exclusion and prophylaxis for infectious diseases
- chickenpox, measles and the hospitalised child
- childhood immunisation
- prophylaxis against infection in asplenic patients
- notifiable infectious diseases (New South Wales).

Universal precautions against transmission of blood-borne viruses

The adoption of universal precautions against blood-borne viruses has the following implications:

- Transmission of all blood-borne virus infections, including HIV, hepatitis B and hepatitis C, should be avoided.
- Specimens and case notes need no longer be labelled 'infection risk' or 'HIV positive' since universal precautions should be applied to all patients and patient specimens.

Principles of universal precautions

- *Avoid penetrating injury*, by:
  - proper disposal of sharp objects such as needles, scalpel blades and glass
  - adequate provision of 'sharps' containers
  - 'sharps' containers being kept out of reach of toddlers

  – no manual re-sheathing of needles (needle guards can be used if necessary).
- *Avoid contact with blood or body fluids*, by:
  – wearing gloves for venipuncture, IV cannulation and aspiration of body fluids, including CSF, particularly if suffering eczema or if any broken skin on hands
  – wearing gloves when dealing with patients who are bleeding
  – wearing goggles, mask and apron as well as gloves when splashing of blood is likely
  – cleaning blood spills immediately using rubber gloves, disposable cloth or paper towels and dilute (0.5%) sodium hypochlorite, which should remain in contact for 30 minutes
  – putting heavily blood-stained linen in a clear plastic bag and securely tying it
  – discarding blood-stained disposable items in yellow 'biohazard' infectious waste bags.

Prompt management of possible exposure

- Blood or body fluids should be washed off the skin with soap and water, or from the eyes with water, immediately.
- If needlestick injury occurs, the wound should be washed and the incident reported to the clinical nurse consultant in occupational health and safety, so that appropriate serology is performed and hepatitis B prophylaxis and other measures can be initiated if indicated.

Needlestick injury

Detailed hospital policies are available for accidental exposure of a child or staff member to blood or blood products. This section summarises the infectious implications.

- If a child or staff member suffers a needlestick injury, it should first be ascertained whether there was genuine exposure to blood and if the source of the blood is known.
- If a child was exposed to blood from an unknown source, it is important to counsel the family that the risk of catching any infection is exceedingly low (less than one in a million).
- If the child or staff member is already immunised against hepatitis B, no booster is required. If not, the child or staff member should be given hepatitis B immunoglobulin (400 IU IM) and

the first dose of a course of hepatitis B vaccine (1 mL), which should be completed 1 and 5 months later.

- Hepatitis C virus infection cannot currently be prevented with immunoglobulin or antivirals.
- Prophylaxis against HIV infection is possible, but toxic, and should be initiated only after consultation with the on-call infectious disease consultant.
- Blood should be taken for immediate serology to hepatitis B, hepatitis C and HIV, and counselling should be given regarding the low risk. The infectious disease team are happy to provide advice.
- Follow-up should be with general paediatrics or infectious diseases, with serology repeated after 3 and 6 months.

Incubation periods, school exclusion and prophylaxis for infectious diseases

Table 12.1 gives a guide to incubation periods, infectious periods, recommended periods of exclusion from school and details of prophylaxis for contacts, where applicable. Public health units may specify different recommendations under particular circumstances.

Chickenpox, measles and the hospitalised child

Chickenpox and measles can cause major outbreaks in hospitals. In addition they can cause severe, potentially fatal disease in immuno-compromised children.

Chickenpox

The management of chickenpox and chickenpox contacts depends upon certain important facts:

- The incubation period is normally 10–21 days, though it may be 10–25 days in a child who has been given zoster immune globulin (ZIG).
- Children are infectious only from one day before the rash appears, up to the time the vesicles have crusted.

Table 12.1 Infectious disease recommendations

Disease	Incubation period	'Infectious' period	Period of exclusion from school	Prophylaxis of contacts
Measles	10–14 days	For 7 days after first symptom	Five days after appearance of rash, or until recovered. Until had rash 5 days or recovered.	If previously unimmunised and over 12 months of age, give MMR. If < 12 months of age and high risk, or if immunocompromised, give normal human immunoglobulin (0.2 mL/kg IM for normal children; 0.5 mL/kg for immunocompromised)
Chickenpox	10–21 days	One day before the rash to when all the vesicles have crusted. Longer for immunocompromised	Exclude until fully recovered. Remaining scabs are *not* an indication for continued exclusion. Isolate hospital contacts from day 8 after first contact to day 21 after last contact (day 28 if given ZIG).	Consider zoster immune globulin (ZIG) for immunocompromised children including newborns. Dose: 0–10 kg: one vial (200 IU) 11–30 kg: two vials (400 IU) > 30 kg: three vials (600 IU)
Mumps	14–21 days	Seven days before to 9 days after parotid swelling is evident	Exclude until fully recovered	None
Pertussis	7–14 days	From onset until 2 weeks after whoop commences, or until 5 days after antibiotics started	For two weeks or until recovered	Erythromycin or clarithromycin for 7 days for family members

Rubella	14–21 days	Seven days before to 5 days after appearance of the rash	Until well	Test immunity of women contacts of childbearing age
Hepatitis A	15–50 days	Several weeks before to 7 days after the onset of jaundice	Exclude until clinical recovery, or on subsidence of symptoms; should be at least 7 days after jaundice onset	Normal human immunoglobulin IM: < 25 kg: 0.5 mL 25–50 kg: 1 mL > 50 kg: 2 mL
Hepatitis B	6 weeks to 6 months	While hepatitis B antigen is present in the serum	None	*Hepatitis B—prophylaxis of contacts:* 1 *Perinatal exposure (mother HbsAg positive):* Hepatitis B vaccine (0.5 mL) given soon after birth, then at 1 month and at 6 months. A single IM dose of hyperimmune hepatitis B immunoglobulin (HBIg) 100 IU is also given soon after birth. 2 *Household contact (postnatal):* Hep B vaccine, 3 doses, 0.5 mL, as above 3 *Needlestick injury:* Combined active and passive immunisation (0.5–1 mL vaccine plus 400 IU hepatitis B immunoglobulin)

continues . . .

Table 12.1 Infectious disease recommendations (*continued*)

Disease	Incubation period	'Infectious' period	Period of exclusion from school	Prophylaxis of contacts
Hepatitis C	15–50 days	While viraemic (low risk)	None	Nil necessary
Diphtheria	2–6 days	2–4 weeks in untreated persons	Re-admit after certificate from medical officer following at least 2 negative throat swabs 48 hours apart.	Persons with positive throat cultures for *C. diphtheriae* should be treated with penicillin or erythromycin and re-cultured after completion of therapy. Immunisation with diphtheria toxoids should be commenced or completed.
H. influenzae type b (systemic infection)		Not infectious after 24 hours of therapy	Exclude until recovered	If the household includes a child less than 4 years of age (other than the patient) then rifampicin is offered to all members of the household. *Dosage: Infants up to 1 month:* 10 mg/kg/day (as a single dose) for 4 days *Children 1 month to 12 years:* 20 mg/kg/day (as a single dose) for 4 days (with a maximum dose of 600 mg/day). *Adults:* 600 mg/day (as a single dose) for 4 days. *Note:* Side-effects of rifampicin include permanent staining of contact lenses and interference with the efficacy of oral contraceptives. Ceftriaxone is recommended for pregnant women.

Meningo-coccal infection		Not infectious after 24 hours therapy	Re-admit on receipt of medical certificate of recovery.	Rifampicin is given to all close contacts: 20 mg/kg/day in 2 divided doses for 2 days, to a maximum of 600 mg/day. Consult Infectious Diseases.
Impetigo		While lesions active	Until appropriate treatment (usually including oral antibiotics) has commenced, providing exposed affected areas are covered by occlusive dressings	None
Diarrhoea (rotavirus, non-typhoid salmonellae, shigella, giardia)	Usually < 4 days	While diarrhoea persists	Exclude from school while diarrhoea persists.	None
RSV	2–7 days	Usually from 7–21 days (longer in immunocompromised)	Until well	None

- ZIG decreases the severity of chickenpox, but does not necessarily prevent infection.
- Spread is by the respiratory route from subjects with chickenpox or shingles (zoster).

Someone is only a chickenpox contact if they were exposed to a person with active varicella zoster virus lesions. The contact is then potentially infectious from 8 days after the first exposure to 21 days after the last exposure.

If there is a definite ward exposure

- Any child with active chickenpox or zoster should be isolated—the clinical nurse consultant in Infection Control will advise.
- Contacts who are immunocompromised should be given ZIG (see Table 12.1).
- A list should be made of all children who have been exposed, including those who have been given ZIG:
    - Those who have had chickenpox in the past are not at risk (although immunocompromised children may have second episodes).
    - Those still on the ward 8 days after their first exposure should be isolated or sent home.
    - If potentially infected children remain on the ward after 8 days, then only children with a history of past chickenpox should be admitted to the ward until all contacts have gone home or are isolated.

Measles

The principles are as follows:

- The incubation period is 10–14 days.
- Children are most infectious in the prodromal period, less so once the rash has appeared.
- Normal human immunoglobulin can prevent or modify measles.
- Unimmunised contacts over 12 months old should be immunised with measles vaccine in preference to using immunoglobulin.

If there is a definite diagnosis of measles in a child in a ward, the clinical nurse consultant in Infection Control should be notified and the infected child isolated.

- A list should be made of all exposed children on the ward.

- Immunise children who are not at risk from the vaccine.
- Children under 6 months old are generally protected by maternal antibodies and not considered at risk.
- Children aged 6–12 months and immunocompromised children should be given IM normal human immunoglobulin (0.2 mL/kg for normals, 0.5 mL/kg for the immunocompromised).
- Unimmunised children over 12 months old without contra-indications should be immunised with MMR vaccine within 72 hours of the contact.

Childhood immunisation

Previous widespread immunisation has led to a marked reduction in cases and deaths for pertussis and the prevention of diphtheria, tetanus and poliomyelitis in those so immunised. Rubella immunisation has been a major factor in the profound lowering of the incidence of rubella embryopathy. Measles, mumps and more recently *Haemophilus influenzae* type b (Hib) vaccines have prevented the high morbidity and significant mortality of those diseases. Nevertheless, many Australian children are unimmunised or inadequately immunised. Consequently, outbreaks of vaccine-preventable diseases such as pertussis, measles and rubella continue to occur. Re-emergence of diphtheria and poliomyelitis is always possible, when there remain susceptible individuals.

Current recommendations on routine childhood immunisation are set out below. For detailed information on both routine and special-situation childhood immunisation, see *The Australian Immunisation Handbook* (8th edition, NHMRC, 2003, or current edition), available from NHMRC, PO Box 100, Woden, ACT 2606.

Every effort should be made to immunise a child. Every visit to this hospital should be used as an opportunity to check and update the child's immunisations. No child should be denied immunisation without serious thought about the consequences for the child and for the community.

Adverse reactions

Immunisation is often followed by mild adverse reactions which *do not* contraindicate further immunisation:

- DTPa is less reactogenic than DTPw, but still causes local reactions in about 10% of children.

Table 12.2 Recommended childhood immunisation schedule (NHMRC, 2003):

Key:
DTPa = acellular diphtheria/tetanus/pertussis toxoid (acellular triple antigen)
IPV = poliomyelitis vaccine (IM)
Hib = vaccines for *Haemophilus influenzae* type b
MMR = measles/mumps/rubella live attenuated virus vaccine
Hep B = vaccines for hepatitis B
BCG = bacille Calmette-Guérin vaccine: a live attenuated bacterial vaccine against tuberculosis
MenC = meningococcal C conjugate vaccine
PnC = pneumococcal conjugate vaccine
VZV = varicella zoster vaccine

	Birth	2 months	4 months	6 months	12 months	18 months	4–5 years	10–13 years	15–17 years
DTPa		✓	✓	✓			✓		✓§
IPV		✓	✓	✓			✓		
Hib‡		✓	✓	✓	✓				
MMR					✓		✓		
Hep B	✓	✓	✓	✓	✓			✓†	
BCG*	✓								
MenC		✓	✓	✓	✓				
PnC		✓	✓	✓				✓†	
VZV						✓			✓

* for high-risk children
† unless immunised earlier
‡ for Aboriginal children use Hib PRP-OMP at 2, 4, 12 months
§ given as dTpa (adult formulation triple antigen)

- After Hib vaccination, 10% develop transient swelling and redness at the injection site.
- MMR vaccine may be followed 7–10 days later by 2–3 days of fever, malaise and occasionally a rash.

DTP does not cause permanent brain damage.

Absolute contraindications

- Immediate severe allergic or anaphylactic reaction to a previous dose of the same vaccine
- Encephalopathy within 7 days of a previous DTP, defined as severe acute neurological illness with prolonged seizures and/or unconsciousness or focal signs (but not simple febrile convulsions)
- Children or adults suffering from malignant or immunosuppressive conditions should not be given oral polio vaccine or MMR vaccine. Their household contacts may receive MMR but not oral polio vaccine.
- Pregnancy is an absolute contraindication to rubella immunisation, and should be avoided for two full menstrual cycles following administration.

Reasons for deferring immunisation (if in doubt contact a paediatrician or public health physician)

- If the child is acutely unwell, with temperature 38.5°C or higher, or has a 'major' illness, defer immunisation several days.
- If the child or household contacts are immunosuppressed, avoid live vaccines (see above).
- While the child is receiving systemic (but not inhaled) corticosteroids, defer immunisation.
- If the child appears to have an evolving neurological disorder (discuss with a neurologist), defer immunisation.

Note: Minor recurrent infections are not a contraindication to immunisation.

Immunisation tips

Before administering any vaccine:

- Check the identity of the ampoule and the expiry date, and record the batch number.
- Be sure that adrenaline injection BP (1 in 1000) is available in case it is needed to treat an allergic reaction.

Record all immunisations in the child's Blue Book.

Routine immunisations should be reported to the Australian Childhood Immunisation Register.

Delayed primary immunisation

In children up to 8 years, give:

- 4 doses of DTP (at 1–2 month intervals, except 6 months between the 3rd and 4th doses)
- 3 doses of polio vaccine at intervals not less than 1 month
- MMR vaccine (followed by a booster dose before commencing school—at age 4–5 years, or at least 1 month after the first dose). Note that a history of measles, mumps or rubella is not a contraindication to MMR.
- Hib vaccine, according to the schedule for standard immunisation.

In children over 8 years of age, give:

- poliomyelitis vaccine and MMR vaccine, as above
- 3 doses of ADT at 1–2 month intervals, followed by a 4th dose after 6 months.

If an immigrant child has no vaccination record and there is no good evidence of vaccination, the standard schedule should be commenced at the first dose. If the child is 12 months or older, the first doses of DTP, IPV, MMR and Hib vaccine can be given at the same visit.

Prophylaxis against infection in asplenic patients

Children with no spleen are at increased risk of infections with capsulated organisms, mainly pneumococcus, but also *Haemophilus influenzae* type b (Hib) and meningococcus. Congenitally asplenic children and children with sickle cell anaemia are at greater risk than those with post-traumatic splenectomy, but all groups are at increased risk, and the risk continues into adult life. Infections, when they occur, can be fulminant.

The following measures (in Table 12.3) will decrease but not abolish the risk of sepsis. Parents should be advised that prophylactic measures are not 100% effective and that medical care should be sought whenever their child has a fever of 39ºC or over.

Table 12.3 Prophylaxis against infection for children with functional or anatomical asplenia

Intervention	Under 24 months	2–5 years	Over 5 years
Antibiotic prophylaxis	Penicillin V 125 mg b.d. or amoxycillin 20 mg/kg once daily essential	Daily penicillin V or amoxycillin prophylaxis recommended	Not recommended, but should wear Medi-Alert bracelet and treat fevers early
Pneumococcal (pneumococcal conjugate, e.g. Prevenar 7-valent, and pneumococcal polysaccharide, e.g. Pneumovax)	Give pneumococcal *conjugate* vaccine primary course and booster.	Single dose of conjugate vaccine essential, then single dose of pneumococcal polysaccharide vaccine at least 1 month later	Single dose of conjugate vaccine essential, then single dose of pneumococcal polysaccharide vaccine at least 1 month later
Hib conjugate vaccine	As per routine childhood schedule	Single dose	Single dose
Meningococcal vaccine (meningococcal conjugate group C vaccine and meningococcal polysaccharide vaccine A, C, W-135,Y)	Give conjugate vaccine at 2, 4, 6 months. Single dose over 1 year of age.	Give single dose of conjugate vaccine, then single dose of polysaccharide vaccine at least 1 month later.	Give single dose of conjugate vaccine, then single dose of polysaccharide vaccine at least 1 month later.

Notifiable infectious diseases

The diseases listed in Table 12.4 are 'notifiable' in New South Wales; regulations may differ in other states. The rationale of notification is to improve infectious disease control. The lists are current for 2003. The notification is done, by telephone, to the local Public Health Unit (from the Children's Hospital at Westmead, contact Western Sydney Public Health Unit, 9840 3603).

Table 12.4 Notifiable infectious diseases—NSW

To be notified by doctors and/or hospital executive	To be notified by laboratories
Acquired immunodeficiency syndrome (AIDS)	Arboviral infection (flaviviruses)*
Acute viral hepatitis	Brucellosis
Adverse event following immunisation	Botulism*
	Chancroid
Botulism	Chlamydia trachomatis
Cholera*	Cholera*
Diphtheria*	Cryptosporidiosis
Food-borne illness in two or more related cases*	Diphtheria*
	Giardiasis
Gastroenteritis among people of any age, in an institution*	Gonorrhoea
	Granuloma inguinale
Haemolytic uraemic syndrome	Haemophilus influenzae type b invasive infection
Haemophilus influenzae type b invasive infection*	Hepatitis A*
Legionnaires' disease*	Hepatitis B
Leprosy	Hepatitis C
Measles*	Hepatitis D (Delta)
Meningococcal disease*	Hepatitis E*
Paratyphoid*	Human immunodeficiency virus (HIV) infection
Pertussis (whooping cough)*	Legionnaires' disease*
Plague*	Leptospirosis
Poliomyelitis*	Listeriosis
Rabies*	Lymphogranuloma venereum
Syphilis	Malaria
Tetanus	Measles*
Tuberculosis	Meningococcal infections*
Typhoid*	Mumps
Typhus (epidemic)*	Mycobacterial infections

Table 12.4 Notifiable infectious diseases—NSW *(continued)*

To be notified by doctors and/or hospital executive	To be notified by laboratories
Viral haemorrhagic fever*	Pertussis (whooping cough)*
Yellow fever	Plague*
	Poliomyelitis*
	Q fever
	Rabies
	Rubella (German measles)
	Salmonella infections
	Syphilis
	Typhus (epidemic)*
	Verotoxin-producing *Escherichia coli* infections*
	Viral haemorrhagic fevers*
	Yellow fever*

*To be notified by telephone to public health units as soon as a provisional diagnosis is made

13

Cardiology

This chapter includes:
- congenital heart disease
- presentation of heart disease
- other issues in children's heart disease.

Congenital heart disease

- This accounts for most paediatric cardiology.
- It occurs at the rate of 7–8 per 1000 live births.
- About one-third of affected children require staged surgical and/or interventional catheterisation, another third require single surgical or catheter procedures and the remainder require little or no intervention.
- A few conditions continue to have a very poor prognosis.
- A good medium-term prognosis occurs in > 90% of children.

Acquired heart disease

Heart disease may also be acquired:

- inflammatory, for example Kawasaki syndrome
- coronary heart disease
- associated with a metabolic disease
- infective, for example SBE, myocarditis
- postinfective, for example rheumatic fever
- associated with arrhythmia
- secondary to severe lung disease.

Making a diagnosis

This will depend upon a comprehensive history, clinical examination and supplementary investigations:

- ECG (note these normal findings: right-sided preponderance, birth to mid-childhood; right precordial T-wave inversion: from 5 days to early adolescence)
- chest X-ray (look for heart size > 55% of thoracic transverse diameter, abnormal heart contour or position, increased or decreased pulmonary vascular markings and evidence of lung disease)
- pulse oximetry (use right arm or leg where possible in neonate)
- blood gases (with hyperoxia test, if necessary)
- echocardiography (this should be seen as part of the overall evaluation, and is not a substitute for clinical assessment)

Presentation of cardiac disease

Signs

Suspect heart disease with:

- cardiac murmur/s
- breathlessness/tachypnoea
- other signs of heart failure
- cyanosis unrelieved by extra oxygen
- unexplained failure to thrive
- phenotypic abnormality
- family history of structural heart disease.

Heart failure

This can occur at any age, including prenatally. Common features are:

- increasing tachypnoea, dyspnoea
- poor feeding, poor weight gain
- diminished exercise tolerance (compared with peers)
- persisting tachycardia
- hepatomegaly
- decreased pulses and perfusion (late signs).

Peripheral oedema or isolated features of right or left heart failure are rarely seen in children presenting with heart failure.

- In newborns, features of heart failure are often rapidly progressive and may signal imminent deterioration.

- With left-to-right shunts (for example, large VSD) symptoms may be delayed until pulmonary vascular resistance drops, at 4–8 weeks of age.
- In older children, heart failure is more likely to be due to acquired conditions or arrhythmias.

Cyanosis

Cyanotic congenital heart disease generally presents in the newborn period. This situation is sometimes a medical emergency, requiring urgent intervention. In 'duct-dependent' lesions, cyanosis coincides with closure of the ductus arteriosus. Cyanosis may be difficult to detect with mild hypoxia (saturation > 85%) or if anaemia is present.

Cyanosis may develop only after weeks or months with some conditions, for example tetralogy of Fallot (with gradually increasing right ventricular outflow obstruction), total anomalous pulmonary venous drainage and truncus arteriosus. Cyanosis may coexist with signs of heart failure in complex admixture lesions.

Differential diagnosis of heart failure and/or cyanosis

Heart failure and/or 'cardiac' cyanosis may be mimicked by many conditions:

- respiratory disease (such as pneumothorax, neonatal RDS, acute viral bronchiolitis, meconium aspiration, tracheo-oesophageal fistula)
- pericardial disease (effusion, tamponade)
- cerebral depression (hypoventilation), for example from maternal opioids
- hypoglycaemia
- methaemoglobinaemia
- polycythaemia
- A-V malformation (cerebral, hepatic or pulmonary).

Management of the child with suspected heart disease

- Attend to airway, breathing, circulation, as required.
- Take full history and do clinical examination.
- Investigate pulse oximetry, chest X-ray and ECG.
- According to the circumstances, investigate blood gases ± hyper-oxia test.

- Discuss with paediatrician/paediatric cardiologist.
- Possibly, further evaluate with paediatric echocardiography following consultation with paediatric cardiology.

Management of heart failure

- Support:
  - oxygen: to maintain saturations > 85% but < 95% (high FiO_2 may lower pulmonary vascular resistance and consequently increase left-to-right shunt, worsening the heart failure)
  - nasogastric feeds, if unable to suck feeds
  - IV fluids at 2/3 maintenance, with supplementary glucose, if the child is unable to feed orally or if there is significant respiratory distress
- Identify the lesion; this usually requires cardiology consultation.
- Lesion and symptom-specific management:
  - left-to-right shunt with myocardial dysfunction (not all required in every case):
    diuretic (for example frusemide 1 mg/kg/dose, once or twice daily)
    digoxin (see the Appendix)
    afterload reduction (usually ACE inhibitor such as captopril)
  - an obstructive lesion may require urgent surgical or catheter intervention
  - an arrhythmia may require immediate termination and consideration of preventative therapy
- Coordinated transfer for early paediatric cardiac assessment: discuss with a paediatric cardiologist before transfer if possible.

Hypercyanotic spells

- These occur particularly in children with tetralogy of Fallot.
- They should be distinguished from transient increases in cyanosis due to crying or exertion, which are expected.
- Attacks usually involve profound cyanosis or pallor and sweating, often with altered consciousness.
- Management:
  - Brief spells usually subside spontaneously.
  - Prolonged attacks require calming the child, the knee-chest posture, oxygen and, if persisting, IV fluids with volume expansion, sedation with morphine (using close monitoring) and beta-blockers.

Long-term outcome in congenital heart disease

The outcome for most children with surgically treated congenital heart disease appears excellent with low rates of important residual abnormalities. Some patients will, however, be at risk of:

- arrhythmia
- ventricular dysfunction
- significant residual lesions
- need for re-operation
- sudden death.

For some forms of complex congenital heart disease the best outcome may be an efficient reorganisation, but not repair, of the heart.

Continuing review of these children is needed through adolescence and adult life, by physicians familiar with the special problems which can be lesion-specific. Prognosis and follow-up are best individualised.

Special issues to be considered may include:

- the need for genetic counselling
- selection of contraceptive methods
- pregnancy planning and management
- job and recreational selection
- reduction of causative factors for degenerative vascular disease.

Other issues in children's heart disease

Innocent murmur

Innocent cardiac murmurs are heard in up to 50% of infants and children, often over months or years. They are more readily apparent during intercurrent illness. They are not associated with any structural or functional heart abnormality. An innocent cardiac murmur, therefore, is a normal physical finding, but the term 'heart murmur' often produces great anxiety for families. Innocent murmurs are:

- usually mid-systolic, and usually not widely heard
- not associated with symptoms or other auscultatory abnormalities
- relatively soft, often with a 'musical' character
- frequently variable with body posture.

Further evaluation

Further evaluation of a cardiac murmur should be considered if it is:

- associated with a situation of increased risk, such as an abnormal phenotype
- particularly loud and persistent
- associated with abnormal or additional heart sounds
- diastolic in timing
- present in an infant less than 12 months of age.

Fever in children with heart disease

- Though uncommon, bacterial endocarditis should be considered in any child with fever and structural heart disease.
- Fever with no obvious focus can be observed, without the use of antibiotics, for up to 3 days if the child is reasonably well.
- If antibiotics are considered necessary on clinical grounds, blood cultures should be taken before commencement.
- Focal bacterial infections are treated in the usual way.
- Persisting fevers after cessation of a course of antibiotics should increase suspicion of infective endocarditis.
- Early echocardiography has a very low yield of positive findings in febrile patients with heart disease.

Antibiotic prophylaxis

Antibiotic prophylaxis to reduce the risk of bacterial endocarditis is suggested for all children with structural cardiac lesions, except those with completely repaired PDA and secundum ASD, with an otherwise normal heart. Antibiotics are chosen according to the predicted sensitivities of the organisms likely to cause bacteraemia.

- Use for potentially contaminated surgery and dental procedures producing major gum trauma.
- Prophylaxis is not recommended for intercurrent illnesses or loss of primary dentition and is not relevant *after* trauma.
- It is given as a single dose before the procedure and may be repeated once or twice at 6-hourly intervals afterwards (depending on circumstances and the antibiotic used).
- Preventative dental care is most important.

The antibiotic used should be appropriate for the potential infective focus:

- *For dental procedures*:
  - non-penicillin-allergic: amoxycillin 50 mg/kg (maximum 2 g) orally, single dose, 1 hour before the procedure
  - penicillin-allergic: clindamycin 10 mg/kg (maximum 600 mg) orally, single dose, 1 hour before the procedure
- *For other procedures*:
  - non-penicillin-allergic: amoxycillin or ampicillin 50 mg/kg (up to 1 g) + gentamicin 2 mg/kg (up to 80 mg)
  - penicillin-allergic: vancomycin 20 mg/kg (up to 1 g) slow IV + gentamicin 2 mg/kg (up to 80 mg)
- Prosthetic valves and bowel surgery may require variations on this regime.

Cardiac surgery and some post-discharge issues

Enormous advances have been made in paediatric cardiac surgery, allowing for the correction or palliation of the vast majority of congenital cardiac lesions. In many cases such surgery is carried out based on high-level paediatric echocardiographic or other non-invasive imaging strategies. Postoperatively, most patients will require some ongoing follow-up with the focus on monitoring and intervening in a timely fashion for expected postoperative variations from normal cardiac anatomy or function.

The 4-week period after cardiac surgery, especially open heart surgery, exposes patients to a special range of potential problems.

Some of the *symptoms* and *signs* indicating a possible, but not exclusively, cardiac aetiology may include:

- fever without focus
- vomiting/nausea/lethargy/new poor feeding
- abdominal pain
- chest pain
- syncope
- headache
- cough
- tachypnoea/respiratory distress
- new redness or swelling of the wound
- chest wall instability
- unexpected degrees of cyanosis.

Cardiac complications which should be considered include (but not exclusively):

- cardiac failure (new)
- pericardial effusion
- cardiac tamponade (signs may be subtle; beware nausea, vomiting)
- bacterial endocarditis
- wound infection, sternal dehiscence
- brady- or tachyarrhythmia (constant or intermittent)
- shunt obstruction
- embolism, stroke
- intercurrent or hospital acquired viral or bacterial infections (such as bronchiolitis, gastroenteritis and urinary tract infection).

Antibiotics should not be commenced in the first 4 weeks after surgery without appropriate investigation (usually including blood cultures) and prior discussion, unless in urgent circumstances (see p. 159, 'Fever in children with heart disease')

If symptoms, signs or the suspected conditions outlined above occur within 1 month of discharge after surgery, contact medical staff from the Cardiology/Cardiac Surgery Service (or the specific surgeon or cardiologist involved) at the Children's Hospital at Westmead.

Cardiovascular risk factors in children

Vascular disease which becomes apparent later in life may begin in childhood, especially where a family history of early adult vascular disease or hypertension exists. This issue is of additional concern where there are pre-existing structural heart lesions.

- Important strategies to introduce early include maintenance of basic fitness and avoidance of obesity, smoking and hyperlipidaemia.
- Test blood lipids in children at age 10 years if there is a family history of early onset of heart disease associated with hyperlipidaemia.
- The most effective dietary and exercise modifications are those shared by the whole family.

Foetal cardiac diagnosis

Improved echocardiographic imaging now allows diagnosis of most important congenital heart lesions as early as 18 weeks gestation. At this stage screening obstetric scans currently identify no more than 15% of diagnosable significant lesions.

- Pregnancies at increased risk for foetal structural heart disease include:
  - a previous child or either parent with congenital heart disease
  - maternal connective tissue disease
  - foetal chromosomal or somatic abnormalities.
- Where required, foetal echocardiography is generally carried out as a 'screening procedure' between 18 and 20 weeks or, as required, later, by a paediatric cardiologist with special expertise in foetal cardiology.
- Some lesions are obscured by foetal circulation and therefore cannot be diagnosed until after birth.

Cardiac catheterisation and catheter intervention

Echocardiography is the main means for diagnosis of heart disease in childhood and frequently is the sole definitive evaluation prior to surgery. However, cardiac catheterisation remains the 'gold standard' for detailed haemodynamic evaluation in complex heart disease and for identification of some structural lesions, for example pulmonary artery abnormalities. There is an increasing role for cardiac catheterisation in therapy. Interventional catheter techniques can often be used to treat abnormalities such as pulmonary artery stenosis, aortic valve stenosis, persistent ductus arteriosus, some forms of atrial septal defect, and re-coarctation of the aorta.

Supraventricular tachycardias and other arrhythmias

Supraventricular tachycardia (SVT) makes up 90% of paediatric arrhythmias. In many cases the episodes are infrequent, brief, self-limiting and benign.

Complex atrial arrhythmias and ventricular tachycardia are rare and most often seen following open heart surgery and in those with complex heart disease.

The long QT syndrome (QTc > 0.44 seconds) with associated ventricular arrhythmias should be considered in patients with syncope or haemodynamic compromise with arrhythmia, and a resting ECG should be carefully examined. Note Bazet's formula: $QTc = QT/\sqrt{RR}$.

Arrhythmia may present as:

- palpitations
- chest pain

- syncope
- heart failure.

A baseline ECG and one recorded in tachycardia can be invaluable.

Re-entrant SVT is often characterised by abrupt onset and cessation, distinguishing it from sinus tachycardia.

Persistent SVT will usually:

- be incessant over a narrow rate range
- have a narrow QRS complex (in > 95% of cases)
- have no atrioventricular dissociation.

Termination of re-entrant SVT may be achieved by:

- Valsalva manoeuvre
- provoking a gag reflex
- ice water to the face
- intravenous adenosine.

Termination of SVT should be documented with continuous monitor strips:

- Eyeball pressure should be avoided.
- Verapamil is not recommended in infants younger than 12 months.

Kawasaki syndrome

See Chapter 11.

14

Respiratory diseases

This chapter includes:

- snoring, stridor and wheeze
- acute upper airway obstruction
- acute asthma
- acute viral bronchiolitis
- acute pneumonia
- cystic fibrosis.

See also:

- neonatal respiratory conditions: Chapter 8
- antibiotic protocols for respiratory infections: Chapter 10.

Snoring, stridor and wheeze

Respiratory disease accounts for about 50% of illness in infants, children and adolescents. The most common problems are infections (particularly viral) and asthma, which remain the most frequent reasons for admission to this hospital. Two other conditions, largely confined to the paediatric age group, are congenital malformations of the respiratory tract and inhaled foreign bodies, especially nuts and plastic toys. A respiratory foreign body should be considered in any child with acute respiratory symptoms, especially between the ages of 1 and 5 years.

Noisy breathing is common in childhood and is due to turbulent airflow caused by obstruction of some part of the airway. The common causes of noisy breathing are listed in Table 14.1.

- Snoring reflects nasal or pharyngeal obstruction. It is characteristically present during sleep (in association with decreased upper airway muscle tone) but, if obstruction is severe, may be present when awake. The presence of obstructive sleep apnoea is an indicator of more severe upper airway obstruction.

Table 14.1 Common causes of noisy breathing

Causes of upper airway obstruction

Above the larynx:
    Choanal atresia or stenosis
    Mid-face hypoplasia (typically, ex-premature infants)
    Pharyngeal cysts
    Retropharyngeal abscess*
    Tonsillar and adenoidal hypertrophy* (the most common cause)
    Epiglottitis (supraglottitis)* (now uncommon)

At the larynx:
    Laryngomalacia
    Laryngeal papillomata*
    Vocal cord palsy
    Laryngeal cysts
    Foreign body*
    Laryngeal diphtheria*
    Laryngeal spasm*

Below the larynx:
    Croup (laryngo-tracheitis)*
    Tracheal compression (vascular ring, mediastinal masses)*
    Tracheal malformations (tracheomalacia, webs, stenosis)
    Tracheal haemangioma
    Foreign body (tracheal, oesophageal)*

Causes of lower airway obstruction

Acute asthma*
Acute viral bronchiolitis*
Chemical bronchitis/bronchiolitis (especially aspiration)*
Suppurative lung disease:
    Cystic fibrosis
    Immune deficiency
    Primary ciliary dyskinesia
    Bronchiectasis (postinfective, idiopathic)
    Chronic lung disease of prematurity
    Bronchial malformations (bronchomalacia, stenosis)

* Conditions which may present acutely.

- Stridor reflects airway obstruction at the level of the larynx or upper trachea. It is predominantly inspiratory and harsh in nature but when severe may have an expiratory component.
- Wheeze reflects lower airway obstruction. It is predominantly expiratory and has a whistling quality. Although the intensity of

165

the wheeze may reflect the severity of the obstruction, wheeze may be absent in severe obstruction due to significant reduction in airflow.

Differentiation of the cause of airway obstruction depends largely on the history and physical examination, aided by X-rays (CXR, lateral airways X-ray, barium swallow), pulmonary function tests (in children > 6 years old), sleep studies and endoscopy.

Acute upper airway obstruction

Croup

The term 'croup' refers to a symptom complex characterised by *harsh barking cough*, with or without *inspiratory stridor*, and with or without *respiratory difficulty*. Causes include the following:

Viral laryngotracheitis

- The most common cause of croup—due to parainfluenza and other viruses.
- Occurs particularly in first 5 years of life, peak incidence 1–2 years.
- Usually preceded by coryzal symptoms.
- Usually self-limiting, but occasionally severe, requiring treatment.

Spasmodic croup

- Appears to be associated with asthma/atopy.
- There is no viral prodrome.
- There is rapid onset and cessation of croup symptoms.
- Often recurrent.

Pseudomembranous croup ('staphylococcal tracheitis')

- May represent secondary bacterial infection following viral infection.
- Thick secretions form a 'pseudomembrane' (less tough and adherent than a diphtheritic membrane).
- Usually affects older children, who are often 'toxic' and very unwell.
- Obstruction tends to be more severe and stridor softer than with viral croup.

Diphtheritic croup

- Should be considered in any unimmunised child.
- Associated with 'toxicity', and often rapidly progressive airway obstruction.
- There is a laryngeal membrane (grey, foul-smelling, bleeds on suctioning and is not easily removed).
- There may be a tonsillar/pharyngeal membrane or exudate.

Management of children with croup

- Initial assessment is aimed at determining the severity of obstruction and the need for hospital admission. The assessment is largely a clinical one—investigations, including lateral airways X-rays, are generally not done. Take particular note of:
  - the general appearance of the child—an alert, interested or sleeping child usually does not have severe airway obstruction; a preoccupied or agitated child may be significantly obstructed and hypoxaemic
  - degree of respiratory difficulty (respiratory and pulse rates, tracheal tug and chest wall retractions, palpable paradox)
  - cyanosis or pallor (generally late signs, suggesting severe obstruction).
- The *need for admission to hospital* is influenced by:
  - a history of severe obstruction prior to admission, or previous severe croup
  - the degree of respiratory difficulty (stridor at rest is an indication for admission)
  - the child's fluid intake
  - the level of parental anxiety, proximity to home and the transport available.
- Oximetry should be part of the initial assessment, with regular monitoring in those with moderate or severe obstruction. However, normal oximetry does not exclude severe upper airway obstruction.
- Oxygen should always be given to relieve hypoxaemia if present (oxygen saturation < 95% or clinical cyanosis). The need for oxygen should be an indication for reassessment by a doctor and for close observation of the patient, with a view to considering other interventions.
- Oral corticosteroid therapy is recommended for all children

167

hospitalised with croup. It should also be given to children presenting to the Emergency Department but not requiring admission, apart from those with trivial croup. A 'stat' dose of oral dexamethasone (0.15 or 0.3 mg/kg) is recommended because it is better tolerated, but prednisolone (0.5 or 1 mg/kg) is a suitable alternative.

- Nebulised adrenaline 1:1000 (0.5 mL/kg, max. 5 mL) can be given to relieve moderate or severe obstruction. Both the need for and response to adrenaline must be assessed by a doctor at the bedside and should always be ordered as a 'stat' dose. The need for repeated doses of adrenaline (for example, > 3) should be an indication for monitoring in ICU.

- Nebulised budesonide (2 mg) may have a role if nebulised adrenaline is contraindicated (such as in tetralogy of Fallot) or if oral steroids are not well tolerated. It may also be used in conjunction with oral steroids.

- Intravenous corticosteroids can be used in the child who is intubated or who requires intravenous fluids.

- Mist therapy and nebulised saline have no place in the treatment of croup.

- Subsequent management decisions, particularly the need for repeated doses of nebulised adrenaline or corticosteroids and the need for admission to ICU, should be discussed with the attending medical officer.

- The decision regarding the need for intubation is largely a clinical one. Clinical signs of impending respiratory collapse include the child appearing tired, agitated, worried or restless, increasing respiratory difficulty and chest retractions, marked use of accessory muscles of respiration and increasing heart rate. Cyanosis, decreased conscious level, extreme restlessness and decreasing respiratory effort along with decreasing stridor and breath sounds are indications of the need for urgent intervention.

Acute epiglottitis

Acute epiglottitis (supraglottitis) is characterised by inflammatory swelling of the epiglottis and aryepiglottic folds. It is most commonly due to infection with *Haemophilus influenzae* type b. This has become uncommon since the advent of Hib immunisation, although it can still occur, due to Hib or other organisms such as group A streptococcus and some viruses. It is a dangerous condition with a high death rate if undiagnosed, or diagnosed late. Both acute epiglottitis and croup may be preceded by a viral prodrome and both occur at similar ages.

Differentiating features from croup

The differentiating features from croup include the following:

- The child is toxic, with high fever.
- The child often sits up, leans forward and drools (because of an inability to swallow).
- The obstruction is more severe and stridor, if present, is soft (not harsh).
- Cough is absent or minimal; it may be muffled, but is not 'croupy'.
- Croup 'bespeaks its name' and the diagnosis is often readily made by lay people; conversely, epiglottitis is uncommon, often insidious, subtle, yet relentlessly progressive, to the point of sudden collapse with complete airway obstruction.

If you suspect acute epiglottitis

- Call the anaesthetic registrar, who should remain with the child.
- Notify the ENT, intensive care and respiratory registrars, who will notify their respective consultants.
- While arranging urgent transfer to the operating theatres for endoscopy and an artificial airway, *do not do anything else unless respiratory collapse occurs*. During this time:
  - Have the parents hold the child, sitting up.
  - Do not try to examine the throat, to insert cannulas or collect blood.
  - Do not attempt lateral airways X-rays.
  - Do not give nebulised adrenaline.
- Cefotaxime is given (following blood cultures ± epiglottic swab). Rifampicin prophylaxis should be considered (see Chapter 12). Hib vaccine should later be given to unimmunised or incompletely immunised children who present with Hib epiglottitis < 2 years of age because of the relatively poor immune response to Hib in this age group.
- The child is cared for during intubation (usually about 24 hours) in intensive care.

Note: Suggested endotracheal tube sizes in acute upper airways obstruction follow:

Age	Size (mm)
0–6 months	3.0
6–24 months	3.5
2–5 years	4.0
> 5 years	4.5

Lateral airways (neck) X-rays

- These have been used as a diagnostic aid in both acute and persistent upper airways obstruction.
- In both situations they have the potential to worsen airway obstruction due to the positioning of the child.
- In severe airway obstruction, lateral airways X-rays should *never* be performed prior to relieving the obstruction (with intubation or other treatment interventions).
- In less severe acute obstruction, lateral airways should not routinely be ordered. If it is felt to be clinically indicated, the emergency registrar should:
  - discuss with the attending physician
  - accompany the child to the X-ray department (with intubation equipment)
  - interpret the X-ray with an experienced individual.

Acute asthma

Assessment of an acute episode of asthma should take into account the previous history including interval symptoms, sleep disruption, exercise-induced symptoms, triggers for asthma episodes, frequency of attacks, regular medications, medications given during the current episode and the clinical signs. Table 14.2 provides an approach to classifying the severity of acute asthma related to the clinical signs, lung function (where applicable) and oximetry.

Treatment

The initial classification of severity can be useful in predicting the need for hospitalisation and the management of the acute episode as illustrated in Table 14.3.

Table 14.2 Initial assessment of severity of acute asthma (adapted from the National Asthma Council *Asthma Management Handbook* 2002 and NSW Health *Paediatric Clinical Guidelines—Asthma*)

Physical sign or test	Mild	Moderate	Severe (*and life-threatening**)
	Acute asthma attack severity		
Altered consciousness	No	No	Agitated (*confused/drowsy*)
Accessory muscle use/recession	No	Minimal	Moderate (*severe*)
Oximetry on presentation (SaO_2)	> 94%	90–94%	< 90%
Talks in	Sentences	Phrases	Words (*unable to speak*)
Pulsus paradoxus	Not palpable	May be palpable	Palpable
Pulse rate/minute	< 100	100–200	> 200 (*bradycardia*)
Central cyanosis	Absent	Absent	Likely to be present
Wheeze intensity	Variable	Moderate to loud	Often quiet
Physical exhaustion	No	No	Yes
Initial PEF or FEV_1 (% predicted)	> 60%	40–60%	< 40% (*unable to perform*)

* Any of these features indicate that the episode is severe. The absence of any feature does not exclude a severe attack.

Oxygen therapy

Oxygen should be used to relieve hypoxaemia (O_2 saturation < 95%) by using face mask oxygen up to 8 L/min. Oxygen should also be used to drive nebuliser therapy in this situation. Oxygen therapy does not cause CO_2 retention in children with acute asthma.

Salbutamol

- May be given via metered dose aerosol + spacer (4–6 puffs < 20 kg/6 years; 8–12 puffs > 20 kg/6 years) or nebulised (salbutamol 2.5 mg nebules < 20 kg/6 years; 5 mg nebules > 20 kg/ 6 years).

Table 14.3 Initial treatment of acute asthma (adapted from the National Asthma Council *Asthma Management Handbook* 2002 and NSW Health *Paediatric Clinical Guidelines—Asthma*)

	Acute asthma severity		
Treatment	**Mild**	**Moderate**	**Severe and life-threatening**
Admission necessary?	Probably not	Probably	Yes—consider ICU
Oxygen	Probably not	Monitor with SaO_2	May need arterial blood gases
Salbutamol† * < 20 kg/6 years ** ≥ 20 kg/6 years	4–6* or 8–12** puffs and review in 20 min	3 doses— 4–6* or 8–12** puffs at 20 min intervals	Nebulised 2.5 mg* or 5 mg** × 20 min or continuous
Ipratropium† * < 20 kg/6 years ** ≥ 20 kg/6 years	No	Optional	3 doses (2*–4** puffs or 250*–500** micrograms) × 20 min, then 6-hourly
Corticosteroids	Consider oral prednisolone	Oral prednisolone 1–2 mg/kg/day	Oral prednisolone 1–2 mg/kg/day IV methylpred or 1 mg/kg 6–8-hourly
Aminophylline	No	No	*Consider in ICU*
IV salbutamol	No	No	Consider IV bolus *or* continuous infusion if poor response to neb. salbutamol (see text for doses)
Observation	For 20 min after dose	For 60 min after last dose (?home ?hosp)	Admit to ward or paediatric intensive care unit—NETS transfer

†*Note*: Use small volume spacers and face mask for children < 4 years, large volume spacers for children ≥ 6 years and either for children between 4 and 6 years.

- Nebuliser therapy is preferred in more severe episodes employing frequent high dose regimes (20-minutely). Continuous nebulised salbutamol (4 mL of neb. solution [5 mg/mL] given at 12 mL/h) can be used for severe and life-threatening asthma.

- Dosage frequency is adjusted according to response and progress.
- Intravenous salbutamol should be considered as an adjunct in severe episodes: 15 micrograms/kg over 10 minutes as bolus, or 5 micrograms/kg/min initially, then 1–20 micrograms/kg/min (max. doses based on 40 kg) according to response as a continuing infusion.

Ipratropium bromide (Atrovent)

- Provides additional bronchodilation when salbutamol used frequently.
- May be given via metered dose aerosol + spacer (2 puffs < 20 kg/6 years; 4 puffs > 20 kg/6 years) or via nebuliser (250 micrograms < 20 kg/6 years; 500 micrograms > 20 kg/6 years).
- May be used up to every 20 minutes × 3 doses in severe episodes and adjusted back to 6-hourly after the initial 3 doses.

Corticosteroids

- Their beneficial role in acute asthma is well established.
- The oral route is generally reliable (prednisolone 1 mg/kg [max. 50 mg] every 12–24 hours for 3–5 days).
- Intravenous steroids may be considered if oral steroids are not tolerated or if there is a severe or life-threatening episode (methylprednisolone 1 mg/kg [max. 50 mg] every 6–8 hours or hydrocortisone 4–5 mg/kg [max. 200 mg] every 4–6 hours).

Theophylline

- Has questionable efficacy in mild-moderate episodes.
- Should be reserved for life-threatening episodes in paediatric intensive care unit.
- Blood levels should be monitored if use prolonged or side-effects (nausea, vomiting, agitation, convulsions) occur.

Other therapy

- IV fluids may be indicated if the patient is not tolerating oral medications and fluids or in a severe episode.
- CPAP or assisted ventilation may be still necessary occasionally despite aggressive medical therapy. Ventilation is usually difficult and is best attempted in a specialised intensive care unit.
- Antibiotics are seldom necessary, as most episodes are viral-induced.

173

- Physiotherapy has no place in the acute phase, but may be of value in the convalescent phase if there is lung collapse.

Assessing response to therapy

Look for:

- increased patient comfort; reduced feeling of 'tightness'
- reduced use of accessory muscles of breathing
- reduction in respiratory rate
- improved air entry
- reduced length of expiratory phase and wheeze
- improved oximetry, reduced oxygen requirement.

Discharge criteria

- Children with acute asthma should be considered ready for discharge when clinically stable on 3rd-hourly bronchodilator.
- Oximetry should not be used as the primary criterion for discharge because it remains unclear what a 'satisfactory' level is—an oxygen saturation > 90% could be considered a minimum 'safe' level.
- Asthma care paths should include a discharge checklist to identify and address potential barriers to discharge.
- At the time of discharge all patients/parents should receive: (1) a discharge summary; (2) an asthma action plan (including a post-discharge plan); (3) discharge medications; (4) follow-up arrangements.

Prevention

An acute episode of asthma should be seen as an opportunity to review the interval severity of asthma and commence or adjust the level of preventive therapy if necessary.

Acute viral bronchiolitis

This is a viral lower respiratory infection which produces small airway obstruction with air trapping and variable respiratory difficulty, from none to severe. Almost all cases occur within the first 12 months of life, most of these in winter. The respiratory syncytial virus (RSV) is the cause in > 90% of infants. RSV also frequently infects older infants, children and adults, but with different patterns of illness.

Aetiology

- RSV in > 90%
- Other respiratory viruses (such as adeno, parainfluenza, rhino viruses)

Clinical presentation

- Most common in first year of life
- Coryzal symptoms → cough → respiratory distress (mild to severe)
- May present with apnoea in early infancy
- Auscultation—fine inspiratory crackles ± wheezing
- Illness peaks at 2–3 days; improves by 5–7 days; continuing cough for up to several weeks
- CXR—hyperinflation with variable opacities
- At risk of more severe illness and death:
  - infants < 3 months old
  - infants with chronic lung disease
  - premature or low-birth-weight infants
  - infants with congenital heart disease

Diagnosis

- Essentially based on history and physical signs (above)
- Nasopharyngeal aspirate immunofluorescence and culture—only in infants sick enough to require hospital admission
- Chest X-ray in infants sick enough to require hospital admission; may help in excluding possible alternative diagnoses:
  - pneumonia, pleural effusion, pneumothorax
  - congenital heart disease, heart failure

Treatment

Mild bronchiolitis

- Clinical features are as follows:
  - The infant feeds normally.
  - There is little or no respiratory difficulty.
  - There is no requirement for extra oxygen (SaO_2 > 95%).
- No specific treatment is required.
- Consider managing at home if:
  - the parents are competent and appropriately informed
  - they have transport and access to after-hours help
  - there is an involved family doctor.

Moderate or severe bronchiolitis

- Treatment is generally supportive and may include:
  - supplementary oxygen (maintain $SaO_2 \geq 95\%$)
  - nasogastric or intravenous fluids, to decrease the risk of aspiration. Note that fluid requirements may be increased.
  - CPAP or ventilatory support.
- *Assessment of deterioration*: Providing timely ventilatory assistance for the very small proportion of infants who require this is crucial. The following indications of deterioration must be looked for and acted upon:
  - appearance of increasing fatigue, increasing chest-wall retractions, nasal flaring and grunting
  - increasing tachycardia and difficulty in maintaining adequate oximetry readings with extra oxygen
  - apnoea, especially if increasing in frequency.

  Note that nurses play a major role in carrying out these observations and alerting medical staff to the possible need for intervention.
- Antibiotics are not routinely used but may be considered in severe disease (especially if there is lobar opacification on CXR), or for children at risk of severe RSV infection.
- Bronchodilators, corticosteroids and ipratropium bromide are of no definite value and generally should not be used. A single-dose trial of nebulised salbutamol might be considered in an older infant where underlying asthma may be an alternative diagnosis. Likewise, corticosteroids may also be used in such circumstances.
- Antiviral agents (such as ribavirin) and passive anti-RSV antibodies are of very limited value and are rarely indicated.
- Safe and effective RSV vaccines have not yet been developed.

Discharge criteria

- Minimal respiratory distress, feeding well
- Oxygen saturations above 90% (note that low 90s are acceptable at this stage) without extra oxygen, except in infants with risk factors for severe disease (see above)
- Parents must be aware of any particular concerns and follow-up arrangements

Acute pneumonia

Aetiology

- Viral (most common)
- Bacterial
  - pneumococcus
  - *Haemophilus influenzae* (untypable or type b)
  - *Staphylococcus aureus*
  - group A streptococcus
- Atypical
  - *Mycoplasma pneumoniae*
  - *Chlamydia pneumoniae*
  - *Chlamydia trachomatis* (neonates)

Clinical presentation

- Nonspecific clinical features:
  - fever, lethargy, anorexia
  - meningism (especially upper lobe)
  - abdominal pain (especially lower lobe)
- Respiratory manifestations:
  - tachypnoea, respiratory distress, grunt
  - cyanosis
  - localised auscultatory signs
  - cough absent unless airway involvement
  - associated effusions and pneumatoceles (especially *S. aureus*)

Diagnosis

- Clinical features and chest X-ray may help distinguish a viral from a bacterial origin.
- Identification of responsible organisms is as follows:
  - Viral:
    nasopharyngeal aspirate (immunofluorescence and culture)
    serology is not useful in babies; useful in older children
  - Bacterial:
    blood culture
    pleural fluid culture
    lung aspiration
    urinary or pleural fluid antigen
  - Atypical: serology/cold agglutinins.

Treatment

Supportive

- Oxygen to maintain $SaO_2 \geq 95\%$
- IV fluids if necessary
- Clinical and radiological monitoring

Antibiotics

- *Birth to 1 week*: IV penicillin and gentamicin (to cover group B strep., etc.)
  Note: Consider HSV pneumonitis if onset is between days 3 and 7.
- *1 week to < 4 months*:
  - if patient afebrile and only mildly ill: oral erythromycin (chlamydia and pertussis)
  - if febrile: IV benzylpenicillin
  - if severe: IV cefotaxime plus flucloxacillin
- *4 months to < 5 years*:
  - mild: oral amoxycillin
  - moderate: IV benzylpenicillin
  - severe: IV cefotaxime plus flucloxacillin
- *5–15 years*:
  - mild: oral amoxycillin plus roxithromycin
  - moderate: IV benzylpenicillin plus oral roxithromycin
  - severe: IV cefotaxime plus flucloxacillin

Complications

- Pleural effusion
  - early diagnostic and therapeutic aspiration (ideally under ultrasound control)
  - large-bore intercostal catheter for large effusions or if fluid 'thick' and loculated. Additional/alternative treatment for loculated effusion is urokinase as a fibrinolyric agent which can be administered via a small 'pigtail' or large bore intercostal catheter. It is recommended that urokinase administration be under the supervision of a respiratory consultant
  - surgical decortication is rarely necessary if early drainage and appropriate antibiotic therapy are used.
- Pneumatoceles:
  - generally managed conservatively

– drainage for pneumothorax or decompression occasionally needed

Sequelae

- Viral infections may predispose to the development of suppurative lung disease.
- Bacterial pneumonias usually have no long-term sequelae (unless there is a predisposing cause).
- Mycoplasma infection may precipitate asthmatic tendency.

Cystic fibrosis

Cystic fibrosis is a hereditary, chronic, life-shortening disease associated with thick, sticky mucus. Suppurative lung disease and pancreatic insufficiency are the major problems in childhood and adolescence. There is a wide variation in clinical severity. Care is provided by a multi-disciplinary team through a hospital specialist clinic. Median life expectancy is now about 30 years.

Genetics

In Australia the incidence of cystic fibrosis is approximately one in 2500 newborns, with a carrier frequency of 1:20 to 1:25. It is an autosomal recessive disorder. It is rare in orientals, negroes and Australian Aborigines. The commonest gene mutation is Delta F508, with over 700 other rarer mutations demonstrated. Commonest genotypes of affected children are Delta F508/Delta F508 (60%), Delta F508/other (30%), and other/other (10%).

Screening

All newborn babies in New South Wales hospitals are screened for cystic fibrosis as follows:

- Primary test: Immunoreactive trypsin (IRT) is done on a day 4 blood spot.
- The 1% of infants with highest IRT then have DNA analysis for the commonest cystic fibrosis mutation, Delta F508 (the secondary test).
- Homozygotes (Delta F508/Delta F508) have cystic fibrosis and should be referred to a cystic fibrosis centre.
- Heterozygotes (Delta F508/NEG) may have cystic fibrosis (where

179

the 'NEG' is another cystic fibrosis mutation) or may be cystic fibrosis carriers. They should have a reliable sweat test performed.
- Note that NEG/NEG may still be cystic fibrosis, due to other cystic fibrosis mutations, missed by the screen.
- Newborn screening will miss 5–10% of children with cystic fibrosis—clinical suspicion ± high IRT should prompt referral to a cystic fibrosis centre for further investigation (sweat test and extended genotype).

Confirmation of diagnosis

Sweat test

Children detected on screening as being homozygotes (Delta F508/Delta F508), heterozygotes (Delta F508/other) and children with symptoms suggesting cystic fibrosis (see 'Clinical Diagnosis', below) require a sweat test. Ideally, patients should have two tests to confirm the diagnosis: abnormal genetic and sweat test or two abnormal sweat tests.

Interpretation of sweat tests

Sweat tests are best performed by pilocarpine iontophoresis in a reference laboratory (for example, at this hospital or Westmead Hospital). 100 mg of sweat is required for a valid test. For infants and young children:

- sweat chloride: > 60 mmol/L—definitely abnormal, indicates cystic fibrosis
  30–60 mmol/L—borderline: repeat and discuss with a consultant
  < 30 mmol/L—normal
- sweat conductivity > 80 mmol/L—indicates cystic fibrosis.

Additional tests

- A pancreatic stimulation test may help when the sweat test result is equivocal.
- DNA studies for Delta F508 and five or six rarer mutations can be provided.

Clinical diagnosis

Clinical suspicion is still very important in the diagnosis of cystic fibrosis, as there is a low but important false-negative rate on screening. 'Classical' presenting symptoms are the combination of recurrent respiratory infections with chronic diarrhoea, leading to failure to thrive. At birth, 40% will have adequate pancreatic function for food digestion; by mid-childhood this drops to 10%. Exclude cystic fibrosis in any infant who is failing to thrive, even without other symptoms.

Where cystic fibrosis is likely

Cystic fibrosis should be strongly considered in:

- infants or children with recurrent wheeze or cough who do not respond well to anti-asthma therapy
- infants and children with a productive cough, especially if failure to thrive is also present
- children with finger clubbing and respiratory symptoms
- children with chest X-rays showing upper lobe changes or generalised bronchial wall thickening.

Where cystic fibrosis is less likely

Non-respiratory presentations of cystic fibrosis include:

- salty when kissed
- hyponatraemia with dehydration
- heat stroke
- prolonged neonatal jaundice (conjugated)
- hypoproteinaemia with oedema
- nasal polyps and/or recurrent sinusitis
- hepatosplenomegaly
- rectal prolapse.

Management

Newly diagnosed cystic fibrosis

- Admit for a minimum of 3 days to meet the cystic fibrosis team, and to educate and reassure the parents.
- Do baseline blood tests (LFTs, FBC, vitamin E and A levels, coagulation tests, bile acids, albumin, EUC), chest X-ray, sputum culture (including *Burkholderia* [previously *Pseudomonas*] *cepacia*) and 3-day faecal fat.
- Commence physiotherapy, pancreatic supplements (pancrease 1 capsule/kg/day, in apple gel for infants) after 3-day fat collection has been completed.
- Give flucloxacillin prophylaxis orally for the first year (dose 30 mg/kg/day in 3 divided doses).

- Organise a gastroenterology consultation.

If the patient is symptomatic, treat until symptoms settle and the chest X-ray clears, using the combination of an aminoglycoside (gentamicin or tobramycin) and flucloxacillin.

Outpatient management of cystic fibrosis patients

Assessment of known cystic fibrosis subjects should include:

- respiratory symptoms and signs
- general and nutritional state, weight and height centiles
- sputum culture, for *Staphylococcus aureus*, *Pseudomonas*, *Burkholderia*, and so on
- chest X-ray
- pulmonary function tests (spirometry) if > 6 years.

These may be combined to form a score such as Schwachmann or NIH for a global assessment. The score can be used to follow progress.

Indications for admission

- Major respiratory exacerbations (see below)
- Minor exacerbations (see below), not responding to home (oral or inhalational) therapy
- Prearranged 'tune-ups' for those with established suppurative lung disease to delay decline
- Fresh haemoptysis
- Pneumothorax
- Acute abdominal pain

Respiratory exacerbations in cystic fibrosis

Assessment of respiratory status

This includes cough, sputum colour and amount, exercise tolerance, wheeze, respiratory distress, chest signs (such as new or increased crackles), significant fall in spirometry (for example, drop of 15%), and decreased O_2 saturation.

Major exacerbation

There is significant deterioration in respiratory status combined with systemic symptoms and signs (such as high fever, anorexia, weight loss).

Management of major exacerbations

- Admit, and get old notes to guide antibiotic choice based on sensitivities.
- Inform the cystic fibrosis team (dietitian, social worker, physiotherapist, consultant).
- Give IV antibiotics (consider insertion of long line), initially tobramycin with ticarcillin–clavulanic acid or ceftazidime for 10–14 days, with oral flucloxacillin (if recent *S. aureus* isolation from sputum culture) for 10–21 days.
- Discharge when respiratory symptoms, especially cough, sputum production, exercise tolerance, lung function, O_2 saturation, and weight return approximately to previous 'best'.

Minor exacerbation

This covers lesser changes in respiratory status. Systemic changes are usually absent. Admission usually not necessary.

Management of minor exacerbations

- Review old notes.
- Check sputum.
- Give an oral antibiotic such as amoxycillin–clavulanic acid, if possible based on recent sputum, in high dose until the symptoms settle.
- Increase physiotherapy.
- Arrange review—cystic fibrosis community nurse/cystic fibrosis clinic/LMO, if not settling in 5–7 days. Depending on the sputum result and progress, change oral antibiotics or add inhaled tobramycin or oral ciprofloxacin.

Specific situations in cystic fibrosis

Pneumothorax

This is more common with increasing age and severity. Effects depend on the pre-existing lung state and the size of the leak. Symptoms vary from asymptomatic to shoulder-tip pain with sudden deterioration.

- *Small/asymptomatic*: Observe only.
- *Symptomatic/large*: Chest tube thoracostomy for 3–5 days (30–50% will recur/persist).

Note: Ensure adequate analgesia to allow effective cough, physiotherapy and mobilisation when the tube is in place. This may require opiates or administration of local anaesthetic via a pleural catheter.

- *Recurrent/persistent leak*:
  - Repeat tube thoracostomy (depending on physical state), or
  - Limited thoracostomy, with apical resection of blebs and mechanical abrasion.
- *In severely ill children*: Consider chest tube with chemical pleurodesis (tetracycline) or putting talc powder into the chest drain.

Haemoptysis in cystic fibrosis

This complication of chronic lung infection is more common with advanced disease in older patients. 60% of cystic fibrosis sufferers > 18 years will have haemoptyses, mostly minor ones.

Assessment

- *Minor*—blood streaking in sputum or small amounts of fresh blood, usually part of respiratory exacerbation
- *Major*—large volume, greater than 200 mL/day, or recurrent: may be life-threatening and may require transfusion.

Management

- Unless the airway is compromised, always follow a conservative approach.
  - Arrange chest X-ray.
  - Exclude underlying cause, for example clotting defects, platelet reduction.
  - Be sure it is haemoptysis, not haematemesis.
  - Give bed rest.
  - Give IV antibiotics, 'tune-up'.
  - Reduce physiotherapy until acute fresh bleeding settles.
  - If the infection is recurrent and/or more than trivial, consider an angiogram (large bleeding vessels can often be embolised).

Abdominal pain in cystic fibrosis

This is common. It has many causes. It can be acute, mimicking surgical emergencies. Concurrent antibiotics and other therapies may mask physical signs, and surgery should not be undertaken lightly.

Consider:

- distal intestinal obstruction syndrome ('meconium ileus equivalent')
- gall stones, renal stones, bile duct stenosis
- oesophagitis, peptic ulcer disease
- terminal ileitis
- pancreatitis (usually pancreatic sufficient patients)
- the possibility of a typical surgical emergency such as appendicitis or intussusception.

Cystic fibrosis-related diabetes mellitus

Cystic fibrosis-related diabetes mellitus (CFRDM) occurs in about 6% of cystic fibrosis children over the age of 10 years, and symptoms are often insidious in onset. Polydipsia and polyuria occur late and ketosis is rare. Children with CFRDM may show poorer nutrition, worse lung disease and higher mortality. Infection or corticosteroid therapy may 'uncover' CFRDM. Annual checks of cystic fibrosis children should include fasting blood sugars and, if abnormal, HbA1C.

Consider CFRDM:
- if there is an unexplained weight loss or decline in respiratory status, particularly in the adolescent age group
- when puberty fails to progress.

Laboratory diagnosis is based on abnormal glucose tolerance, suggested by:
- fasting blood glucose (FBG) > 7 mmol/L on two or more occasions
- FBG > 7 mmol/L and random glucose > 11 mmol/L
- random glucose > 11 mmol/L with symptoms on two or more occasions.

CFRDM is confirmed by 2-hour oral glucose tolerance test (OGTT) glucose > 11 mmol/L.

Treatment
- Dietary management
- Insulin therapy, if control is not achieved by dietary means

15

Endocrinology and diabetes

This chapter includes:
- acute adrenal insufficiency
- ambiguous genitalia
- pituitary emergencies
- hypoglycaemia
- hypocalcaemia
- hypercalcaemia
- acute thyroid disorders
- diabetes mellitus
- diabetic ketoacidosis
- fasting and surgery in diabetes
- hypoglycaemia in diabetes
- sick day management.

Acute adrenal insufficiency

Presentations
- In known adrenal insufficiency, with an intercurrent illness
- New presentation: think of this with any severely ill child
- In patients withdrawing from glucocorticoid therapy

Causes
- Primary adrenal diseases (associated with elevated ACTH levels), for example Addison's disease, congenital adrenal hyperplasia, adrenal aplasia/hypoplasia, adrenoleukodystrophy, adrenal destruction
- Secondary adrenal insufficiency due to ACTH deficiency, pituitary disorders, hypothalamic disorders
- Secondary causes include the adrenal insufficiency which follows withdrawal from prolonged treatment with corticosteroids (2 weeks or more)

Clinical features

- Muscle weakness, lethargy, vomiting, anorexia, depression (due to cortisol deficiency, electrolyte disturbances)
- Weight loss (due to anorexia, volume depletion)
- Pigmentation (in primary cases only, from ACTH excess)
- Hypoglycaemia (due to decreased hepatic glucose production)
- Hypotension, shock (from loss of vasomotor tone and volume depletion)

Biochemical features

- Low Na^+, high K^+ (due to aldosterone deficiency)
- Elevated serum urea and creatinine (due to associated dehydration)
- Hypoglycaemia (due to lack of glucocorticoid)
- Elevated plasma renin activity (as an index of volume depletion)
- Elevated plasma ACTH (only in primary adrenal deficiency; in hypothalamic-pituitary disorders mineralocorticoid function is unaffected)
- Low cortisol before and after adrenal stimulation, for example by Synacthen

Therapy of adrenal crisis (acute adrenal insufficiency)

- Therapy is urgent! Consult Endocrinology.
- Give hydrocortisone by IV or IM injection. *Dose*: 100 mg/m^2 body surface area, or if < 6 months 25 mg, 6 months to 2 years 50 mg, 2 to 10 years 100 mg, > 10 years 150–200 mg.
- Repeat dose if there is a poor response after IV fluid resuscitation.
- If there is hypotension/shock/poor perfusion give 0.9% saline 10 mL/kg bolus. Repeat as necessary.
- If the patient is hypoglycaemic, give 10% glucose 2 mL/kg over several minutes.
- Continue fluid replacement with 0.9% saline with 5% glucose added initially. Electrolytes and clinical progress guide subsequent fluid choice. Do not add potassium if serum potassium is high.
- Continue stress doses of hydrocortisone at 100 mg/m^2/day, divided into 4–6-hourly IV doses, until the situation is improved.

Maintenance therapy in adrenal insufficiency

- Replacement hydrocortisone—12–15 mg/m^2/day, usually in 3 divided doses (8–10 mg/m^2/day in ACTH deficiency). The requirement for glucocorticoids increases with stress (fever, vomiting, diarrhoea, surgery, anaesthesia).
- Replacement mineralocorticoid in primary adrenal disease: fludrocortisone 0.05–0.2 mg per day (total dose, *not* per kg or m^2), given in 1 or 2 divided doses. The dose is adjusted according to BP, electrolytes and plasma renin activity.

Management of patients peri- and postoperatively

Patients with adrenal insufficiency, or possible adrenal insufficiency following glucocorticoid therapy for longer than 2 weeks, are at risk of adrenal crisis and need glucocorticoid cover for surgery.

For most minor surgery

At induction of anaesthesia, give a single dose of IV hydrocortisone as recommended for acute adrenal insufficiency (see above). Then, if recovering normally, give additional oral hydrocortisone for 24 hours at three to four times the usual oral dose.

For major surgery

At induction of anaesthesia, give the IV dose of hydrocortisone recommended for acute adrenal insufficiency (see above). Subsequently, give 100 mg/m^2/day IV divided into 4 to 6 doses until the major stress of the postoperative period is resolved.

Management of patients with, or at risk of, adrenal insufficiency during intercurrent illness

Children with or at risk of adrenal insufficiency *must be given* increased doses of replacement hydrocortisone for stress. Parents have these guidelines:

- If the child is moderately unwell and/or temperature is 38–39°C, give three times the usual doses of hydrocortisone.
- If the child is more unwell and/or temperature > 39°C, give four times the usual doses of hydrocortisone.
- If the child has gastroenteritis or any cause of diarrhoea, give four times the usual dose of hydrocortisone.
- If a dose is vomited, give the increased dose again in 30 minutes.

If this is vomited, then immediately contact LMO or take the child to Emergency.

- If there is any delay, parents are to administer their own intramuscular hydrocortisone (25–200 mg, depending on age).
- Patients who are at risk of adrenal insufficiency but not requiring everyday replacement therapy (for example, for partial ACTH deficiency) should take doses of hydrocortisone of 60–100 mg/m²/day in 3 divided doses in such circumstances for the duration of the physiological stress.
- The child should wear a Medical Alert identification.

Note: Increase only the dose of hydrocortisone (not fludrocortisone).

When the stress or illness is over, revert to the previous hydrocortisone dose without tapering.

Ambiguous genitalia

The birth of a baby with ambiguous genitalia is a social and medical crisis. Life-threatening conditions such as congenital adrenal hyperplasia (CAH) need to be diagnosed and treated quickly.

Causes of ambiguous genitalia (intersex)

These can be broadly categorised as follows:

- virilised females or 46XX sex reversal (female pseudohermaphroditism)—the main possibilities are congenital adrenal hyperplasia, aromatase deficiency, maternal androgen ingestion or maternal androgen secreting tumour
- undervirilised males or 46XY sex reversal (male pseudohermaphroditism)—a wide variety of testicular disorders and defects of androgen formation or action
- chromosomal defects—a variety of possible effects, such as mixed gonadal dysgenesis
- other rare causes or morphological (non-endocrine) causes.

Management of a child with sexual ambiguity

- It may take several days until a definitive diagnosis can be made.
- Be honest—say you don't know the sex of the baby. Don't guess, but reassure parents that investigations will clarify the situation.
- Instruct all staff to refer to child as 'baby' and not 'he', 'she' or 'it'.

- Note the phallus size, position of urethral and other orifices, degree of labioscrotal fusion, any gonads palpable and any pigmentation.
- Make an urgent paediatric endocrine consultation.
- Test for karyotype (peripheral blood, request urgent processing).
- Do ultrasound and X-ray studies of genital tract (genitogram) to delineate internal anatomy.
- Investigate for CAH in virilised female (measure 17-OHP, Synacthen test).
- Do hormone studies to assess testicular/ovarian/pituitary function.
- Assign sex (especially take into account the ability of the male to be functional).
- Do therapy to achieve successful sex assignment (surgery, hormones).
- Counsel and involve parents in all stages of decision-making.

Pituitary emergencies

There are several situations in which pituitary disease or dysfunction can require urgent attention.

Adrenal crisis due to secondary adrenal insufficiency

See the adrenal section on p. 186.

Acute diabetes insipidus

Possible occurrences

- In patients with known diabetes insipidus (DI) and intercurrent illness or other decompensation
- After neurosurgery, especially involving the pituitary region
- As a new presentation—especially after head trauma, or newly presenting pituitary disease

Clinical features

- Thirst and polydipsia (in conscious patients)
- Polyuria (without glycosuria)
- Dehydration. May be difficult to detect. Skin may have a doughy consistency.
- Weight loss, lethargy
- Seizures, CNS depression may occur

Biochemical features

- Hypernatremia, hyperosmolality, elevated urea and creatinine
- Inappropriately dilute urine (on specific gravity or osmolality)

Management

- The basis of management is accurate fluid and electrolyte replacement.
- Accurate fluid balance is important.
- Antidiuretic hormone (ADH) may be administered by several routes, but is used with great caution in acute DI, especially post-operatively or after trauma. Expert consultation is required.

Syndrome of inappropriate ADH secretion

Possible occurrence

- Following neurosurgery, head trauma
- In other CNS disorders, such as encephalitis, abscess, meningitis
- With certain drugs (such as vincristine, carbamazepine, phenothiazines, clofibrate, chlorpropamide)
- In rare situations—secretion by tumours, obstructive lung disease, ventilation

Clinical features

- Usually related to fluid overload and cerebral oedema—nausea, headaches, malaise, confusion, coma, seizures
- Oliguria, weight gain

Biochemical features

- Hyponatraemia, low serum osmolality
- Small volumes of inappropriately concentrated urine (on specific gravity or osmolality)

Management

- This requires expert consultation.
- The basis of management is fluid restriction, accurate electrolyte replacement and accurate fluid balance.
- Hypertonic saline is required rarely—expert consultation is required.

Hypoglycaemia

Neonatal hypoglycaemia is covered in detail in Chapter 8.

Definition

- Consider if blood glucose level (BGL) is < 2.2 mmol/L (capillary or whole blood) or < 2.6 mmol/L (plasma or serum).
- Plasma or serum levels are 10–15% higher than capillary or whole blood.
- Most healthy children and adults maintain BGL > 3.5 mmol/L.

Basal glucose requirements

Neonates 5–6 mg/kg/min, infants and children 3–5 mg/kg/min, adults 2–3 mg/kg/min

Causes

Hypoglycaemia arises when there is an imbalance between influx and efflux of glucose in the circulation.

Broad categories are:

- decreased influx from food, for example starvation, vomiting
- decreased influx from preformed glycogen stores, for example intrauterine growth retardation, maternal starvation, prematurity, smaller of twin pregnancy in the neonatal period, starvation in the older child, ketotic hypoglycaemia
- decreased influx from gluconeogenesis and glycogenolysis, for example glycogen storage disease, galactosaemia, fructose intolerance, GH deficiency (hypopituitarism), adrenocortical insufficiency (primary adrenal disorder or secondary due to ACTH deficiency), fatty acid oxidation disorders
- increased efflux into stores, for example hyperinsulinism as seen in the infant of a diabetic mother, excess maternal IV glucose, persistent hyperinsulinaemic hypoglycaemia of infancy (PHHI), nesidiocytosis, nesidioblastosis, Beckwith-Wiedemann syndrome, islet cell adenoma, drugs, erythroblastosis
- increased efflux due to increased energy expenditure or increased use of glucose as fuel, for example sepsis, shock, asphyxia, hypothermia, RDS, polycythaemia/hyperviscosity, fever.

Clinical features

- *Neurogenic*: tremors, sweating, pallor, tachycardia, anxiety, weakness, hunger
- *Neuroglycopenic*: apnoea, cyanosis, hypotonia, coma, seizures, poor feeding, headache, lethargy, irritability, confusion, visual disturbance

Investigations

- Glucose utilisation rate as estimated from IV glucose needs will separate hypoglycaemic condition into:
  - excessive utilisation (> 8–10 mg/kg/min)—hyperinsulinism and occasionally in severely asphyxiated neonates
  - normal glucose utilisation—due to all other causes of hypoglycaemia.
- The sample taken at the time of hypoglycaemia is critical and usually diagnostic, and used to measure the following:
  - *hormones*: insulin, GH and cortisol
  - *metabolic fuels*: glucose, FFA, ketones, lactate
  - *urine screen*: collect a sample for testing for inborn errors of metabolism and test urine with dipstick for ketones.
- Sample collection requirements for the critical sample:
  - 5 mL of blood (2 mL in neonate) into a lithium heparin tube and, if available, 0.5 mL into a perchlorate tube (for ketones and lactate)
  - 10–20 mL of urine into a clean jar; freeze if not sent immediately to the laboratory
- A fasting study may need to be done at a later date to induce hypoglycaemia for diagnostic purposes.

Treatment

- *Prevention*: prenatal and postnatal feeding, avoidance of iatrogenic causes (drugs)
- *Treat cause* if possible, for example sepsis, RDS, hypothermia, polycythaemia, hyperinsulinism, endocrine deficiency, metabolic disorder
- *Glucose IV*:
  - bolus of 2 mL/kg 10% glucose
  - maintenance IV glucose to provide a starting rate of 4–8 mg/kg/min

193

- the rate must be adjusted to achieve and maintain a minimum blood glucose 3–4 mmol/L
- *Hydrocortisone* 3–5 mg/kg/day. This is usually used as a treatment for hypoglycaemia in the neonatal period only where there may be multiple factors operating and before a definitive diagnosis.
- *Glucagon*: continuous intravenous infusion is preferable, at 5–20 micrograms/kg/hour. A loading dose of 20 micrograms/kg (maximum 1 mg) may be given if needed. Note that glucagon will elevate the blood glucose acutely in hyperinsulinism only when there are good glycogen stores. Glucagon infusions also have a place in neonatal hypoglycaemia
- *Specialised treatments for hyperinsulinism*: depend on cause, for example diazoxide, octreotide (Sandostatin), surgery

Hypocalcaemia

Definition

- Total serum calcium < 2.0 mmol/L (normal range 2.1–2.7 mmol/L) in term infants and children, or ionised calcium of < 1.0 mmol/L (normal range 1.15–1.30 mmol/L).
- A lower level of total serum Ca of 1.8 mmol/L is sometimes applied to preterm neonates.
- Low serum albumin will give a falsely low total calcium level, with the total serum calcium declining by 0.1 mmol/L for every 5 g/L decrease in serum albumin below 40 g/L. Measuring serum ionised calcium overcomes this problem.

Causes

Age is important in determining likely causes:

- early neonatal—prematurity, low Ca intake, birth asphyxia, infants of diabetic mothers, maternal hyperparathyroidism
- late neonatal—high dietary phosphate load, calcium malabsorption, hypomagnesaemia, hypoparathyroidism, maternal hyperparathroidism, di George (velocardiofacial) syndrome
- infants and children of any age—hypoparathyroidism, vitamin D deficient rickets, vitamin D dependent rickets, hypomagnesaemia, pseudohypoparathyroidism, malabsorption, renal tubular disorders, bisphosphonate therapy.

Clinical features

- May be subtle or asymptomatic in neonates—tremulousness, apnoea, poor feeding, irritability, seizures
- In older patients—paraesthesiae (extremities or circumoral), carpopedal spasm, tetany, irritability, fatigue, malaise, seizures, laryngeal spasm, Chvostek's sign (facial nerve hyperexcitability), Trousseau's sign (carpal spasm with BP cuff inflated 20 mmHg above systolic for 3 min).

Investigation

- Measure total serum calcium and albumin. If available, measure ionised calcium.
- Also measure serum glucose (hypoglycaemia may mimic hypocalcaemia in neonates), electrolytes, creatinine, phosphate, magnesium, alkaline phosphatase, PTH, 25-hydroxyvitamin D and 1,25-dihydroxyvitamin D, urine spot Ca:Cr ratio, ECG—prolonged Q-T interval.
- Other studies for cause as indicated, such as CXR for thymic shadow, chromosomes for 22q11 deletion, and so on.

Treatment of acute severe hypocalcaemia

Severe symptoms (seizures, tetany, laryngeal spasm) require urgent therapy with IV calcium. Use either:

- Ca chloride (10%) (27.2 mg/mL or 0.68 mmol/mL of calcium) 0.2 mL/kg over 2–3 minutes or more (dilute at least 1 in 10); followed by infusion of 1.2–2.4 mL/kg/day

or

- Ca gluconate (10%) (9.4 mg/mL or 0.25 mmol/mL of calcium) 0.5 mL/kg over 2–3 minutes (dilute at least 1 in 10); followed by infusion of 3–6 mL/kg/day.

Note: IV calcium is very irritant and extravasation can result in severe burns and tissue necrosis. A central line or long line should be used. If it is necessary to use a peripheral vein in emergencies, use a large vein with careful observation. Note that 1 mmol Ca = 40 mg elemental calcium.

Other therapy

- Treat any precipitating factors.
- Mild or asymptomatic hypocalcaemia can be treated with an increase in calcium infusion in neonates.
- Oral therapy to treat hypocalcaemia should be used in most situations except for acute emergencies as above. Use calcitriol 40–60 ng/kg/day in 2 to 3 divided doses, and calcium salts to provide elemental calcium 50–100 mg/kg/day in 4 to 6 divided doses initially.
- Direct maintenance therapy at the cause as necessary, for example calcitriol in hypoparathyroidism and acute management of vitamin D deficient rickets, ergocalciferol in vitamin D deficient rickets after the acute phase.

Hypercalcaemia

Hypercalcaemia is relatively uncommon in infants and children, but may require urgent therapy.

Definition

- Total serum calcium > 2.7 mmol/L or ionised calcium > 1.4 mmol/L
- Falsely elevated readings can result from elevated serum albumin (correction as above) or stasis during collection.

Causes

- *Neonatal*—phosphate deficiency, hypervitaminosis D, hyperparathyroidism, idiopathic infantile hypercalcaemia (Williams' syndrome), subcutaneous fat necrosis, Ca-sensing receptor gene mutations, some tumours
- *Childhood*—idiopathic infantile hypercalcaemia, hyperparathyroidism, Ca-sensing receptor gene mutations (including familial hypocalcuric hypercalcaemia), vitamin D intoxication, vitamin A toxicity, immobilisation, malignancy, renal failure, Addison's disease

Clinical features

- Rarely symptomatic until total serum Ca > 3.0 mmol/L
- Gastrointestinal—nausea, vomiting, constipation, anorexia, abdominal pain

- CNS—lethargy, depression, ataxia, psychosis, coma
- Neuromuscular—weakness, proximal myopathy
- CVS—hypertension, bradycardia, short QT interval
- Renal—stones, polyuria, decreased GFR
- Systemic—metastatic calcification

Investigation

- Measure total serum calcium and albumin. If the test is available, measure ionised calcium.
- Also measure electrolytes, creatinine, phosphate, magnesium, alkaline phosphatase, PTH, 25-hydroxyvitamin D and 1,25-dihydroxyvitamin D.
- Measure urine calcium, phosphate, creatinine.
- Take other tests as indicated—PTH-related peptide (tumours), urine cAMP, X-ray hands and wrists, renal ultrasound, and so on.

Therapy

- Acute treatment is indicated for symptomatic patients or those with serum Ca > 3.25 mmol/L.
- Rehydration is the universal first step, using intravenous normal saline at 3000 mL/m^2/day (double maintenance). Frusemide may also be given, 1 mg/kg every 4 to 6 hours, once circulating volume is restored, to speed the excretion of calcium.
- Cease any vitamin D or calcium supplements.
- Other therapies, depending on the cause, may include glucocorticoids, bisphosphonates and parathyroid surgery (requires endocrine consultation).

Acute thyroid disorders

Congenital hypothyroidism

Definitions

- Primary hypothyroidism: causes high TSH levels on newborn screen
- Secondary hypothyroidism: low TSH not detected on newborn screen, usually associated with other pituitary hormone deficiencies

Clinical features

- Detected on newborn screening performed at day 2 to 5.
- Requires urgent evaluation (within 48 hours).

- Important history includes maternal diet, drugs or autoimmune disease.
- Examine for clinical features including coarse facial features, large tongue, umbilical hernia, constipation, poor feeding, intellectual and developmental delay as well as goitre, jaundice, growth parameters and other congenital problems (for example, heart disease).

Investigation

- Include thyroid function tests (TSH and free T4), plasma bilirubin if indicated and a diagnostic thyroid scan (usually technetium 99).
- With a history of maternal autoimmune disease, maternal and baby thyroid antibodies measurements are indicated.
- Thyroid ultrasound is indicated if there is no uptake on the thyroid nuclear scan.
- Test for bone age.

Therapy

- Commence thyroxine (10 micrograms/kg daily) as soon as diagnosis is confirmed.
- Repeat thyroid function tests at 1–2 weeks, 6 weeks, 3 months and thereafter 2- to 3-monthly until 3 years and then 4- to 6-monthly.
- Treatment is aimed at keeping the free T4 concentration in the upper third of the normal range and TSH suppressed into the normal range.
- If dyshormonogenesis is suspected, hearing tests should be performed regularly for at least the first year of life and development monitored.

Thyrotoxicosis

Clinical features

- Symptoms and signs may include tachycardia, tremor, sweating, restlessness, poor sleeping, weight loss, diarrhoea, eye signs (Graves' disease), proximal muscle weakness or arrhythmia.
- If severe, this can cause life-threatening thyrotoxic crisis or thyroid storm.
- Early specialist referral is required.

Investigation

- TSH, FT4, FT3 and thyroid antibodies (usually thyroid stimulating immunoglobulin, thyroid peroxidase Ab and thyroglobulin Ab).
- Thyroid imaging is not commonly indicated in typical Graves' cases, but is helpful in other situations.

Therapy

- Antithyroid drug treatment (carbimazole or propylthiouracil) is the common first-line treatment, sometimes combined later with thyroxine in a 'block and replace' regimen.
- Radioactive iodine treatment may be used in older children or adolescents.
- Thyroidectomy surgery is rarely used.
- Thyroid storm will require additional measures such as iodine or steroid therapy and general supportive measures.

Neonatal thyrotoxicosis

- Occurs in 2% of babies of mothers with a history of Graves' disease, due to the transplacental transfer of thyroid stimulating antibodies.
- High maternal TSI and suppressed cord TSH are predictive.
- Measure TSH, free T4 and free T3 from day 2 and twice weekly until the course is clear.
- Thyrotoxicosis will usually manifest by day 9.
- Untreated neonatal thyrotoxicosis has high morbidity and mortality.
- Endocrinology consult is advisable.
- Treatment is with beta-blockers and antithyroid drugs (alone or in a 'block and replace' regimen with thyroxine).
- Additional measures such as iodine or steroid treatment can be required in severe cases.
- Antibody levels decline and treatment can usually be tapered and stopped by 12 weeks.

Sick euthyroidism

- This is an abnormality in thyroid function in patients with severe non-thyroidal illness.
- Commonly, there is a low free T3, low to normal free T4 and normal TSH.
- Free T4 may be lower in more severe illnesses.

- Transient mild elevation of TSH (up to 20 mU/L only) may occur in the recovery period.
- Usually there is no benefit from thyroid hormone treatment.

Patients undergoing total thyroidectomy

- This is uncommon surgery in children.
- Indications include thyroid cancer, risk of familial thyroid cancer, thyrotoxicosis or large multi-nodular goitres.
- Surgical risks include haemorrhage, airway obstruction, recurrent laryngeal nerve damage and infection.
- Endocrine risks include hypoparathyroidism (usually transient, but permanence is possible) and the need for long-term thyroxine replacement.
- All patients are at risk of hypocalcaemia from transient hypoparathyroidism and should be commenced on calcium supplementation within 12 hours of surgery.
- Begin thyroxine, 100 micrograms/m^2 daily, on the first postoperative day unless the surgery was for thyroid cancer, in which case this is delayed pending nuclear scanning.

Diabetes mellitus

Presentation

Type 1 (insulin dependent) diabetes mellitus (IDDM or T1D)

- This is the most common type of diabetes in children.
- *Classical presentation*: increasing polydipsia, polyuria, malaise and weight loss over 2–6 weeks.
- *Atypical presentations*: vomiting illness, dehydration or shock, secondary enuresis, vaginal candidiasis especially in a prepubertal girl, weight loss or failure to gain weight, tachypnoea or signs of sepsis in a toddler, irritability and decreasing school performance, recurrent superficial skin infections (especially staphylococcal)

Type 2 (non-insulin-dependent) diabetes (NIDDM or T2D)

- Increasingly diagnosed in adolescents and some older children.
- Common clinical features include obesity, acanthosis nigricans, high-risk ethnic groups and positive family history.
- Ketosis is often absent but may occur and type 2 diabetes can even present with DKA.

Diagnosis

This is based on symptoms of diabetes and laboratory confirmation:

- Do urinary dipstick testing for glucose and ketones.
- Random plasma glucose > 11.1 mmol/L or fasting plasma glucose > 7.0 mmol/L confirms the diagnosis. Glucose tolerance tests are infrequently required in children.
- Remember that stress hyperglycaemia (not representing diabetes) may occur in acutely unwell infants and children, especially those treated with glucocorticoids.
- At diagnosis collect blood for C-peptide and type 1 diabetes related antibodies (GAD, ICA, IA-2 and IAA) which will help classify the type of diabetes. Also collect blood for thyroid function tests, thyroid antibodies and endomysial antibodies to examine for coexistent autoimmune disease.

Diabetic ketoacidosis

Diabetic ketoacidosis (DKA) may:

- be the initial presentation of type I diabetes mellitus
- recur if insulin is omitted (recurrent DKA in adolescence is almost always due to insulin omission)
- occur as a result of an intercurrent illness.

Clinical features

- Severe dehydration
- Decreased perfusion or shock (rapid pulse rate, low blood pressure, poor peripheral circulation, mottling and peripheral cyanosis)
- Frequent vomiting
- Continuing polyuria despite the dehydration
- Weight loss due to fluid loss and loss of muscle and fat
- Flushed cheeks due to the ketosis
- Acetone detected on the breath
- Hyperventilation of DKA (Kussmaul respiration), characterised by high respiratory rate and large tidal volume, giving a sighing quality
- Disordered sensorium (disoriented, drowsy or, rarely, comatose)

Management of DKA

- Once the diagnosis of DKA has been made, the following sequence of events should occur:
  1 Resuscitate.
  2 Take baseline laboratory measurements.
  3 Commence regular clinical monitoring.
  4 Assess fluid, sodium and potassium replacement.
  5 Start rehydration and maintenance fluids.
  6 Start insulin infusion and adjust as needed.
- Close clinical and biochemical monitoring and individualisation of therapy is essential.
- Management in ICU is essential for severe DKA (pH < 7.1) or if the child is hypernatraemic, and preferable for milder DKA in young children or if there are associated problems.
- Consider a possible precipitant, such as occult infection.
- Cerebral oedema is an ever-present risk of diabetic ketoacidosis and can occur despite careful attention to the rate of rehydration, choice of fluids and attention to electrolyte management.

Resuscitation

- If signs of shock (hypotension, severe peripheral shut-down, oliguria) are present, resuscitate with boluses of 10 mL/kg of 0.9% saline. It is rare that more than 1 or 2 boluses are required.
- Avoid repeated boluses unless there is continuing shock/hypovolaemia, as this may increase the risk of cerebral oedema.
- Remember that acidosis contributes to decreased peripheral perfusion, which will correct only gradually as the acidosis is reversed.
- In shock, oxygen by face mask should be given.

Laboratory measurements

Insert a sampling cannula if possible.

- Baseline blood glucose, electrolytes, calcium, phosphorus, venous pH and acid-base status (arterial if signs of shock are present), full blood count, urea and creatinine, triglycerides, microurine, urine test for ketones, investigation for infection if indicated
- Hourly blood glucose measurement
- 2–4-hourly electrolytes and venous pH, depending on severity and progress

Clinical observations

- Hourly pulse rate, respiratory rate, blood pressure, neurological observations
- Hourly blood glucose measurement while on an insulin infusion
- Accurate fluid balance (indwelling urinary catheter may be required)
- 2–4-hourly temperature
- Test all urine for ketones until negative.
- Strict fluid balance is essential. Reassess fluid status every few hours.

Continuing polyuria may worsen the dehydration if a positive fluid balance is not being achieved. The patient initially should be 'nil by mouth' except for ice to suck.

Rehydration and maintenance fluids

Dehydration is frequently in the order of 7.5–10% in significant ketoacidosis.

- Calculate the initial fluid rate to correct fluid and electrolyte deficits over 48 hours.
  - Give maintenance fluid volumes plus calculated replacement volume.
  - If the corrected serum sodium value is in the hypernatraemic range (> 150), even slower rehydration may be considered.
- Initial rehydration fluid should be 0.9% saline. KCl should be added at the commencement of rehydration unless the patient is known to have renal failure. Some centres use a combination of potassium chloride and potassium phosphate.
- Regular reassessment of fluid balance is required. If there are ongoing urine losses due to osmotic diuresis and the metabolic status of the patient is not improving, it may be necessary to partly replace these so that positive fluid balances are achieved.

Electrolyte replacement

Sodium

- Replacement is based on biochemical monitoring.
- The serum sodium may be falsely lowered by the dilutional effect of the coexistent hyperglycaemia and hyperlipidaemia.
- An approximate corrected sodium can be calculated as follows: corrected sodium = sodium + 0.3 (glucose − 5.5) (all values in mmol/L)

- If corrected sodium is greater than 150 mmol/L, a hypernatraemic as well as an independent glucose hyperosmolar state exists and correction of the dehydration and electrolyte imbalance over 48–72 hours is advocated to minimise the risk of cerebral oedema. Consider using half-normal saline after expert consultation.
- Hyponatraemia during treatment is also of concern and usually reflects overzealous volume correction and insufficient electrolyte replacement.

Potassium

- Commence replacement (5 mmol/kg/day or 0.2 mmol/kg/hour) as soon as resuscitation is completed and prior to commencing the insulin infusion.
- If renal failure is suspected, withhold potassium until electrolytes are available and an indwelling urinary catheter is inserted.
- Check serum potassium 2 hours later and then 4 hourly.
- If hypokalaemic, then more potassium may be given (with cardiac monitoring) but serum levels will need to be measured more frequently.
- Beware of the patient with low or low to normal serum potassium at presentation. In the face of acidosis this indicates severe potassium depletion.

Bicarbonate

- Even with optimal therapy, serum bicarbonate only gradually normalises over 12 to 24 hours (often lagging behind improvement in pH) and in general bicarbonate therapy is not required.
- Bicarbonate may be considered after consultation in shock with severe acidosis (arterial pH < 7.0 and/or HCO_3 < 5 mmol/L).
- Cardiac monitoring is required if bicarbonate is given; hypokalaemia and exacerbation of hypernatraemia are risks.
- Bicarbonate should be given by an intravenous infusion over 30 minutes and the dose can be calculated by the formula:
  Bicarbonate dose for total repair of base deficit = 1/3 (base deficit × body weight in kg) but only 1/4 of this dose should be given at any one time and the response noted before repeating.

Insulin infusion

- Start after resuscitation is completed and rehydration and KCl replacement are under way.

- Add 50 units of short-acting insulin (such as Actrapid or Humulin R) to 500 mL of 0.9% saline, so that 10 mL of solution will contain 1 unit of insulin.
- The infusion may be run as a side line with the rehydrating fluid, providing a volumetric pump is used.
- Insulin infusion must be labelled clearly so as not to confuse it with the rehydrating fluids.
- In general, commence the infusion at 0.075–0.1 units/kg/h.
- A lower starting dose of 0.05 units/kg/h may sometimes be used if there has already been a rapid initial BGL fall with IV fluids alone or in very young patients. This will usually need to be increased later (with increased glucose infusion if needed) to facilitate clearance of acidosis and ketones.
- It is not necessary to give a priming bolus of insulin.
- Aim to produce a fall in blood glucose of 4–5 mmol/L per hour over the first 2 hours; however, rehydration alone will result in a fall in blood glucose and a larger fall can be accepted at this time without a reduction in the insulin infusion rate.
- When the blood glucose falls to 12 mmol/L, the IV solution can be changed to 0.45% saline and 5% glucose (this can be prepared by adding 25 mL of 50% glucose to 500 mL of 0.45% saline and 2.5% glucose). Should hyponatraemia be a problem, then IV fluid with a higher sodium concentration may need to be given.
- The glucose infusion concentration should be adjusted to keep the blood glucose between 8 and 12 mmol/L. The insulin infusion rate can also be adjusted but remember that adequate insulin is needed to clear the ketonaemia and reverse the acidosis.
- If the patient still requires IV fluids after 24 hours, use either 0.225% saline and 3.75% glucose or 0.45% saline adjusted to 5% glucose.

Cerebral oedema

- This can be a sudden and unpredictable complication in the first 24 hours of treatment of diabetic ketoacidosis.
- All patients should be monitored for signs and symptoms of raised intracranial pressure.
- Risk factors and warning signs include severe dehydration and shock, severe acidosis and low serum potassium indicating severe total body loss of potassium, hypernatraemia indicating a hyper-

osmolar state, hyponatraemia, severe lipaemia and a deteriorating conscious state during therapy.

- If suspected it requires immediate treatment with mannitol 1–2 g/kg by IV infusion over 30 minutes.
- Transfer to an intensive care facility and arrange a neurological assessment and CT scan.

Management of the ketoacidosis recovery phase

When to start oral fluid

- Keep nil by mouth, except for ice to suck, until metabolically stable (blood glucose < 12 mmol/L, pH > 7.30 and HCO_3 > 15 mmol/L).
- Low joule or low calorie fluids can then be given by mouth to see if they are tolerated.

Use of insulin infusion to cover meals and snacks

- It is useful to maintain the insulin infusion until the child has had at least one meal.
- For snacks the basal infusion rate is doubled at the start of the snack and continued for 30 minutes afterwards, before returning to the basal rate.
- For main meals the basal infusion rate should be doubled at the start of the meal and continued for 60 minutes after the meal, before returning to the basal rate.

When to stop the infusion

- It is most convenient to change to subcutaneous insulin just before mealtime.
- Subcutaneous insulin is given 30 minutes before the meal and insulin infusion is continued at the current rate throughout the meal and stopped 90 minutes after giving the subcutaneous insulin.
- The half-life of intravenous insulin is only 4.5 minutes, so it is important that the subcutaneous insulin is given before stopping the infusion.

Subcutaneous insulin regimen

- Total daily dose required is usually around 1 unit/kg/day but may need to be adjusted on the basis of previous insulin dosages and serial blood glucose levels.

- This can be given as 6-hourly short-acting insulin—one regimen is to start with 2/7 of the total daily dose being given before breakfast, lunch and the evening meal and 1/7 without food at midnight.
- A more common regimen is a combination of short- and intermediate-acting insulin at a dose of 1 unit/kg/day, with 2/3 given before breakfast (split 2/3 intermediate, 1/3 short-acting) and 1/3 before the evening meals (split 2/3 intermediate, 1/3 short-acting).
- Some patients (usually adolescents) will continue on pre-meal short-acting insulin with an intermediate- or long-acting dose before bed (usually about 30–40% of the total daily dose).

Fasting and surgery in diabetes

- The optimal method of maintaining metabolic control during surgery or fasting is by an insulin infusion, started when fasting commences.
- Simpler regimens are possible for minor procedures under sedation or with short general anaesthetic.
- Surgery in children with diabetes should be undertaken only in paediatric hospitals or other hospitals with expert staff (medical, anaesthetic, surgical and nursing) and facilities for the care of children with diabetes.

Emergency surgery

Unless absolutely necessary, emergency surgery should be delayed in any patient with ketoacidosis until diabetes control has improved and the diabetes stabilised. Diabetic ketoacidosis may by itself cause an acute abdomen which resolves with treatment of the ketoacidosis.

Elective surgery

This should be performed only if diabetes is under good control. If control is uncertain or poor, admit 1–3 days beforehand for assessment and stabilisation. If control remains poor, surgery should be cancelled and re-booked.

Scheduling of surgery

Schedule operations early in the morning if possible. If not possible, schedule first on the afternoon list. This allows postoperative stabilisation during the day.

Maintaining metabolic control

Any patient with diabetes who is fasting requires:

- continuous intravenous glucose
- adequate insulin replacement
- hourly blood glucose monitoring. Aim to maintain blood glucose levels of 5–12 mmol/L.

Short or minor procedures with general anaesthetic or sedation

Patients on twice or three times daily insulin regimens

Procedure first on morning list

- Consider the need for reduction (20–30%) of evening intermediate insulin if there is a pattern of low blood glucoses in the mornings.
- Give a reduced morning insulin dose at about 7 a.m.—50–60% of the usual intermediate-acting insulin dose, with no short-acting insulin unless the blood glucose level (BGL) is high.
- Commence IV fluids at same time—N/4 (0.225%) saline adjusted to 5% glucose at maintenance volumes (this can be prepared by adding 12.5 mL of 50% glucose to 500 mL of N/4 dextrose saline—0.225% saline and 3.75% glucose).
- Perform hourly BGLs. Increase glucose concentration if needed.
- Postoperatively, stop IV once oral intake resumes and give additional doses of short-acting insulin if required (start with a dose of 10% of the total daily insulin dose). The usual dose of evening insulin can be given if the patient has recovered and is eating normally.

Procedure first on afternoon list

- Breakfast will usually be allowed, so insulin needs to cover this. Give a reduced morning insulin dose prior to breakfast: 30–40% of the usual intermediate-acting insulin dose and 50% of the usual short-acting insulin, depending on BGL.
- Commence IV fluids 2 hours after breakfast: 0.225% saline with 5% glucose at maintenance volumes.
- Perform hourly BGLs. Increase glucose concentration if needed.
- Postoperatively, stop IV once oral intake resumes and give additional doses of short-acting insulin if required (start with a dose

of 10% of total daily insulin dose). The usual dose of evening insulin can be given if the patient has recovered and is eating normally, otherwise a reduced dose will be needed.

Patients on basal-bolus insulin regimens

Procedure first on morning list

- Consider the need for reduction (20–30%) of evening intermediate insulin if there is a pattern of low blood glucoses in the mornings.
- About 7 a.m., give 40 to 50% usual short-acting insulin (or about 10% of total daily dose).
- Start IV fluids 0.225% saline, 5% glucose at maintenance.
- Perform hourly BGLs.
- Increase glucose to 7.5% or 10% if required.
- Give extra mid-morning short-acting insulin if needed (10–25% total daily dose).
- Usually resume normal food and insulin from lunch.

Procedure first on afternoon list

- The patient is usually allowed breakfast.
- About 7 a.m. give 50 to 60% usual short-acting insulin.
- Start IV fluids 0.225% saline, 5% glucose at maintenance 2 hours after breakfast.
- At 12 noon give about 10% of total daily dose short-acting insulin.
- Perform hourly BGLs.
- Increase glucose to 7.5% or 10% if required.
- Postoperatively, give additional short-acting insulin, usually 10% of total daily dose as needed 4-hourly.
- Give the usual insulin and food at dinner and supper.

Patients on insulin pumps

- The diabetes team will determine the approach depending on the individual patient and procedure.
- *Minor procedures*: The pump can be continued at basal rate, keeping glucose infusion to a minimum. Monitor BGL hourly. Correction doses can be given preoperatively and postoperatively as needed and carbohydrate boluses when the patient is ready to eat. Alternatively, the pump can be discontinued preoperatively and a basal-bolus regimen instituted with adjustment as above.

- *Major surgery*: The subcutaneous (sc) insulin pump is discontinued and an IV insulin infusion used.

Major surgery or surgery where oral intake not possible for a prolonged period

- This is most easily managed using an insulin infusion (50 units of short-acting insulin in 500 mL 0.9% saline—equivalent to 1 unit of insulin per 10 mL saline) run through a volumetric pump. The initial maintenance rate is 0.02 units/kg/h via a line separate to the hydration fluid.
- Administer IV fluids at maintenance rates (usually 0.225% saline with 5% glucose).
- Maintain BGLs between 5 and 12 mmol/L by adjusting the rate of the insulin infusion up or down by increments of 10–25%, as needed.
- If the patient is hypoglycaemic (BGL < 4 mmol/L), cease insulin infusion for 15 minutes, then resume at a lower rate while continuing maintenance saline/glucose (IV insulin has a half-life of only 3 to 4 minutes).
- If the patient is severely hypoglycaemic, a medical officer should be present and an additional bolus of 2 mL/kg of 10% glucose or equivalent may be required.
- Perform hourly BGLs while on an insulin infusion.
- Give replacement potassium if IV fluids continue for more than 12 hours.
- The insulin infusion therapy is continued until oral food intake has been established and subcutaneous insulin therapy is possible. When changing to subcutaneous insulin, continue the intravenous insulin infusion for 90 minutes after the first subcutaneous insulin injection.

Hypoglycaemia in diabetes

Hypoglycaemia is the most frequent acute complication of IDDM.

Symptoms, counter-regulatory hormone responses and cognitive deficits may be detected at plasma glucose values between 3.5 and 4.0 mmol/L. Thus, it is advisable to maintain blood glucose values above 4.0 mmol/L in children and adolescents with diabetes.

Symptoms

- *Neurogenic symptoms*: Cholinergic (sweating, hunger, tingling around the mouth); adrenergic (tremor, tachycardia, pallor, palpitations and anxiety)
- *Neuroglycopenic symptoms*: Weakness, headache, visual disturbance, slurred speech, vertigo, dizziness, difficulty in thinking, tiredness, drowsiness, change in affect (for example depressed, angry, argumentative), mental confusion, coma, convulsions

Causes

- Inadequate or missed meals or snacks
- Exercise (unplanned or more prolonged than usual) without appropriate food intake
- Insulin errors
- Alcohol ingestion which causes impaired hepatic gluconeogenesis
- Idiopathic (no obvious cause discernible)

Confirmation of hypoglycaemia

Although it is useful to have the hypoglycaemia confirmed by a blood glucose measurement, treatment is urgent and should not be withheld if undue delay is likely.

Treatment

Mild to moderate hypoglycaemia

- Give 7.5 to 15 g (1/2 to 1 exchange) of a rapidly digested form of carbohydrate (for example 125 to 200 mL orange juice or ordinary soft drink, 7 jelly beans, 2–3 teaspoons of sugar or honey).
- Follow with a snack of a more slowly digested carbohydrate (for example 1 slice of bread, 1 apple, 300 mL of milk, 2 plain sweet biscuits) to maintain normoglycaemia until the next meal or snack.
- The child will usually be feeling better within 10 minutes, but it may take 10 to 20 minutes to see a measurable rise in BGL.

Severe hypoglycaemia

- For severe hypoglycaemia, therapy is urgent if the patient is unconscious, fitting or unable to swallow.
- Nothing should be given by mouth.
- Check airway, and position in the coma or recovery position.

Outside hospital

- Glucagon by subcutaneous or intramuscular injection: dose 0.5 units (0.5 mg) for age < 5 years, 1 unit (1 mg) for all older age groups.
- If the parent or caregiver is not available to attend to a severe hypoglycaemic episode, and if a doctor or appropriate health professional cannot be found quickly, then an ambulance should be summoned immediately.

In hospital

- Either IV glucose (preferred) or glucagon (sc or IM, dose as above) can be used.
- IV glucose: dose 2 mL/kg of 10% glucose given over a few minutes, followed by IV fluids containing 5–10% glucose.
- The diabetes team should be consulted to guide management.

Follow-up of treatment of hypoglycaemia

Many children vomit persistently after severe hypoglycaemia and it is important to ensure that the hypoglycaemia does not recur.

- Monitor blood glucose levels frequently.
- Ensure that food is tolerated (either as frequent small amounts of sugary drinks or as an adequate amount of quickly digested starch such as bread).
- Arrange supervision by a relative or friend who should accompany the child home.
- Arrange contact with the diabetes team for a review of the diabetes management.
- If food is not tolerated then hospitalisation for a continuous infusion of glucose/saline and frequent monitoring is necessary.

Sick day management

Impact of illnesses on diabetes

In general, children and adolescents with well-controlled diabetes cope with illnesses well. Illnesses may have little effect on the diabetes, or may cause high blood glucose levels or low blood glucose levels:

- Mild URTI is an example of an illnesses causing little effect on the diabetes.

- High blood glucoses and ketones are more common responses to systemic illness, usually infections, and are largely due to insulin resistance. Treatment is urgent as without extra insulin this state may progress into ketoacidosis. Infections may have a silent prodromal phase which may cause unexplained high glucose levels for several days before the illness declares itself.
- Illnesses causing low blood glucose levels are usually illnesses with nausea, vomiting and diarrhoea but *not* accompanied by a fever or systemic features. There is inability to absorb or retain food.

General principles of sick day management

The essential principles in sick day management are:

- *Treatment of the underlying illness*: This is no different in the child with diabetes. However, medical assessment should be sought earlier in case antibiotic or other therapies are required.
- *Symptomatic relief and rest*: If a fever, headache or aches and pains are present, paracetamol can be given.
- *Sugar-free medications*: Many sugar-free medications are available, but those not sugar-free are satisfactory as the amount of sugar present in each dose is too small to cause a problem.
- *Hydration*: Encourage plenty of fluids. Losses may be higher due to fever and osmotic diuresis. If the blood glucose is > 15 mmol/L, water or low-joule drinks should be offered so as not to raise the blood glucose further.
- *Monitoring*: Blood glucose should be monitored more frequently and the urine or blood tested for ketones if blood glucose is > 15 mmol/L.
- *Insulin therapy*:
  - Additional insulin given at home can frequently avert hospitalisation in illnesses associated with hyperglycaemia and ketosis. Short-acting insulin is given every 2–4 hours in a dose equal to 5–20% of the total daily insulin dosage.
  - In general, 20% of the total daily dosage is used for the additional injections if the patient is very sick, has a blood glucose in excess of 15 mmol/L and has moderate or large amounts of ketones in the blood or urine.
  - Once the blood glucose is less than 15 mmol/L but above 12 mmol/L, repeated doses are usually 10% of the total daily dose, given every 4 hours.

Persistent hypoglycaemia

- These illnesses are marked by semi-starvation due to extreme anorexia, often associated with vomiting and diarrhoea.
- Blood glucose is tested frequently and frequent sips of glucose-containing drinks (not diet drinks) or small portions of glucose-containing foods are given.
- Insulin doses should be reduced but must not be suspended. Insulin doses may need to be reduced by 20–50%, especially the short-acting doses.

Indicators for patient to be admitted to hospital

Sick day management at home should be abandoned and admission to hospital arranged if:

- vomiting persists, especially if it becomes bile-stained
- hyperventilation occurs, suggestive of Kussmaul respiration
- ketones are present and are increasing
- blood glucose continues to rise despite treatment
- the child becomes more unwell, drowsy, disoriented or confused
- the nature of the illness is not understood
- abdominal pain is severe or localised
- the caregivers are uncertain about how to handle the situation
- the caregivers become exhausted
- other diseases coexist (such as cystic fibrosis)
- the patient is very young (for example, under 2 years).

Management in hospital

Low blood glucose levels

- If BGL cannot be maintained by oral intake, IV fluids are commenced, usually as 0.225% saline with 5% glucose or 0.45% saline with 5% glucose as guided by electrolytes.
- BGLs are checked 1–2-hourly initially and reduced insulin doses given as guided by monitoring.

High blood glucose and ketones

If BGL is > 15 mmol/L and there are moderate or large ketones but with no or only mild ketoacidosis (venous pH > 7.20):

- Commence IV fluids—0.9% saline initially at maintenance plus replacement of estimated deficits over 24–48 hours.

- Extra doses of short-acting sc insulin (10–20% of total daily insulin given as short-acting) are given every 2–4 hours until BGL < 15 mmol/L and ketones are cleared.
- Once BGL falls below 12–15 mmol/L glucose should be added to IV fluids. Grade to oral intake when possible.
- The diabetes team should be consulted to guide management.

16

Gastroenterology

This chapter includes:

- acute gastroenteritis
- gastro-oesophageal reflux
- acute gastrointestinal bleeding
- acute (fulminant) liver failure
- fever in chronic liver disease
- fever in the patient with a central line
- problems in liver transplant patients.

Acute gastroenteritis

Acute gastroenteritis is characterised by the sudden onset of vomiting and/or diarrhoea and/or fever.

Any morbidity and mortality are usually related to dehydration and electrolyte imbalance. The main focus of therapy is replacement of fluid and electrolytes.

Aetiology

Table 16.1 shows the major causes of acute gastroenteritis in infants and young children. In hospitalised patients, viruses are the cause in about 50% and bacteria in 15–20%. In the remainder, the cause is unclear despite the best laboratory facilities.

Differential diagnoses

It is important to think of other diagnoses, since vomiting and diarrhoea can occur in other diseases particularly in the very young:

Table 16.1 Major causes of acute gastroenteritis

Rotavirus	20–40%	C. jejuni	8–10%
Adenovirus	6–8%	Salmonella species	4–8%
Small round viruses	2–4%	Other bacteria	2–5%

- surgical: acute appendicitis, intussusception, peritonitis, volvulus
- infective: urinary tract infection, septicaemia, pneumonia, meningitis
- metabolic: diabetes mellitus (with ketoacidosis), inborn errors
- others: anaphylaxis, chronic gastrointestinal disease, inflammatory bowel disease.

Some symptoms suggest an alternative diagnosis:

- Protracted bilious vomiting with or without surgical signs in the abdomen is surgical until proven otherwise.
- Acute appendicitis is a major diagnostic challenge in under 2 year olds.
- Temperature above 39°C suggests systemic infection.
- Growth failure suggests the presence of chronic underlying disease.
- Haematemesis or organomegaly (particularly of the liver) suggest an alternative diagnosis.
- Infants under 6 months provide a real challenge—beware.
- Headache or altered consciousness—think CNS or metabolic.

Assessment of dehydration

Dehydration is the main clinical complication of acute gastroenteritis and provides the basis of therapy. Major symptoms are thirst and oliguria, though the latter can be very difficult to assess in an infant with watery diarrhoea. The 'eyeball test' (just looking at the child) is usually a good indicator of unwellness. Table 16.2 shows the way to

Table 16.2 Assessment of dehydration

Symptom/sign	Mild (< 5%)	Moderate (5–10%)	Severe (> 10%)
Thirst	+	++	+++ (may be obtunded)
Oliguria	+	++	Anuric
Dry mouth, eyes, decreased skin turgor	–	+	++
Tachypnoea (due to acidosis)	–	+	++
Tachycardia	–	+	++
Shock	–	–	+

assess dehydration most commonly used in Australian hospitals but it slightly overestimates the degree of dehydration (by about 2%).

If the history obtained from the parents suggests a more severe problem than the assessment, believe the history. Signs of dehydration may lag behind the onset of symptoms. Physical signs are unreliable in the obese infant.

Is resuscitation required?

If the patient is shocked or severely dehydrated, with anuria, fluid expansion is needed urgently. This can be performed via IV line or, where IV cannulation is not immediately possible, by intra-osseous cannula. Replacement is about 20 mL/kg stat and is repeated until the patient has a reasonable blood pressure. Replace with crystalloid such as Hartmann's solution or normal saline, as the cause of shock usually is loss of water and electrolytes. Decisions about investigations and ongoing treatment can wait until the patient is stable.

Investigations

- Stool bacterial cultures should be done:
  - if the patient has bloody stools and/or high temperature
  - if other family members have diarrhoea and vomiting, or if the child attends day care centre or has recently travelled overseas
  - if there are leucocytes on microscopy—in an infant this often indicates a bacterial cause.
- Where the child is sick enough to require hospital admission, both bacterial and viral cultures should be requested
- Serum electrolytes should be done in any child with moderate or severe dehydration, on admission, repeated after 6–8 hours (see Chapter 7).
- Septic work-up should be done in any sick infant or in any sick, febrile toxic infant or child.

Common electrolyte disturbances

Hypokalaemia (K < 3.5 mmol/L) and hyponatraemia (Na < 135 mmol/L)

These usually occur because of electrolyte loss in the stool. Sodium is usually lost because of osmotic diarrhoea. Potassium is lost because of the action of aldosterone on both the small and the large intestine and in the kidneys.

Acidosis

In gastroenteritis, acidosis is usually due to bicarbonate loss in the stool. The resulting picture is one of low HCO_3 and high Cl (a low anion gap). Acidosis can occur from lactic acidosis (shock), keto-acidosis (diabetes), a previously unrecognised inborn error, or ingestion of drugs such as salicylate. The latter have a high anion gap—low HCO_3 and low Cl with unmeasured anions. Acidosis usually responds to treatment of dehydration.

Hypernatraemia (Na > 145 mmol/L)

This results from osmotic water loss in excess of electrolytes. It can be caused by severe carbohydrate intolerance or the use of hyper-osmolar feeds, for example undiluted carbonated drinks or concentrated infant formulae. Note that despite the high serum Na, the total body sodium is depleted. Care is required in rehy-drating such patients, since osmolytes in CSF equilibrate much more slowly than in blood; this can result in fluid shifts into the brain and consequent cerebral oedema. Rehydration is carried out over 48 hours.

Treatment

The mode of replacement will depend on the degree of dehydration. As a rule of thumb, children with mild dehydration (< 5%) can be managed via the oral route.

Children with > 5% dehydration should be treated in hospital. Oral rehydration therapy can often be used successfully in this group, but IV therapy is more commonly utilised, especially where vomiting is frequent and/or diarrhoea is profuse.

Fluid replacement calculation

Assess the *deficit*: volume (mL) = % dehydration × weight (kg) × 10

For example, 5% dehydration in a 10 kg infant: 5 × 10 × 10 = 500 mL

Calculate the *maintenance* requirements and make an estimate of likely *ongoing losses*. Write your calculations in the calculation section of the IV Fluid Sheet.

Add deficit + maintenance + ongoing losses and give over 24 hours, but always reassess at 6–8 hours. (See Chapter 7.)

Oral rehydration therapy (ORT)

A commercially prepared oral rehydration solution (ORS) is the treatment of choice. These solutions contain glucose/sodium in proportions designed to stimulate glucose-coupled sodium absorption. Gastrolyte is an example. It contains 2% glucose, Na 60 mmol/L, K 20 mmol/L, Cl 60 mmol/L and HCO_3 10 mmol/L. ORS can be delivered safely via a nasogastric tube. It needs to be clear to parents that ORS is not a treatment for vomiting and/or diarrhoea, but therapy for treatment or prevention of dehydration.

Oral rehydration solutions are salty and children don't enjoy the taste. Use a flavoured variety. Offer it frequently. Children who are dehydrated will usually drink any fluid, so will tolerate ORS. Non-dehydrated children can be treated with diluted sweet drinks such as carbonated beverages and fruit juice. These are hyperosmolar in full strength and need to be diluted with water at least 1 in 4. Oral rehydration is used in both home and hospital management of children with gastroenteritis. It should be used with greater caution in children aged < 12 months. Frequent clinical reassessment is necessary. When used at home, parents must be given a written management plan, including advice on when to seek further medical advice.

IV therapy

The choice of IV fluid replacement therapy will depend on any electrolyte disturbance present. Normally, N/2 dextrose saline with added potassium (20 mmol/L) will replace losses from diarrhoea and/or vomiting. *Do not use N/4 saline for fluid replacement therapy as this exacerbates or induces hyponatraemia and may result in cerebral oedema.* The deficit should be replaced over 8–12 hours with repeat electrolytes at that time. Hypernatraemic dehydration should be treated over a longer time with close monitoring of electrolytes. Half-normal saline with added potassium is the preferred treatment as it will slow the rate of decline of sodium and serum osmolarity and protect against cerebral oedema. It is not usually necessary to administer bicarbonate unless there is a life-threatening acidosis (pH < 7.0) as this will correct with correction of dehydration and electrolyte disturbances (see Chapter 7).

Medications

There is *no indication* for the use of *antivomiting*, *antimotility* or *antidiarrhoeal agents* in the treatment of childhood gastroenteritis.

These therapies can worsen the outcome because of side-effects and do not prevent dehydration. *Antimicrobials* are indicated in some settings:

- invasive infections such as *Shigella* dysentery, *Salmonella* bacteraemia and in infants < 6 months with bacterial gastroenteritis
- parasitic infections such as *Giardia* or *Strongyloides*.

Diet

Breastfeeding should not be discontinued. Extra fluids should be provided between feeds. Normal dietary intake should be continued in formula-fed infants and other children taking normal diets not later than 24 hours after start of fluid therapy. It is not necessary to dilute infant formulae. Give extra fluids to compensate for ongoing diarrhoea. Secondary lactose intolerance should be treated with a lactose-free formula rather than with continued 'clear fluids'. A normal diet should be offered to toddlers and older children. They know when they are well enough to eat.

Traps for the unwary

Haemolytic uraemic syndrome is an uncommon syndrome with haemolytic anaemia, thrombocytopenia and renal failure. In Australia it is usually caused by enterohaemorrhagic *E. coli* and patients often have a diarrhoeal prodrome. Measure the blood pressure and check FBC if patient is pale.

Children with short gut syndrome and/or ileostomy or colostomy are at dire risk of dehydration if they develop infectious gastroenteritis. They should be admitted to hospital even if they do not appear to be particularly unwell.

Young infants, particularly under 3 months, can be a real diagnostic challenge. Treat them with the utmost respect.

Children requiring gastrostomy or NG feeds may have difficulty in self-regulating water intake and maintaining normal homeostasis. Development of acute gastroenteritis in these patients may lead to severe dehydration if nasogastric feeds continue at normal maintenance rates.

For more detail refer to *Acute management of young children and infants with gastroenteritis. Clinical practice guidelines*, New South Wales Department of Health, 2002. This document can be downloaded from the NSW Health website: www.health.nsw.gov.

Gastro-oesophageal reflux

Gastro-oesophageal reflux (GOR) occurs physiologically at all ages, but much more frequently in infants up to 15 months. It causes frequent regurgitation in up to a third of young infants. Only a small proportion of these suffer complications which, by implication, render the GOR pathological. GOR causes effortless regurgitation, but not vomiting.

Where significant vomiting is occurring, a cause other than GOR should be sought. Vomiting is a nonspecific symptom with a multitude of structural and organic causes; important surgical causes are considered in Chapter 31.

An infant with no more than uncomplicated GOR will normally be thriving and happy, and will have normal physical signs.

Complicated gastro-oesophageal reflux

- Problems associated with excess gastric acid in the oesophagus, causing oesophagitis, are:
  - excessive crying and irritability, in infants with regurgitation
  - haematemesis (rare)
  - oesophageal stricture (very rare).
- Problems associated with contact of refluxed acid/milk with the airways are:
  - tracheobronchial aspiration, with or without bronchospasm, persistent cough, aspiration pneumonia or 'bronchitis'
  - laryngospasm, sometimes with respiratory arrest and even cardiac arrest
  - apnoea and bradycardia, especially in premature infants and infants and children with neurological diseases.
- Often a combination of anorexia (from oesophagitis), caloric loss (from frequent regurgitation) and the extra work of breathing (from respiratory complications) may cause failure to thrive.

Investigation and management of gastro-oesophageal reflux

- Where an adequate history and normal physical examination are consistent with uncomplicated GOR, no investigations or treatment are warranted. Antacids and drugs aimed at promoting gastric emptying should not be used.
- In infants considered to have milder symptoms investigations are

rarely of value. Simple measures such as lateral posturing with head-up elevation of the cot and thickening of feeds (with corn-flour or commercial products) are often used, without clear evidence of benefit or harm. A trial of small doses of alkali antacids after feeds is often used.

- Infants and children considered to have serious manifestations of reflux may warrant imaging investigations, to exclude anatomical abnormalities of the upper gastrointestinal tract (such as hiatus hernia). Oesophageal pH studies are most useful when episodic manifestations, such as pain behaviour or apnoea, are thought to be manifestations of GOR. Gastroscopy and oesophageal biopsy are necessary to positively confirm oesophagitis. Lateral postur-ing and feed thickening (as above) are generally used and consideration is given to the use of H_2-receptor agonists (cimeti-dine or ranitidine) or proton pump inhibitors (omeprazole) for treatment of oesophagitis.

- In infants and children with respiratory conditions possibly due to GOR, barium swallow and/or milk scan may help in differen-tiating between reflux with aspiration and aspiration at the time of swallowing (for example from bulbar palsy or pharyngeal discoordination).

- In infants and children with persistent oesophagitis, repeated aspiration episodes or other serious complications of GOR, and where conservative measures (as above) have been unsuccessful, fundoplication requires consideration. This is a major surgical procedure with significant morbidity.

Acute gastrointestinal bleeding

Upper gastrointestinal tract

Bleeding can range from trivial to life-threatening. Causes include oesophagitis, gastritis (allergic, drug-induced—particularly aspirin, *H. pylori*), Mallory-Weiss tear, duodenal ulcer disease, vascular malformations and oesophageal varices. Think of epistaxis and vomiting of swallowed blood.

Mild

A small amount of fresh blood and/or 'coffee ground' vomitus occurs.

Approach

- History and physical examination usually provide the diagnosis.
- Investigations will depend on the clinical setting, though endoscopy is usually the fastest route to an accurate diagnosis. This will need to be discussed with the gastroenterology unit.
- Withhold treatment with H_2 antagonists until the diagnosis is established.
- Proton pump blockers should not be used without an accurate diagnosis.

Severe (life-threatening)

This is most often due to variceal haemorrhage. Splenomegaly may not be present before resuscitation and may become evident later.

Approach

- Stabilise (correct hypovolaemia, if present).
- Check Hb, coagulation screen, cross-match blood.
- Transfer the patient to Intensive Care.
- Notify the gastroenterologist on call (upper gastrointestinal bleeding is not usually a surgical condition in the first instance).
- Endoscopy will usually be required but not until the patient is stable. Endoscopic intervention (for example, banding, sclerotherapy, thermal coagulation) may stop bleeding.
- Intravenous somatostatin may be required to control portal hypertensive bleeding.
- Shunt surgery or transjugular intrahepatic portosystemic shunt (TIPS) may be needed to prevent re-bleeding.

Lower gastrointestinal

Mild

- Usually trivial and, if not associated with diarrhoea, is usually caused by anal fissure or juvenile polyp (in the young child). Check for fissure and, if present, treat with stool softener.
- Bloody diarrhoea is usually due to bacterial gastroenteritis—check stool microscopy and cultures. Antibiotic therapy is usually not indicated in uncomplicated cases. If cultures are negative, consider inflammatory bowel disease.

Severe (shock and/or dropping haemoglobin)

This is usually due to Meckel's diverticulum but can be caused by vascular malformations and Crohn's disease.

Approach

- Stabilise (correct hypovolaemia, if present).
- Arrange radionuclide scan.
- Notify surgeons as this is usually a surgical problem.

Acute (fulminant) liver failure

The onset of coagulopathy and encephalopathy occurs within 8 weeks of onset of illness. Patient may or may not have overt jaundice. Usual causes are:

- viruses (hepatitis B, C, etc. or presumed viral hepatitis)
- drugs (such as paracetamol)
- metabolic disorders (Wilson's disease, inborn errors of metabolism such as hereditary fructose intolerance, respiratory chain and fatty acid oxidation disorders, urea cycle abnormalities).

Acute liver failure can be caused by acute decompensation of chronic liver disease which may not have been previously recognised:

- Wilson's disease
- choledochal cyst
- autoimmune hepatitis
- cryptogenic cirrhosis
- α-1 antitrypsin deficiency
- viral hepatitis.

Approach

- Examine the patient, looking for signs of chronic liver disease.
- In addition to the usual blood tests check *coagulation screen* and *albumin* (markers of liver synthetic function) and NH_3.
- Think of paracetamol poisoning (check paracetamol level and urinary metabolic screen). If paracetamol poisoning is suspected, consider N-acetyl-cysteine.
- The on-call gastroenterologist must be notified at the time of admission. The child should be admitted to Intensive Care.

Few liver diseases are curable and many are potentially fatal if untreated. The exceptions are Wilson's disease, choledochal cyst and hereditary fructose intolerance—if the diagnosis is made early enough.

Fever in chronic liver disease

Infants and children with chronic liver disease are more prone than the normal child to sepsis. Ascending cholangitis occurs in children with disorders of the biliary tree or postbiliary surgery. Examples include:

- biliary atresia
- sclerosing cholangitis
- gallstones
- following choledocho-jejunostomy
- following liver transplantation.

Gram-negative sepsis is often associated with fulminant hepatic failure, especially in infants (for example, galactosaemia). Pneumococcal infection can occur, particularly in children with ascites.

Infants or children with chronic liver disease presenting with fever should have the following performed:

- full blood count and differential white cell count
- liver function tests
- blood cultures.

Discuss abdominal tap (in patients with ascites) and the use of antibiotics with the on-call gastroenterologist. *If bacterial sepsis is suspected antibiotics should be commenced before the test results are available.*

Fever in the patient with a central line

Central lines are commonly used in this hospital for:

- monitoring severely ill patients (usually in Intensive Care)
- improved venous access
- delivery of medications (antibiotics, chemotherapy)
- delivery of total parenteral nutrition (TPN).

Fever in such patients can be due to bacterial and/or fungal infection of the central line. In such patients the following should be undertaken:

- full blood count and differential white cell count
- blood cultures—peripheral and through the central line
- assessment of other potential sites of infection (such as micturating cystourethrogram, CXR).

Discuss the use of antibiotics with the consultant on call.

Taking blood cultures from a central line requires disconnection of the line. This requires sterile technique and is often performed by nursing staff. Refer to the relevant protocol in the policy and procedures manual in the intranet.

Problems in liver transplant patients

Children who have had liver transplantation can have significant medical problems which resident staff may encounter.

These include:

- fever
- respiratory compromise
- fluid balance
- ascites.

Fever

Post-liver-transplant patients are immunosuppressed and at risk for sepsis. They also often have central venous catheters *in situ*. Any liver transplant patient with a fever of 38.0°C or more should be assessed for possible causes of sepsis. These may include central venous line (CVL) infection, wound infection, peritonitis, cholangitis or generalised septicaemia. Cultures should be taken from all lumens of the CVL, as well as peripheral blood cultures, along with FBC, electrolytes, renal and liver function. Ascitic fluid should be sent for microscopy and culture. Other investigations are performed according to the clinical scenario. The on-call gastroenterologist should be consulted and a decision made as to whether antibiotics should be started, or CVL removed.

Respiratory compromise

Causes of post-transplant respiratory difficulty include pleural effusion, collapse/consolidation, diaphragmatic splinting from abdominal distension/ascites, fluid overload or septicaemia. A full clinical assessment, saturation monitoring and chest X-ray should be performed. The on-call gastroenterologist should be consulted and the case discussed. Treatment options include supplemental oxygen, tapping of either pleural or peritoneal effusions, and diuretic therapy.

Fluid balance and ascites

Post-transplant patients often have problematic fluid dynamics, with hypoalbuminaemia, ascites and pleural effusions, and poor urine output. Assessment of these patients includes daily (and sometimes twice-daily) weights, accurate fluid balance charts with urine outputs, recording of vital signs, and blood electrolyte and albumin measurements. Management options include judicious use of diuretics, concentrated albumin infusions (usually 1 g per kg daily for 3 days of 20% albumin) and, sometimes, tapping of ascitic collections. Cases should be discussed with the on-call gastroenterologist.

17

Neurology and neurosurgery

This chapter includes:

- epilepsy
- febrile convulsions
- rapid onset of limb weakness
- emergency management of head injury
- hydrocephalus and shunt problems.

See also:

- coma (Chapter 3)
- meningitis (Chapter 11).

Epilepsy

Epilepsy is a chronic disorder producing a wide variety of signs and symptoms which result from excessive neuronal discharges from the brain. It is important to define the type of seizure disorder in each child.

Classification of epileptic seizures

Partial seizures

These have a focal onset.

- In *simple partial seizures* there is no impairment of consciousness. The seizure begins from and is confined to a relatively small area of the brain. Examples include Jacksonian seizures (focal clonic seizures with march) and auras.
- In *complex partial seizures* there is impairment of consciousness. These may begin with an aura (a simple partial seizure) but as the seizure spreads to involve more of the brain, the characteristic alteration of consciousness occurs. The child often looks 'vacant' and may carry out simple, repetitive actions during the seizure.

Post-ictal drowsiness often occurs and is an important clinical feature differentiating complex partial seizures from absence seizures and daydreaming.

- In *partial seizures with secondary generalisation* the seizure begins focally but then spreads to involve both hemispheres, resulting in generalised tonic-clonic seizures.

Generalised seizures

These arise from both hemispheres simultaneously. They are bilaterally symmetrical without focal onset.

- *Absence seizures* ('petit mal') are sudden seizures with abrupt onset and termination. Typically the child stares, but automatisms and blinking are frequently seen. Generally they last less than 30 seconds and there is no aura or post-ictal drowsiness. The characteristic EEG is generalised 3 per second spike and wave activity which is particularly provoked by hyperventilation.
- *Generalised tonic-clonic seizures* ('grand mal') involve sudden loss of consciousness with initial tonic stiffening, followed by clonic jerking and post-ictal confusion and/or sleep.
- *Myoclonic seizures* are abrupt, shock-like jerks of the limbs and trunk of brief duration.
- *Atonic seizures* cause sudden loss of tone in a group of muscles or the whole trunk, resulting in a fall.

Epileptic syndromes in the paediatric age range

- *Infantile spasms* almost always commence in the first year of life. Typically, there is a sudden flexion of the arms and head in a brief spasm (salaam seizure) but extensor or asymmetrical posturing may occur. Characteristically the episodes occur *in runs* when the child is drowsy. Hypsarrhythmia is typically seen on the EEG but is not essential to the diagnosis.
- *Lennox-Gastaut syndrome* usually starts in the preschool years and is characterised by a variety of seizures, including drop attacks, atypical absences, myoclonic seizures, nocturnal tonic seizures and generalised tonic-clonic seizures. There is associated intellectual decline. Slow spike and wave discharges (2–2½ Hz) are typically seen on the EEG.
- *Benign focal epilepsy of childhood* (benign rolandic epilepsy) usually begins in the 5–10 year age group. The seizures most frequently

occur during sleep in an otherwise healthy child. Often they start with the child making a gurgling or clucking noise and this is followed by a clonic seizure involving one side of the body. The child may be awake but is unable to speak—a very frightening experience. The seizure may then become secondarily generalised. Centro-temporal spikes typically are seen on the EEG.

- *Juvenile myoclonic epilepsy* usually develops in the early teenage years. Myoclonic jerks occur on awakening. Absence seizures and generalised tonic-clonic seizures also are seen. The generalised tonic-clonic seizures typically occur early in the morning after sleep deprivation. A history of *early morning myoclonus* should always be sought in teenagers who present with their first generalised seizure as often this information is not volunteered spontaneously and it is an important clue to the diagnosis. Rapid polyspike and wave discharges typically are seen in the EEG.

Conditions confused with epilepsy

A precise description of the sequence of events before, during and after a 'turn' should always be obtained as this may establish that the child has a non-epileptic paroxysmal disorder.

- *Syncope* is usually a vasovagal response provoked by stressful stimuli such as an emotional upset, seeing blood, standing in a crowded room, and so on. The child feels light-headed, nauseated and clammy, and may describe a progressive fading out of vision. Loss of consciousness is secondary to cerebral hypoxia and may be accompanied by stiffening and clonic jerks. Rarely, syncope may be due to arrhythmia associated with the prolonged QT syndrome. Consider this, and ask for an electrocardiogram, especially if the episodes occur with exercise.
- *Breath-holding attacks* are always provoked by an unpleasant stimulus, typically a mild bump to the child's head, but they may also be provoked by an emotional upset, such as being scolded. They usually begin in the first two years of life.
  - In a *cyanotic breath-holding attack*, vigorous crying commences, followed by breath-holding in expiration and loss of consciousness, often with tonic stiffening. Clonic jerking can be seen following both forms. In both, the child usually recovers quickly, returning to normal within a few minutes.

231

- In a *pallid breath-holding attack*, after a short cry there is loss of consciousness, marked pallor and often tonic stiffening.
- *Hypoglycaemia* must always be considered in the differential diagnosis of epilepsy.

Investigations

Although many investigations are now available, a precise history remains by far the most important step in the diagnosis of epilepsy.

Investigations attempt to confirm the clinical impression of seizures, and may be helpful in differentiating partial from generalised seizures, localising the site of origin of partial seizures, predicting outcome, and so on.

- *Electroencephalogram (EEG)*: This may show a characteristic pattern in certain epilepsy syndromes as described above. It must be remembered that the awake EEG may be normal in children with both partial and generalised seizures. A record performed after sleep deprivation and which includes sleep increases the yield. The EEG should never be performed in the hope of excluding epilepsy. Routine 'follow-up' EEGs have no value, nor is there a role for the EEG in the investigation of simple febrile seizures.
- *Metabolic studies*: Fasting blood sugar, electrolytes, calcium, magnesium and urine metabolic screen may be useful, depending on the clinical setting.
- *Neuroimaging*: CT scan or MRI scan is indicated when an anatomical lesion is suspected. If there are partial seizures, focal neurological signs, focal EEG (except in benign focal epilepsy of childhood) or difficult-to-control seizures, with a normal CT scan, MRI scan should be done.

Drug treatment of epilepsy

Monotherapy is the goal of treatment of epilepsy and is possible in the majority of patients. However, it must be recognised that some children need multiple antiepileptic drugs (AEDs) to achieve even modest control.

- In general the dose of AEDs in children is determined on a weight basis.
- A basic principle of treatment is 'go low, go slow'—unless the seizures are very frequent, start with a low dose and gradually increase.

- If the seizures continue, the drug dosage is generally pushed to the maximum that can be achieved without causing side-effects.
- Most AEDs are given in a twice-daily divided dosage.
- Drug levels are useful for dosage adjustment with carbamazepine, phenytoin and phenobarbitone, and as a guide to compliance with any AED.
- If the child is not having seizures, regular checking of AED levels is unnecessary. If the child is rapidly growing, the dose can be adjusted on a weight basis.
- It is important to remember that *rashes* induced by AEDs may be accompanied by fever and hepatic and bone marrow dysfunction. This should not be assumed to be evidence of a viral infection—the AED should be stopped.
- Many of the AEDs have teratogenic potential and this needs to be considered in teenage girls. Carbamazepine may render the 'low-dose' oral contraceptive pill ineffective.

Antiepileptic drugs commonly used in children

Carbamazepine

Carbamazepine is available in 100 mg and 200 mg tablets as well as a 100 mg/5 mL suspension. A controlled-release form is available with tablets of 200 mg and 400 mg, which can be broken in half. The controlled-release form provides a more even serum level throughout the day and is useful in those children who have side-effects soon after a dose. Carbamazepine is useful in simple and complex partial seizures and in generalised tonic-clonic seizures.

Starting dose: 5 mg/kg/day in 2 divided doses, increasing to 10 mg/kg/day after approximately 5 days. Subsequent dosage adjustments are guided by seizure control and toxicity. Doses of 20 mg/kg/day or more may be required.

With higher doses, drowsiness, diplopia, dizziness and hyperactivity may occur. The most common potentially serious side-effect is a morbilliform rash which occurs in the first 2 months of treatment. This can progress to Stevens-Johnson syndrome if the drug is not stopped immediately. Other serious side-effects include bone marrow depression and hepatitis. Erythromycin should be avoided in children taking carbamazepine as it inhibits its metabolism and produces toxic carbamazepine levels.

Sodium valproate

Sodium valproate is available in 200 mg and 500 mg enteric coated tablets which should be taken whole, and in 100 mg crushable tablets. There is also a liquid preparation of 200 mg per 5 mL.

Starting dose: 10 mg/kg/day in 2 divided doses, increasing to 20 mg/kg/day after approximately 5 days. Doses of 40–60 mg/kg/day may be tolerated.

Common side-effects include gastrointestinal upset, weight gain, hair loss and tremor, all of which are reversible after stopping treatment. Fatal hepatic failure has been reported rarely and is more common in the first 6 months of treatment in children under the age of 2 years who are on multiple drugs. Pancreatitis, encephalopathy and, in higher doses, thrombocytopenia may occur. Polycystic ovarian disease has been reported with valproate in obese teenagers.

Valproate is often stopped before planned neurosurgical procedures such as temporal lobectomy or spinal surgery as excessive bleeding can occur in the face of normal coagulation studies.

Vigabatrin

Vigabatrin is available in 500 mg tablets and sachets. The dose is generally between 50 and 150 mg/kg/day. It is useful in the treatment of complex partial seizures and infantile spasms. An exacerbation of seizures may occur, particularly if the child has myoclonus. Marked behavioural problems may also be precipitated. Vigabatrin can cause visual field loss, which limits its use. Regular, 6-monthly visual field monitoring is essential in children old enough to comply.

Lamotrigine

Lamotrigine is available in 2 mg, 5 mg, 25 mg, 50 mg, 100 mg and 200 mg tablets. It is useful in generalised and partial seizures. It must be started very slowly, particularly if the child is already on sodium valproate. Maximum doses are generally 5 mg/kg/day in 2 divided doses if the child is on sodium valproate and 10–15 mg/kg/day if the child is on other AEDs. The major side-effect is a rash which can progress to Stevens-Johnson syndrome, but is rare if the drug is introduced gradually. Insomnia and behavioural changes can occur.

Benzodiazepines

Benzodiazepines can be very effective in a variety of seizures. Although relatively free of systemic toxicity, they can cause drowsiness, learning difficulties and hyperkinetic behaviour. Ataxia and bronchial and salivary hypersecretion may also occur.

- *Clobazam* is available in 10 mg tablets. It is not currently listed in the Pharmaceutical Benefits Scheme system as an AED, so is more expensive than clonazepam but side-effects may be fewer.
- *Clonazepam* is available in 0.5 mg (orange) and 2 mg (white) tablets and drops (0.1 mg per drop).
- *Nitrazepam* is available in 5 mg tablets.

Phenytoin sodium

This is available in capsules (30 mg and 100 mg), chewable tablets (50 mg) and suspension (6 mg per mL). *Note*: Some children may be prescribed Dilantin Forte which has a strength of 20 mg per mL. The dose can vary widely but is generally between 5 and 10 mg/kg/day.

Phenytoin is useful in generalised tonic-clonic and complex partial seizures. Although now a second-line drug in childhood because of its frequent side-effects, it can on occasions be effective where the other AEDs have not worked. In general it is better to avoid the suspension because of dosage variation due to precipitation. Overdosage causes nystagmus, ataxia, diplopia, nausea, vomiting and drowsiness. Occasionally, seizure control worsens if the plasma levels become too high. Side-effects include gum hypertrophy (made worse by poor dental hygiene), increased hair growth on the trunk and limbs, coarsening of facial features, hepatitis and a morbilliform rash.

Ethosuximide

This is useful in typical absence seizures. It is available in 250 mg capsules and a liquid 250 mg per 5 mL. The dose is 10–40 mg/kg/day. Rash, nausea, abdominal pain, drowsiness, dizziness and headache may occur. Aplastic anaemia and SLE are rarely seen.

Phenobarbitone

This is available in 30 mg tablets and 15 mg per 5 mL liquid. The dose is usually 3–5 mg/kg/day. Excessive dosage causes drowsiness and ataxia. Side-effects include hyperactivity, aggressiveness, learning difficulties, depression, morbilliform rash and exfoliative rash.

Newer AEDs

The role of newer AEDs such as topiramate, gabapentin and tiagabine is currently being evaluated. Topiramate is likely to have a role in children with intractable conditions such as Lennox-Gastaut syndrome. Side-effects include drowsiness, renal stones, behaviour disorders and weight loss.

Duration of treatment

This varies with the severity of the seizures and the age of the patient. In general, the minimum requirement is freedom from seizures for 2 years. Withdrawal of the drug should proceed very slowly, generally over a 4–6 month period. Patients with juvenile myoclonic epilepsy may need life-long treatment with sodium valproate or lamotrigine.

Treatment of status epilepticus

This is an emergency situation and the seizures should be stopped as soon as possible. Seizures continuing for more than 30–60 minutes may cause permanent neurological damage.

All patients should have *full cardiac monitoring* and facilities for rapid resuscitation and *assisted ventilation* must be available.

Acute control of the seizure

- *Diazepam* 0.2 mg/kg IVI, repeated as necessary, but observing carefully for respiratory depression. Rectal diazepam 0.5 mg/kg is an effective but slower alternative when intravenous access is hard to obtain. Diazepam should not be given by intramuscular injection, though intramuscular midazolam (0.2 mg/kg) is an alternative. If diazepam does not control the seizure, or for more prolonged anticonvulsant action, phenytoin or phenobarbitone can be used.
- *Phenytoin* 15–20 mg/kg should be given in normal saline intravenously over 20–30 minutes with *full cardiac monitoring*. This is followed by 3 mg/kg IVI or oral every 6 hours for 48 hours and then maintenance doses of 5–10 mg/kg/day. Phenytoin levels should be checked on a daily basis initially as the levels can be quite unpredictable.

- *Phenobarbitone* 10 mg/kg, maximum 500 mg, can be given intra-muscularly or intravenously diluted in normal saline or dextrose and given over a 20-minute period. Respiratory depression is a particular risk when combined with benzodiazepines.

If the above has failed to stop the seizures within half an hour, then generally the patient should be admitted to Intensive Care and a midazolam or thiopentone infusion started.

Other drugs which may be useful for status epilepticus include *paraldehyde* 0.15–0.3 mL/kg rectally up to 10 mL. The intramuscular route may produce abscesses and should be avoided.

Once the acute seizures have been controlled, it is important to try to determine the cause of the seizures and ensure that regular AED therapy has been prescribed.

Usual drugs of first choice in common forms of epilepsy

- Partial seizures and generalised tonic clonic seizures:
  - carbamazepine
  - sodium valproate
- Absence epilepsy:
  - ethosuximide
  - sodium valproate
- Juvenile myoclonic epilepsy:
  - sodium valproate

Febrile convulsions

Febrile convulsions usually occur between the ages of 3 months and 6 years. They are associated with fever but not with intracranial infection or a metabolic cause. Two to 4% of children under 5 years of age have at least one febrile convulsion. The convulsion is often the first sign of the illness. Susceptibility to febrile convulsions is genetically determined.

Fever and convulsions in this age group may also be due to:

- intracranial infection, for example meningitis, encephalitis, brain abscess
- epilepsy coinciding with an unrelated febrile illness.

An accurate description from the parents is important.

- Note especially the duration of the convulsion and the presence of any focal element, including Todd's paresis (transient focal paralysis).
- Try to differentiate between the tremulousness and twitching commonly seen in acutely febrile children and definite seizure activity. Rigors (for instance, in an infant with UTI) may be misinterpreted as febrile convulsions. Loss of consciousness in a generalised seizure is a distinguishing feature.

Management

- If a febrile convulsion continues for longer than 10 minutes, give diazepam 0.2 mg/kg, intravenously.
- If IV injection is not immediately possible, give the intravenous solution rectally in a dose of 0.5 mg/kg. As a general rule, children 3 years and under can be given 5 mg rectally, and children over 3 years can be given 7.5–10 mg rectally. Intramuscular diazepam is poorly absorbed and is not recommended.
- Look for and, if necessary, treat the *cause* of the fever.
- Although paracetamol is widely used in children with fever, it is often ineffective in reducing fever and does not reduce the incidence of febrile convulsions.
- Likewise, evaporative cooling (tepid sponging) is ineffective in preventing febrile convulsions.

Investigations

- Physical signs may suggest the need for tests for the cause of the fever.
- *Lumbar puncture*: A seizure with fever may be an early sign of meningitis. Consider doing a lumbar puncture, even if signs of meningitis are absent:
  - in infants < 12 months of age
  - if the seizure lasted more than 10 minutes
  - if the post-ictal period was longer than 30 minutes
  - if the infant was pale and unwell before the seizure
  - if the patient is already being treated with antibiotics
  - if you are unsure.
- *Electroencephalogram (EEG)*:
  - An EEG is not a helpful prognostic indicator in febrile convulsions.

- Even the finding of paroxysmal epileptogenic activity does not predict the subsequent development of epilepsy and should not be used as an indication for the prescription of antiepileptic drugs.
- In general EEGs should not be done in children with febrile convulsions (simple or complex).
- *Neuroimaging*:
  - Neither CT nor MRI scanning is necessary in a neurologically normal child with febrile convulsions.
  - However, if recurrent focal seizures from the same site occur or if a neurological abnormality develops, neuroimaging should be undertaken.

Features that increase the risk of subsequent epilepsy

Epilepsy is more likely to develop in children with febrile convulsions if they have any of the following:

- a prolonged seizure (more than 15 minutes), or a focal seizure
- an underlying neurological or developmental abnormality
- more than one seizure on the same day
- a residual neurological abnormality as a result of the seizure
- a family history of epilepsy in a parent or sibling
- very frequent febrile convulsions.

If none of these is present, the risk of epilepsy is no greater than in other children.

Preventive therapy

- Phenobarbitone and sodium valproate, but not diazepam, reduce the frequency of recurrence of febrile convulsions, but they are not recommended because the potential side-effects outweigh the benefits of treatment.
- When there has been a previous prolonged febrile convulsion, instruct the parents on the use of rectal diazepam (0.5 mg per dose) to treat subsequent seizures.
- The most useful part of management is giving a thorough explanation and reassurance to the parents. They should be taught the acute management of a seizure.

Rapid onset of limb weakness

Rapid onset of limb weakness carries a wide differential diagnosis. Children with this problem must always be carefully monitored as they may develop respiratory failure.

- *Guillain-Barré syndrome* (GBS) is the most common cause. Typically, the weakness evolves over several days and can be proximal, distal or both. Meningism, limb and back pain can be pronounced. The tendon reflexes are usually depressed or absent. Some younger children present with apparent ataxia, suggesting a cerebellar problem but careful examination will usually reveal weakness and areflexia. The presence of facial weakness and/or sixth-nerve palsies helps to differentiate GBS from spinal cord lesions.
- *Spinal cord lesions* must always be excluded as there is a risk of permanent paraplegia. A careful search should be made for a motor or sensory level and sphincter dysfunction. Fever and a history of back pain or stiffness of weeks or months duration are other important clues. If there is any doubt, a spinal MRI scan must be performed urgently. Lumbar puncture is dangerous if there is spinal cord compression.
- *Envenomations*:
  - *Tick bite* paralysis closely resembles GBS. A thorough search should always be made for the engorged tick which is often behind the ear. Fixed dilated pupils are common in tick paralysis but rare in GBS. There is commonly a rapid progression of the weakness in the 24–48 hours after the removal of the tick and the child should be admitted and carefully observed even if there is only relatively mild weakness.
  - *Snake bite* is a rare but important cause of progressive weakness. Bites may be unrecognised or unreported. Transient unconsciousness with or without seizures may occur soon after snakebite. The bite site may appear no more than a scratch, without local swelling. Abnormal clotting studies should suggest snakebite as a possibility. Note, however, that neuropathy without coagulopathy occurs with bites of some snake species. Use of the Venom Detection Kit (from the Commonwealth Serum Laboratories) on a swab from a possible bite site, or on urine, may facilitate diagnosis. See Chapter 27.

- *Poliomyelitis* and other paralytic conditions due to enteroviruses are usually distinguishable by the presence of fever, asymmetry of weakness, lack of sensory involvement, CSF findings (pleocytosis and raised protein) and the results of other laboratory investigations.
- *Acute viral myositis* may cause the impression of weakness, but the principal problem is leg pain, particularly of the calves. The serum creatine kinase is elevated.
- *Infantile botulism* must be considered in children under 1 year of age. Neither GBS nor tick paralysis are common in this age group. Preceding constipation and pupillary and/or eye movement abnormalities are important clues.

Emergency management of head injury

Head injury is the leading cause of death in children older than 1 year. It is the third most common cause of death in infants aged less than 1 year. Boys suffer head injury twice as often as girls and are four times as likely to suffer a fatal head injury.

Immediate priorities

Establish:

- A—Airway
- B—Breathing
- C—Circulation
- C—Cervical spine stability.

Assess each of these and treat, as necessary, in every instance of head trauma. Poor outcome following head injury correlates closely with persisting hypotension and hypoxaemia.

The Glasgow Coma Scale

The paediatric version of the Glasgow Coma Scale (GCS) used at the Children's Hospital at Westmead is shown in Chapter 3. The GCS is useful in scoring the severity of the head injury at the initial assessment, and is even more useful in monitoring progress during the acute phase of the injury.

Mild head injury (GCS 13–15)

This is the most common form of head injury, accounting for over 85% of paediatric head injuries.

Assessment

- Assessment is largely dependent upon the history and physical examination.
- If the child is neurologically normal and there is nothing to suggest the possibility of a skull fracture, no imaging is required.

Indications for skull X-ray

- Obvious injury to scalp or skull
- History of focal impact to head
- Mechanism of injury unclear
- If CT scan needs to be done (see below) it is usually not necessary to do a plain skull X-ray as well.

Indications for CT scan

- Neurological deterioration or failure to improve to a GCS of 15
- Focal neurological deficit
- Skull fracture in association with an abnormal GCS
- Possible penetrating skull injury
- CSF rhinorrhoea, otorrhoea or other suspicion of skull base fracture

Admission for observation

Strongly consider admission for observation if there is:

- any history of loss of consciousness
- post-traumatic seizure
- skull fracture or other abnormality on CT scan
- neurological deficit
- failure to improve to GCS of 15
- persistent headache, nausea or vomiting
- suspected child abuse
- absence of a suitable caretaker to observe child at home, or if the child is unable to return for further care if needed.

Moderate head injury (GCS 9–12)

The child will require admission under a neurosurgeon to either a high dependency unit or an intensive care unit.

Assessment

- ABCC review and stabilisation are essential.
- Obtain venous access and send blood for clotting studies, urea and electrolytes, Ca, LFT and glucose.
- Assume that the neck is broken and nurse the child in a hard collar until a fracture is excluded radiologically and clinically.
- Continuously monitor pulse, respiration, blood pressure and oxygen saturation.
- The Glasgow Coma Score should be reassessed each 15 minutes in the emergency room.
- A CT scan is always required; if the child is unco-operative, intubation will be needed. *Do not sedate the child unless he or she is intubated.*

Severe head injury (GCS 3–8)

The child will always require intubation, ventilatory support and admission under the care of a neurosurgeon to the intensive care unit.

Assessment

- Review ABCC; the child must be intubated, ventilated and prepared for immediate CT scan.
- Simultaneously, obtain venous access and send blood for FBC, clotting studies, urea, electrolytes, Ca and sugar; cross-match blood.
- Assume that the neck is broken and nurse the child in a hard collar until a fracture is excluded, both radiologically and clinically.
- Ventilate for end-tidal CO_2 of 35–40 mmHg and oxygen saturation of 100%. Excessive hyperventilation (end-tidal CO_2 < 30 mmHg; $PaCO_2$ < 25 mmHg) reduces cerebral flow.
- Continuously monitor pulse, respiration, blood pressure, oxygen saturation and end-tidal CO_2.
- Notify the operating theatres—most patients will require the insertion of an intracranial pressure monitor and many will require the evacuation of an intracranial mass lesion.

Mannitol

This is an osmotic diuretic, effective in reducing intracranial pressure.

- *Dosage*: 0.5–1.0 g/kg given intravenously over 20 minutes.

Indications for use in the emergency department prior to a CT scan are:

- evidence of herniation (such as pupillary dilation, bradycardia)
- evidence of mass effect (such as hemiparesis)
- sudden deterioration prior to a CT scan.

Contraindications to the use of mannitol are:

- hypotension/haemodynamic instability
- renal failure.

Post-traumatic seizures

Post-traumatic seizures occur in about 6% of children with minor head injury and become more common as the severity of the head injury increases. Seizures are associated with twice the risk of poor outcome following a head injury.

Timing of seizures

- 20% are impact seizures.
- 98% occur in the first 24 hours.
- ~ 1% occur between 1 and 7 days.
- ~ 1% occur after 7 days.

Type of seizure

- 70% are generalised tonic-clonic seizures.
- 23% are focal motor seizures.
- 7% are atypical seizures.

Post-traumatic seizures are usually benign, self-limited and rarely progress to epilepsy or recurrent seizures. Indications for drug treatment are rare but include:

- prolonged seizures
- recurrent seizures
- seizures occurring after the first week.

Skull fractures

Skull fractures are common in children. The vast majority require no specific treatment. Skull fractures are more common with increasing severity of the head injury. They are associated with a twofold increase in the risk of poor outcome and a twentyfold increase in the likelihood of requiring some form of operative intervention. With any skull fracture, consider the possibility of non-accidental injury. Have an even higher index of suspicion with 'branching' or multiple fractures, or where the history is inconsistent with the severity of the injury.

Management of linear undisplaced skull fractures

- Strongly consider admission for any child with a skull fracture.
- If the child is well and without neurological deficit, no further imaging is required and the child may be admitted for observation.
- If the child has persistent symptoms, a decreased level of consciousness, a neurological deficit or evidence of a skull base fracture, a CT scan will be required.
- The fracture itself rarely requires treatment but serves as a marker for the potential presence of an intracranial mass lesion.

Possible late complications of a linear skull fracture

- Subgaleal or subperiosteal haematomas
- Growing skull fracture (leptomeningeal cyst)

Child abuse

At least 10% of children < 10 years of age presenting to hospital with alleged accidents have been victims of abuse. Factors raising the suspicion of abuse include:

- retinal haemorrhages
- bilateral chronic subdural hygromas
- multiple skull fractures; other fractures of different ages
- often absent external signs of trauma (shaken babies).

Hydrocephalus and shunt problems

Cerebrospinal fluid (CSF) shunts are used in the management of hydrocephalus. They divert CSF from the cranium (usually the ventricle) to a distal site (usually the peritoneal cavity, less commonly pleura or right atrium) for reabsorption. This section covers only the signs of common shunt problems and initial investigations. The two most common problems are shunt malfunction (obstruction) and infection.

The child's parents are almost always right; if they think that there is a problem with the shunt, further evaluation is always necessary.

Shunt malfunction/obstruction

The shunt malfunction rate is ~ 17 % during the first year following shunt placement in the paediatric population. Approximately 45% of shunts are revised within the first 5 years.

Symptoms and signs of shunt malfunction

- Headache
- Lethargy or decreased level of consciousness
- Nausea or vomiting
- Diplopia, upward gaze palsy or visual obscuration
- Papilloedema
- Ataxia
- In infants—apnoea, bradycardia or irritability
- Seizures—new-onset or a change in the pattern of seizures
- Bulging of anterior fontanelle, prominent scalp veins
- Excessive rate of head growth, splitting of skull sutures
- Fluid along the course of the shunt

Most shunt blockages require an urgent operative procedure to revise the shunt and replace the malfunctioning component.

Shunt infection

- The shunt infection rate is ~ 7 % per procedure. Fifty per cent of infections occur within 2 weeks of the surgical procedure and 70% occur within 2 months.
- Eighty per cent of infections are due to *Staphylococcus* species.

Signs of shunt infection

- Fever
- Nausea, vomiting, lethargy, anorexia, irritability
- May mimic acute abdomen if infected CSF shunted into peritoneal cavity
- Erythema or tenderness along shunt tubing
- Wound infection
- Meningitis
- Peritonitis
- Shunt malfunction (as above)

Most shunt infections require treatment with intravenous antibiotics and surgery to remove and subsequently replace infected hardware.

Initial investigations of shunt malfunction or infection

- CT head scan
- Shunt series (skull, chest and abdominal X-rays)
- FBC, EUC, urinalysis, ESR, CRP
- CSF sampling from shunt or Rickham reservoir
- Isotope shunt study

Keep the child nil by mouth.

Consult the neurosurgeon before ordering investigations. If in doubt, admit the child for observation.

18

Renal medicine

This chapter includes:

- urinary tract infection
- nephritis
- nephrotic syndrome (NS)
- isolated proteinuria
- acute renal failure (ARF)
- haemolytic uraemic syndrome (HUS)
- hypertension.

Urinary tract infection

- Urinary tract infection (UTI) is the most common serious bacterial illness in febrile infants and children.
- Infants younger than 6 months old have a significant risk of bacteraemia.
- Early and accurate diagnosis allows appropriate management.
- Any child with an unexplained fever for more than 1 day should have a urine culture performed.

Presentation

- Infant—fever, vomiting, anorexia, irritability
- Child—fever, loin pain, frequency, dysuria, secondary enuresis

Acute pyelonephritis can be considered the likely diagnosis in any child with the above symptoms, along with significant bacteriuria and a temperature > 38°C. A DMSA renal scan is not necessary to confirm the diagnosis.

Diagnosis

- $\geq 10^8$ organisms/L on urine culture (single organism)
- Any bacteria on suprapubic aspiration (SPA) or catheter urine

Method of collection of urine

- Midstream clean catch *or* catheter *or* suprapubic aspiration
- A clear bag urine will exclude a diagnosis of UTI.

Urinalysis

A presumptive diagnosis of UTI is suggested by:

- microscopy—bacterial rods or cocci (negative microscopy does not exclude UTI).
- dipstick—nitrite and leucocyte esterase positive (a negative nitrite test and absence of pyuria do not exclude UTI).

Urinalysis may support the diagnosis of UTI and allow prompt initiation of treatment, but confirmation of UTI requires urine culture.

It is common in febrile illnesses other than UTI to see up to $100 \times 10^6/L$ white blood cells in urine; do not treat empirically as UTI without organisms and without other reasons to diagnose UTI.

Urinary pathogens

First UTI

- *E. coli*, *Klebsiella*, *Enterobacter*, enterococci
- Group B streptococcus in infants
- *Staphylococcus saprophyticus* in adolescents

Subsequent UTIs

More likely to be due to organisms other than *E. coli* (such as *Pseudomonas*), especially if the patient is on prophylactic antibiotics.

Treatment

- Prompt antibiotic treatment is required for a febrile UTI.
- Children aged less than 6 months old have an increased risk of bacteraemia and require IV antibiotics.
- For children older than 6 months if febrile (but not very unwell):
  - 'stat' dose (for example, IM gentamicin or cephalosporin)
  - oral antibiotics for 10 days (cephalexin, trimethoprim sulpha-methoxazole, amoxycillin–clavulanic acid).
- Children who are toxic, or are not tolerating oral fluids or medication, require IV fluids and IV gentamicin and ampicillin.
- A vomiting child should receive $1\frac{1}{2} \times$ maintenance fluids unless renal function is impaired.

- Continue IV antibiotics until the child is afebrile for 24–36 hours.
- Change to the oral antibiotic to which the organism is sensitive and give for 7–10 days.
- Repeat urine culture at the conclusion of treatment.
- Continue prophylactic antibiotics until renal imaging is completed.
- Children with a non-febrile UTI may be treated with a 2–4 day course of oral antibiotics.

Investigation of febrile UTIs

Aim to identify children at risk for renal damage. Risk factors include:

- renal tract obstruction
- severe vesicoureteric reflux (VUR)
- neurogenic bladder.

All children with a febrile UTI should have a *renal ultrasound* performed within the first few days. It identifies obstruction, hydronephrosis, absent or dysplastic kidneys, and pyelonephrosis.

Further investigation depends on the age of the child:

- *Micturating cystourethrogram*
  - < 2 years—once the urine is clear. Antibiotic prophylaxis is recommended to prevent infection at the time of the procedure.
  - 2 years or older—only if abnormalities are demonstrated on ultrasound, or if scarring is present on later DMSA scan.
- *DMSA scan*
  - A renal scan should be performed more than 6 months after the acute infection to determine the presence of permanent renal damage.
  - Small renal scars detected on DMSA scan do not alter patient management as their significance is uncertain.
  - Moderate to severe renal scarring in a child over 2 years may be an indication for micturating cystourethrogram.

Long-term considerations

Long-term prophylactic antibiotics are indicated in moderate to severe VUR and for children with frequent symptomatic UTIs. The usual indication for surgical correction of VUR is breakthrough infections occurring while on prophylactic antibiotics. Children with severe VUR may have small scarred kidneys secondary to dysplastic changes occurring in utero rather than as a consequence of UTI.

Preschool children may have recurrent UTI related to bladder instability and constipation, and treatment of these is important regardless of whether VUR is present. Any child with severe pyelonephritis may develop renal scarring even when VUR is not associated. An annual BP is recommended for all children with moderate to severe renal scarring.

Children likely to develop renal impairment are those children with dysplastic kidneys (± VUR), obstructive lesions and neuro-pathic bladder abnormalities.

Nephritis

Presentation

- Haematuria
- Oliguria
- Oedema
- Hypertension
- Reduced renal function

Investigations

- Urine:
  - Red blood cells (number and morphology)
  - Casts (red cell, white cell, granular)
  - Proteinuria
- Blood:
  - Full blood count, ESR
  - Renal function tests
- Serum ASOT, anti-DNase B
- Serum C3, C4
- Double-stranded DNA (ANA)
- Swabs:
  - Throat swab (if history of pharyngitis)
  - Skin swab (if impetigo)

Differential diagnosis

Postinfectious glomerulonephritis (GN)

Poststreptococcal GN

- Previous pharyngitis or skin lesions (may be no history)
- ASOT and/or anti-DNase B elevated
- Low C3, C4 normal or slightly low
- Hypertension—secondary to salt and water overload
- *Treatment:*
  - Hypertension: frusemide 1–5 mg/kg/dose, ± calcium channel blocker, such as nifedipine 5–10 mg orally
  - No added salt diet; limited fluid intake
  - Penicillin if *Streptococcus* is still present
- *Follow-up:*
  - Repeat C3 in 8–12 weeks to confirm return to normal.
  - Consider mesangiocapillary GN if C3 is persistently low.
  - Note that abnormal urinary red blood cells and protein may last 12 months or longer.

Other postinfectious GN (usually have low C3)

- Secondary to infected ventriculoperitoneal shunt
- Associated with bacterial endocarditis

IgA nephritis

- There is an intercurrent viral infection at the time of presentation.
- The patient may have recurrent episodes of macroscopic haematuria.
- Microscopic haematuria may persist between episodes.
- Increasing proteinuria is a poor prognostic sign.
- Nephrotic syndrome ± reduced renal function is a bad prognostic sign.

Rarer differential diagnoses

- Rapidly progressive GN, suggested by deteriorating renal function
- Systemic lupus erythematosis (usually low C3, C4)
- Mesangiocapillary GN (usually low C3)
- Hereditary nephritis (Alport's syndrome)—consider with increasing proteinuria and decreasing renal function in the second decade, in males

Indications for renal biopsy

- Concern over rapidly progressive course
- Doubt about the diagnosis
- Presence of nephrotic syndrome and reduced renal function

Nephrotic syndrome (NS)

Presentation

- Oedema
- Proteinuria
- Hypoalbuminaemia
- Hyperlipidaemia

The majority of children have steroid-responsive, minimal-change nephrotic syndrome. The course may be characterised by multiple relapses but the NS eventually resolves and renal function remains normal. Transient hypertension, microscopic haematuria and azotaemia may be consistent with minimal change GN.

Investigations at presentation

- Serum albumin < 25g/L, urine protein > 50 mg/kg/day or > 40 mg/m²/day or urine protein/creatinine ratio > 0.35
- Renal function tests
- Hepatitis B surface antigen test if child is older or a migrant

Complications

- Thrombosis—secondary to haemoconcentration and urinary loss of antithrombin III. This can involve any vessels, but most often the renal veins or sagittal sinuses.
- Infection:
  - Secondary to loss of factor B—necessary for opsonisation of encapsulated bacteria
  - Increased risk of sepsis from pneumococci, *Haemophilus* and *E. coli*
- Acute renal failure—secondary to hypovolaemia
- Hyperlipidaemia (raised cholesterol, triglycerides, LDL, VLDL)

Management

Manage oedema and hypovolaemia—most children with minimal change NS are euvolaemic. However, in children with rapid onset of

NS, sudden fall in plasma oncotic pressure and massive oedema, plasma volume is low. Additional fluid losses increase the risk of hypovolaemia. Urinary sodium < 5 mmol/L indicates maximum sodium conservation secondary to hyperaldosteronism.

Treating hypovolaemia

Use albumin infusion with frusemide.

- Give albumin 20%—1 g/kg as a slow IV infusion, over 3–4 hours *plus* frusemide 1 mg/kg halfway through, then repeated at the end of the infusion.
- Albumin is used only with minimal change NS and with normal renal function. It is not appropriate for other causes of NS.
- Intravenous albumin should always be given with a diuretic unless there is severe intravascular depletion. Too-rapid movement of fluid into the vascular space may cause hypertension and convulsions. Children should be monitored (BP, RR, HR) every 30 minutes during infusion.
- Diuretics should generally not be given without albumin as this increases the risk of hypovolaemia and hypercoagulation.
- *Antibiotics*: Prophylactic penicillin should be given while the child is nephrotic.
- *Pneumococcal vaccines*: Pneumococcal conjugate vaccine (7vPCV) is recommended for all children with NS aged below 5 years. Currently, pneumococcal polysaccharide vaccine (PPV23) is recommended for children aged 5 years or more. Vaccines may be given during prednisolone therapy. They do not protect against all strains of pneumococcus.

Immunosuppression regimens for steroid sensitive NS

- Prednisolone
  - *At initial presentation*: 60 mg/m^2 (approx. 2 mg/kg) for 1 month. Alternate day regimen starting at 60 mg/m^2 and reducing the dose slowly over 6 months.
  - *Subsequent relapses*: 60 mg/m^2 but taper the dose once protein-free (urine protein/creatinine ratio < 0.02) for 3 consecutive days.
  - *Frequent relapses*: Low dose alternate day treatment: aim for 2.5 mg above the dose at which the last relapse occurred. If maintenance prednisolone of more than 0.5 mg/kg alternate

days is needed, or if there are marked Cushingoid side-effects (especially slowing of growth rate) consider alternative immunosuppression.

- Cyclophosphamide: 2–3 mg/kg/day for 8–12 weeks. FBC should be carried out fortnightly during treatment and the child should be given trimethoprim/sulphamethoxazole as prophylaxis against pneumocystis.
- Cyclosporin A: This is reserved for frequently relapsing NS where cyclophosphamide has failed to provide a prolonged remission or is considered contraindicated (for example, in a child who has not had chickenpox).

Indications for renal biopsy

- Steroid resistance—no response within 4–6 weeks of full dose prednisolone
- Clinical features suggesting that the NS may not be due to minimal-change GN

The aim of the biopsy is to confirm or exclude focal segmental glomerulosclerosis (FSGS) or other causes of NS which may have a different prognosis to minimal-change GN. During adolescence the risk of focal segmental glomerulosclerosis and membranous GN approaches that of the adult population, with minimal-change GN in only 30–40%.

Isolated proteinuria

Proteinuria is usually detected on urine dipstick analysis. '0–trace' is seen in healthy children. Up to '2+' may be seen in normal children following exercise, and may be associated with macroscopic haematuria.

Assessment of proteinuria

Assessment of proteinuria may be by:

- protein/creatinine ratio (g/mmol)
  - children < 2 years—normal < 0.05
  - children > 2 years—normal < 0.02
  - nephrotic range > 0.35
- 24-hour urinary protein:
  - *Normal value* is < 150 mg or 4 mg/m^2.

- *Nephrotic range* is > 3 g/24 h or > 40 mg/m^2/day.
- *Normal adolescents* may excrete 300–400 mg/day due to a change in body habitus.
- The commonest cause of isolated protein excretion of less than 1 g/day is orthostatic proteinuria.
- An early morning specimen for protein/creatinine ratio or timed overnight urine collection will help identify orthostatic proteinuria as the underlying cause.
- Renal biopsy is usually considered if more than 1–1.5 g/24 hours is excreted.

Acute renal failure (ARF)

This term refers to an acute change in renal function resulting in the inability to excrete a renal solute load. Commoner causes of acute renal failure are:

- prerenal:
  - hypovolaemia (for example, due to severe dehydration)
  - shock (from whatever cause)
- renal:
  - haemolytic uraemic syndrome
  - acute tubular necrosis (ATN)
  - vascular—venous or arterial disease
  - acute severe GN
  - tumour lysis syndrome
- post-renal:
  - lower urinary tract obstruction.

Investigations

- Blood:
  - FBC, differential white cell count
  - Electrolytes
  - Urea, creatinine, Ca, Mg, PO$_4$, bicarbonate
  - Serum albumin, C3, C4
- Urine:
  - White cells, red cells, casts
  - Osmolality
  - Sodium
  - Microscopy, culture and sensitivities

- Imaging:
  - Renal ultrasound

The following tests differentiating pre-renal ARF from ATN:

- Urinary sodium:
  - < 10 mmol/L: suggests prerenal ARF
  - > 20 mmol/L: suggests established ATN
  - *Note*: Urine is collected before the diuretic and saline are given.
- Diuretic and fluid challenge:
  - If there is hypovolaemia, give 10–20 mL/kg colloid and 1–2 mg/kg frusemide IV.
  - If there is normovolaemia or hypervolaemia, give 1–2 mg/kg frusemide IV.
  - If there is no response, treat as ATN.

Management

- Fluids:
  - 150–200 mL/m^2/day = insensible loss *plus* previous day's fluid output (that is, urinary and gastrointestinal losses)
  - Aim to lose 0.1–0.2 kg/day.
- Treating complications:
  - *Hypertension*: If sodium and water restriction are insufficient, add calcium channel blockers or clonidine. (*Note*: avoid beta-blockers if there is fluid overload, and avoid ACE inhibitors as they cause potassium retention.)
  - *Acidosis*: Sodium bicarbonate 2 mmol/kg IV.
  - *Hyperkalaemia*: See Table 18.1.
  - *Hypocalcaemia*: calcium gluconate 10% 0.5 mg/kg IV (with cardiac monitor)
  - *Hypomagnesaemia*: magnesium sulphate IM (see p. 451)
  - *Hyperphosphataemia*: oral calcium carbonate, until urine output re-established (see p. 422)
- *Drug dosage*: A decrease in the frequency of administration of antibiotics (especially aminoglycosides) is required in ARF (see *Therapeutic Guidelines: Antibiotic*); cardiac glycoside doses should also be lowered.
- Indications for dialysis:
  - If the clinical course suggests a prolonged period of oliguria is likely

Table 18.1 Treatment of hyperkalaemia—alternatives

Drug/dose to treat hyperkalaemia	Action	Duration
Salbutamol 4 mg/kg IV over 20 min or nebulised 2.5 mg (< 25 kg); 5 mg (> 25 kg)	30 min Over 10 min	4–6 hours
Sodium bicarbonate 1–2 mmol/kg IV	10–30 min	2 hours
Glucose 0.5–1 g/kg IV ($\pm$ insulin 0.1 U/kg)	30 min	2 hours
Calcium gluconate 10% 0.5–1 mg/kg IV	1–3 min	30 min
Ion exchange resin (Resonium) 1 g/kg orally or rectally	1–2 hours	4–6 hours

- – Presence of salt and water overload producing hypertension or pulmonary oedema
- – Hyperkalaemia (> 6 mmol/L)
- – Uncontrolled acidosis
- – Uraemia
- – If blood transfusion is required
- Forms of dialysis:
  - – Peritoneal
  - – Haemofiltration
  - – Haemodialysis

Haemolytic uraemic syndrome (HUS)

Haemolytic uraemic syndrome (HUS) is the commonest cause of ARF in childhood. Haemolytic anaemia with fragmented red blood cells and thrombocytopenia is often identified on peripheral blood films.

Epidemic or diarrhoea-associated HUS

- Toxin-producing *E. coli* is isolated in more than 75% of cases. The most common serotype in Australia is 0111, rather than 0157, seen overseas. Other organisms that are rarely involved include *Shigella*, *Campylobacter* and *Pneumococcus*.
- One week after the diarrhoea, ARF, microangiopathic haemolytic anaemia and thrombocytopenia develop.

- The disease is notifiable and can be associated with large outbreaks.
- The microangiopathic process may involve other organs rarely, producing cardiomyopathy, cerebral infarcts or haemorrhages, bowel perforation and diabetes.
- Treatment is supportive, with early dialysis and blood transfusion as indicated. Platelets are usually not required as these children rarely bleed due to thrombocytopenia. Platelet transfusion is required only if there is acute haemorrhage, as extraneous platelets are usually consumed in the microangiopathic process. Blood transfusion is contraindicated if *Pneumococcus* is the causative agent.
- The long-term prognosis for renal function is generally good.

Atypical or sporadic HUS

This is uncommon.

- There may be an insidious onset or a preceding URTI. Severe hypertension is common and irreversible renal failure occurs more frequently. This disease may be familial (autosomal recessive or rarely dominant). Recurrent episodes are common. There is overlap with TTP with some patients having CNS involvement.
- Plasma exchange is indicated in addition to supportive dialysis and blood transfusion.
- The renal prognosis for atypical HUS is poor, with a 50% risk of disease recurrence after renal transplantation.

Hypertension

Most acute hypertension in childhood is due to glomerulonephritis. Chronic hypertension is most commonly associated with renal parenchymal disease but a small proportion will have renovascular hypertension, phaeochromocytoma or coarctation of the aorta.

Measurement

Blood pressure readings are unreliable in anxious or crying children. The bladder cuff should completely encircle the arm, and should be wide enough to cover approximately 75% of the upper arm between the top of the shoulder and the elbow. Using a cuff that is too small results in a falsely high reading. High readings should be confirmed with two or three additional measurements in circumstances designed to relieve the child's anxiety.

Normal range

See Table 18.2. Levels above the 95th percentile require further evaluation. Blood pressure levels persistently more than 10 mmHg above the 95th percentile warrant detailed investigation and consideration of therapy.

Table 18.2 Percentile blood pressure (mmHg) at various ages

Age (years)	50th percentile		95th percentile	
	Systolic	Diastolic	Systolic	Diastolic
1	90	60	110	75
5	95	60	115	75
10	105	65	125	80
15	115	65	135	85
18	120	70	140	90

Diagnostic evaluation of the hypertensive child

Initial evaluation

- Full blood count
- Renal function tests
- Urinalysis
- Urine culture
- Renal ultrasound

Additional tests as indicated

- Echocardiography
- Plasma renin
- Cholesterol, triglycerides, LDL, VLDL, HDL
- Calcium, phosphorus, uric acid
- Doppler ultrasound of renal arteries
- Plasma and urinary catecholamines
- Measurement of plasma and urinary steroids
- Renal arteriography (only after urinary catecholamines have excluded phaeochromocytoma)

Hypertensive emergencies

When seizures, severe headaches, eye changes or cardiac failure occur with hypertension, immediate blood pressure reduction is required (see Tables 18.3a and 18.3b). Intravenous treatment should be started with IV sodium nitroprusside or labetolol infusion if available. Bolus doses of clonidine or hydralazine can be given initially where an infusion is unavailable. It is recommended that children with longstanding hypertension have a 20–30% reduction in their mean arterial pressure over 60–90 minutes.

Drugs for maintenance therapy

The aim of treatment is reduction of blood pressure to a level below the 95th percentile. Therapy is usually initiated with either an ACE inhibitor or a calcium channel blocker because of their efficacy and fewer side-effects. Diuretic therapy should be considered in patients with renal disease who are salt- and water-overloaded. Weight reduction, salt restriction and exercise should be encouraged in obese adolescents.

Beta-blockers are available if multiple medications are required for control of the hypertension or the tachycardia produced by calcium channel blockers. Beta-blockers should be avoided in children with asthma, cardiac failure or heart block. Children tend to become drowsy when centrally acting drugs are used. Phenoxybenzamine or labetolol are the drugs of choice for phaeochromocytoma.

Drugs for maintenance oral therapy

See Table 18.4.

Table 18.3a Drug treatment of hypertensive crisis

Medication	Dose	Max. dose	Side-effects
Sodium nitroprusside 50 mg/vial	0.3–0.8 micrograms/kg/min via continuous IV infusion	10 micrograms/kg/min. If ineffective in 10 min, stop.	Caution regarding cyanide toxicity (should only be used for 48 hours in renal failure)
Labetolol 100 mg/20 mL	1 mg/kg/h by continuous IV infusion ↑ by $^{1}/_{4}$–$^{1}/_{2}$ mg/kg/h every $^{1}/_{2}$ hour until reaching desired level	3 mg/kg/h	Hypotension; bradycardia (not for use with cardiac failure, asthma, severe bradycardia)
Clonidine 150 micrograms/mL	3–6 micrograms/kg in 10 mL 0.9% saline over 5 min Repeat every 4 hours	900 micrograms/day	Sedation, dizziness, dry mouth, nausea and vomiting, bradycardia
Hydralazine solution 1 microgram/mL	Initial dose 0.15–0.8 mg/kg/dose /IV 4–6-hourly	25 mg/dose IV	Flushing, headaches, vomiting, drug-induced lupus

Table 18.3b Oral drug treatment of acute hypertension requiring immediate therapy

Medication	Dose	Max. dose	Side-effects
Nifedipine tablets—10 mg, 20 mg	0.5–1.0 mg/kg/dose 4–6 hourly	20 mg	Tachycardia, headache, flushing
Clonidine tablets—150 micrograms	3–6 micrograms/dose 4–6-hourly	300 micrograms	Sedation, rebound hypertension

Table 18.4 Oral antihypertensive for maintenance therapy

Medication	Dose	Max. dose	Side-effects
Calcium-channel blockers			
Nifedipine Tablets: 10 mg 20 mg Long-acting: 30 mg (daily dose)	Initial: 0.5 mg/kg/day in 2 divided doses Maintenance: 1–1.5 mg/kg/day	10–30 mg/dose	Tachycardia, headache, flushing
Amlodipine Tablets: 5 mg 10 mg Can be dissolved	Initial: 0.1–0.2 mg/kg/day single dose Maintenance: 0.1–0.3 mg/kg/day single dose	15 mg/day	Long half-life Adjust dosage every 3–5 days Decrease dose in hepatic impairment
ACE inhibitors			
Captopril Tablets: 12.5 mg 25 mg 50 mg Can be dissolved	Initial: 0.1–0.3 mg/kg/dose 8-hourly Maintenance: 0.3–4 mg/kg/day in 3 doses	6 mg/kg/day	Hyperkalaemia, cough, rash, angioneurotic oedema (ARF with renal artery stenosis)

continues . . .

Table 18.4 Oral antihypertensive for maintenance therapy
(continued)

Medication	Dose	Max. dose	Side-effects
Enalapril Tablets: 2.5 mg 5 mg 10 mg 20 mg	Initial: 0.2 mg/kg/day single dose Maintenance: 0.2–1.0 mg/kg/day single dose	40 mg/day	As above
Lisinopril Tablets: 5 mg 10 mg 20 mg Can be dissolved	Initial: 0.1 mg/kg/day single dose Maintenance: 0.2–0.4 mg/kg/day single dose	40 mg/day	As above
Beta-blockers			
Metoprolol Tablets: 50 mg 100 mg	1–4 mg/kg/day 1–2 doses	400 mg/day	May exacerbate asthma, cardiac failure and heart block
Atenolol Tablets: 50 mg	1–4 mg/kg/day single dose	200 mg/day	As above
Labetolol Tablets: 100 mg 200 mg	2–4 mg/kg/day in 2 divided doses	600 mg/day	As above
Centrally acting drugs			
Clonidine Tablets: 150 micro- grams	3–15 micrograms/kg/ day in 3 divided doses	900 micro- grams/day	Rebound HT may occur with sudden cessation
Methyldopa Tablets: 125 mg 250 mg	10–45 mg/kg/day in 3 divided doses	2250 mg daily	Sedation, abnormal LFTs

19

Psychiatry

This chapter includes:

- situations requiring immediate psychiatric consultation
- non-urgent referral
- non-accidental self-harm
- psychiatric assessment for non-psychiatrists
- managing the disruptive child
- depression
- medical presentations of psychiatric conditions and vice versa.

Situations requiring immediate psychiatric consultation

- A child or adolescent presenting as a *danger to themselves or others* (see 'Non-accidental self-harm', p. 266, and 'Depression and suicidality', p. 287)
- A child or adolescent who appears to have a *major psychiatric disorder*
- Before admitting any child whose *primary problem* is a psychiatric disorder
- Before admitting a medical or surgical patient who is *likely to be very disruptive* in the hospital
- Before prescribing major psychiatric medications, such as antipsychotics and newer antidepressants. Use of many of these is restricted, within the hospital, to psychiatrists.

Note: Initial contact should be by telephone. In normal working hours, contact the Department of Psychological Medicine; outside normal working hours, contact the child psychiatry registrar via the hospital switchboard.

Non-urgent referral

- The Department of Psychological Medicine gives priority to the psychiatric needs of medical and surgical in-patients of the hospital.
- The Department of Psychological Medicine is often involved with children suffering complex, long-term illnesses.
- Out-patient services are provided for children with emotional and psychiatric problems beyond the scope of the referring practitioner.
- Outreach services are provided, in part via telemedicine, to many district centres in New South Wales.

Referral is via letter to the intake psychiatrist in the Department of Psychological Medicine.

Non-accidental self-harm

This term encompasses a range of situations from *dangerous suicide attempts* to *lesser degrees of self-harm*, which may indicate a widely variable degree of psychiatric disturbance and/or family disarray. Non-accidental self-harm is a 'marker' that the young person perceives a severe problem in his or her life and has ineffective ways of coping with the problem.

Common underlying problems predisposing to non-accidental self-harm

- Chronic physical illness
- Drug and alcohol problems in self and/or family
- Poor school achievement and poor peer relationships
- Family conflict and/or psychiatric illness
- Unusual life stresses such as sexual abuse

Assessment of obvious or possible non-accidental self-harm

- Every instance of suicidal ideation or intention, with or without actual self-harm, requires assessment.
- What was the nature and potential lethality of the suicide attempt? Did the person *intend* the self-harm to be fatal?
- Has there previously been self-harm (including suicide attempts)?

- Are there underlying predisposing problems (see above)?
- Are there disruptive precipitating social events, including death (especially suicide) of a family member or peer? Are these still current?
- Was there concealment of the seriousness of the suicide attempt?
- With injuries claimed as accidental, is the history bizarre or are the injuries inconsistent with the history?

Management of an instance of non-accidental self-harm

- The first priority is medical treatment for the injury or ingestion.
- Every instance that is considered serious should be discussed initially by telephone with the psychiatric registrar on call.
- Asking about suicidal thoughts in those at risk will not in itself encourage suicidal behaviour and may bring out helpful information.
- The need for hospital admission or other care arrangements will be decided in conjunction with the psychiatric registrar.
- The five key questions are:
  1 Is suicidality still present?
  2 Is there an underlying treatable psychiatric condition?
  3 Is there a social predicament to be addressed?
  4 Is there a place of safety with appropriate people to help/ supervise?
  5 Is the young person likely to be disruptive or attempt to run away?
- Some patients who are mentally disordered and a risk to themselves or others may require scheduling, which must be done in accordance with New South Wales legal requirements and only after psychiatric consultation.
- Develop a plan of action which will include an emergency plan for any subsequent crisis.

Non-accidental self-harm assessment interview: a summary

- *Establish contact*. See the parents and the child separately as well as together. Listen to the young person. Be calm and take control. Show realistic hopefulness.
- *Understand the attempt*. Get details of what occurred.
- *Explore suicidal ideation*. For how long, how intense?

- *Explore suicidal plans.* Is there evidence of premeditation, planning, anger at being found?
- *Assess previous attempts.*
- *Find out about current problems.* Make a list for 'solving'.
- *Explore coping methods.* 'How do you react to finding out …?', etc.
- *Clarify safety issues* with the legal guardian and the young person. Where can the young person go? From whom will he or she accept support, protection and supervision?
- Conclude with giving *a plan of action* which will now be followed.

Questions to ask
Suicidality

- Have you ever just wanted to get away from it all?
- Do you ever feel like going to sleep and not waking up?
- Have you ever wished that you could die?
- Have you ever wanted to hurt yourself?
- In what ways have you thought about hurting yourself?
- Do you want to hurt yourself now?
- Do you want to die now?

Support

- Who is worried most about what you have done?
- Who knows best how to make you feel better when you feel bad?
- Who would have missed you most if you had succeeded?

Coping

- Can you think of any reasons for going on living? If 'no', have you always felt this way?
- Can you think back to when life was OK?
- What was different then? If your problems could be sorted out, would you still want to hurt yourself?
- Tell me about the part of you that wants to keep living.

Psychiatric assessment for non-psychiatrists

The following brief guide will assist in assessing a child where a significant emotional or psychiatric condition is suspected. Avoid the common error of being medically unsystematic when dealing with children with psychiatric disorders.

- Start with a standard, comprehensive *medical history* and *physical examination*.
- Ask about the *presenting* (?emotional/psychiatric) *complaint*: what was the duration? what was the severity? what makes it worse? what helps? what effect has it had on the family? what would the parents like to see happen?
- Extend the family history to include:
  - physical and psychiatric *family history* (including suicide or other deaths)
  - personality, upbringing and schooling of *parents and siblings*
  - drug and/or alcohol abuse; criminal history.
- Take special note of:
  - problems during *pregnancy* with that child
  - how the mother felt towards that child before/after birth and subsequently
  - any problems in development
  - problems reported by preschool teachers, teachers and peers.
- Ask about interpersonal relationships:
  - with family members, peers
  - any physical or sexual abuse
  - sexual orientation, anxieties, practices, problems with puberty
- Ask specifically about (if appropriate):
  - *attentiveness*: activity level, clumsiness, weakness, tics, gait
  - *sleep*: nightmares, night terrors, sleepwalking
  - *habits*: including nail biting, thumb sucking, head banging/rocking, repetitive habits, comforting behaviours and favourite routines
  - *speech*: normal progression, delay, comprehension
  - *vision and hearing* including hallucinations, frightening dreams while awake
  - *thought processes*: concentration, daydreaming, delusions, muddled thoughts
  - *personality and behaviour*: emotional expression, worries, fears, phobias, aggression, excitability, adaptability, disobedience
  - *antisocial behaviour*: lying, stealing, fighting, alcohol/drugs, trouble with school authorities/police/courts
  - *fantasy life*: games played and their content, imagination, imaginary friends, transitional objects, times when 'in a world of their own'
  - *attack disorders*: breath-holding, fits, fainting.

- *Mental state examination*: in addition to your neurological examination, note:
  - *appearance and behaviour*: attire, cleanliness, self-care, appropriateness of clothing, general health, injuries, nonverbal communication, language, motor function, interaction with interviewer
  - *speech*: rate, quantity, pattern, perseveration, articulation, vocabulary, ability to read and write
  - *thought*: content, avoided subjects, preoccupations, thought flow, unusual use of language, hallucinations, delusions, obsessions, phobias, paranoia
  - apparent *intellectual ability*
  - *mood and affect*: is the child happy? sad? fearful? angry? suicidal? Observe the child for appropriate affect: is he/she blunted? labile? perplexed? suspicious?
  - *attitude* to family, friends and school; fantasy life (the child's three magical wishes, the three most wanted people on a deserted island).
  - *observed play*: content, concentration, distractability, imagination; significance or symbolism demonstrated?
  - Consider use of the mini mental state examination.

Managing the disruptive child

Disruptive children and adolescents in the Emergency Department or wards can be very difficult to assess and contain safely in the hospital setting. Disruptive behaviour can be secondary to psychosis, substance abuse, head injury, developmental delay or family chaos or disarray. Making an accurate diagnosis is essential. However, only immediate management steps are included below.

Five 'Don'ts'

1 Don't accept the assessment and admission of a disruptive patient over the phone without consulting the on-call psychiatric registrar.
2 Don't admit disruptive patients because they have been abandoned by their parents; for these, the Department of Community Services should be notified immediately.
3 Don't admit disruptive patients to the wards in order to solve an Emergency Department problem.

4 Don't admit disruptive patients without considering oral, IM or IV sedation.

5 Don't deal with difficult interactions with multiple 'spectators', such as in waiting areas.

Five 'Do's'

1 Do warn staff if a known potentially disruptive patient is to be admitted.

2 Do make sure others are around when you interview, and consider alerting security staff.

3 Do avoid confronting, 'make or break' interactions and shouting.

4 Do have one person in charge and avoid others 'putting their oar in'.

5 Do get children and non-involved families out of the way.

Management

- Seek a quiet location where there is no audience.
- Avoid confinement, at least initially.
- Ask individuals who may inflame to leave and individuals who calm to stay.
- Consider what examinations *must* be done and what examinations *can* be done. Do what can be done initially and define what must be done later.
- If restraint is necessary it must be planned, decisive, effective and speedy.
- The person carrying out sedation or investigation must not be trying to restrain as well.
- Use of sedative or any other medication would usually be considered only after discussion with a psychiatrist and/or a senior emergency physician.
- If the child agrees to take oral medication the following can be considered:
  - *risperidone* syrup: 0.25–1 mg depending on the child's size
  - *olanzapine* wafer 5 mg or tablet 2.5 mg.
  The above can be combined with oral *diazepam*, 2.5–10 mg depending on the child's size.
- If IM sedation is required, consider either droperidol or midazolam or a combination. *Do not give diazepam by intramuscular injection.*
  - *Droperidol* 0.1–0.3 mg/kg/dose to a maximum dose of 10 mg
  - IM droperidol is very effective in 20 minutes

- *Midazolam* 0.2 mg/kg to a maximum of 10 mg
- If IV sedation is required, consider droperidol followed by diazepam. Monitor vital signs. Give *droperidol 0.1–0.3 mg/kg/dose* diluted with water *to a maximum of 10 mg*, over 5 minutes. Give *diazepam 0.2 mg/kg/dose* diluted with water until clear *to a maximum of 20 mg*.
- Rarely, dystonias including laryngeal spasm causing respiratory obstruction may occur using droperidol, requiring benztropine 0.5–2 mg IM.
- Physical restraint may be needed, while awaiting the onset of action of medication.
- Arrange for a psychiatric assessment after you have dealt with the crisis, if you have not already done so.
- Recheck to see if you have missed any medical issues or issues that the psychiatry team should know about.

Depression

From age 6 years children often express sadness and by 7–8 years of age express negative feelings about themselves. Significant depression affects at least 2% of children from this age, and at least 4% of adolescents. (See also 'Depression and suicidality', p. 287.)

Presentation

- Symptoms may include low mood, tearfulness, sleep and appetite disturbance, poor concentration, deterioration in school performance, loss of interest in previously enjoyed activities and suicidal thoughts.
- *Developmental variations*:
  - In pre-adolescents, somatic complaints (such as headache and abdominal pain) and separation anxiety may predominate; mood irritability may be more prominent than sadness. The child will often appear sad, inactive, tearful and bored.
  - Adolescents generally follow 'adult' patterns, with inability to enjoy pleasurable activities, hypersomnia, hopelessness, and reduction in energy and concentration. Drug abuse might occur, to obtain relief, and suicidal thought might be implied or expressed. In adolescents, parents often complain of the tetrad of increased irritability, social withdrawal, drop-off in school performance and combativeness.

Comorbidity is common, especially involving anxiety and behaviour disorders.

Assessment

- Elucidate symptoms and signs; non-communicativeness is a clear sign.
- Get information from more than one source. Include the school and, if possible, a friend.
- See the parents and child separately, as well as together.
- Assess the suicide risk (see 'Non-accidental self-harm', p. 266).
- Assess coping at school, with friends and at home.
- Look for 'acute' events and long-term 'stressors', especially parental marital discord.
- Assess medical problems, drug and alcohol use/abuse.
- Assess sexual history, including the possibility of pregnancy and recent break-ups.
- Assess important relationships and identify 'key' helpers and detractors.

Action

- If the child is suicidal, refer at once to psychiatry (see above).
- For non-suicidal out-patients, refer to psychiatry for an early appointment.
- Principles of management include:
  - explaining, educating and reassuring about the generally good prognosis of depression in childhood and adolescence
  - minimising suicide risk. This includes *not* prescribing tricyclic antidepressants. This group of drugs is generally contraindicated for treatment of depression in adolescents. Use newer antidepressants, family work, cognitive or other psychotherapy, as indicated.

Medical presentation of psychiatric conditions and vice versa

- Almost any medical symptom may be evoked, made worse, prolonged, elaborated or obscured by psychological factors (see Table 19.1).

- Children with medical problems may have unrelated psychological problems and vice versa.
- Children with protracted medical problems will almost always have some emotional sequelae, which may predominate or outlast the original problem.
- Conversion disorder is very uncommon before the age of 7 years.

Table 19.1 Some examples of symptoms and signs which may indicate both medical and psychiatric conditions

Symptom/sign	Usually suggests	May be an indication of
Acute stridor	Croup	Hysterical stridor (in a child of 7 years or older).
Hyperventilation	Anxiety	Asthma. *Note*: This could be due to either, or both, in a child or adolescent with asthma.
Acute abdominal pain	Many potential medical and surgical causes	Aerophagy due to anxiety
Recurrent abdominal pain (older child)	Idiopathic abdominal pain of later childhood	Peptic ulceration, renal disease, gallstones
Acute vomiting	Gastroenteritis, other medical/surgical conditions	Somatisation of psychological symptoms
Chronic pain	Wide variety of medical problems	Underlying depression
Seizures	Epilepsy	'Pseudoseizures', associated with psychological problems; may occur in known epileptics
Amenorrhoea	Gynaecological cause	Anorexia nervosa
Diffuse muscle pain	Systemic disease	Hyperventilation due to long-standing anxiety
Limb paralysis	Acute neurological problem	Conversion disorder

Table 19.1 Some examples of symptoms and signs which may indicate both medical and psychiatric conditions *(continued)*

Symptom/sign	Usually suggests	May be an indication of
Confusional state	Drug overdose, acute neurological condition	Hysterical fugue
Carpopedal spasm	Hypocalcaemia	Hyperventilation from anxiety
Complex partial seizures	Epilepsy variant	Masturbatory habit disorder, in 3–5 year olds
Deafness	Glue ear, congenital deafness	Autism spectrum disorders
Mutism	Organic cause	Selective mutism
Inanition, inability to walk, speak	Major systemic illness	Pervasive refusal disorder

20

The adolescent patient

This chapter includes:

- normal adolescent development
- puberty
- history and examination
- problems of growth and physical development
- nutritional problems
- orthopaedic problems
- chronic illness and disability
- depression and suicidality
- adolescent sexuality and sexual health
- sexually transmitted diseases
- the symptomatic adolescent.

Normal adolescent development

Adolescence is a time of physical, psychological and emotional transition from childhood to adulthood. Prerequisites of good medical assessment and care include:

- a comfortable, confidential approach by the physician
- recognition that adolescents have neither the naivety of the child nor the awareness or experience of the adult
- knowledge of presentations of conditions affecting adolescents.

Substages of adolescence

Early adolescence (10–14 years)

Predominant issues are the new bodily sensations, changes of puberty and a preoccupation with normality. The same-sex peer group becomes all important and separating from parents begins. High levels of physical activity and mood swings are common.

Mid-adolescence (14–17 years)

Major conflicts are over independence. The peer group sets behaviour standards as parents begin to exert less authority. There is enjoyment of new intellectual powers. Efforts to establish a functional sexual identity have a narcissistic quality.

Late adolescence (17–20 years)

The emphasis is on functional role definition in work, lifestyle and relationship plans. A degree of emancipation, a realistic body image and gender role identification will have been established. Relationships tend to involve mutual caring and responsibility.

Puberty

Definition

Puberty is the attainment of secondary sexual characteristics and reproductive capacity. The age of onset for girls is 8–13.5 years; for boys 9.5–14 years.

Events of puberty

These follow a sequence, but timing is very variable.

- The average duration is about 3 years.
- The Tanner Staging System (Tables 20.1 and 20.2) is based on breast, genital and pubic hair changes, with Stage 1 being prepubertal and Stage 5 adult.
- Height velocity and weight velocity increase and peak during the adolescent growth spurt.
- In girls, peak height velocity (PHV) occurs early (Stages 2–3), while menarche is a late event (Stage 4).
- In boys, first ejaculation (semenarche) normally occurs around mid-puberty (Stage 3); PHV is achieved later than in girls (Stage 4).
- Sensitivity about aspects of normal growth and development are common and require reassurance.

Table 20.1 Classification of genital maturity stages in girls

Stage	Pubic hair	Breasts
1	Preadolescent	Preadolescent
2	Sparse, lightly pigmented, straight, medial border of labia	Breast and papilla elevated as small mound; areolar diameter increased 'bud' stage
3	Darker, beginning to curl, increased amount	Breast and areola enlarged, no contour separation
4	Coarse, curly, abundant but amount less than in adult. Filled-in pubic triangle	Areola and papilla form secondary mound: 'mound on a mound'
5	Adult feminine triangle, may spread to medial surface of thighs	Mature; nipple projects, areola part of general breast contour (secondary mound has disappeared)

Adapted from Tanner, J. M., *Growth and Adolescence*, 2nd edn, Oxford, Eng., 1962, Blackwell Scientific Publications. William A. Daniel Jnr, *Adolescents in Health and Disease*, The C. V. Mosby Co., Saint Louis, 1977 (used with permission).

Table 20.2 Classification of genital maturity stages in boys

Stage	Pubic hair	Penis	Scrotum (testes)
1	None	Preadolescent	Preadolescent (2–5 mL)
2	Scanty, long slightly pigmented	Slight enlargement	Enlarged, scrotum pink, texture altered (5–10 mL)
3	Hair spreads sparsely, darker, coarser	Elongates (pencil penis)	Increased growth testes (10–15 mL)
4	Resembles adult type, but less in quantity; coarse, curly	Larger; glans and breadth increase in size	Larger, scrotum dark (15–20 mL)
5	Adult distribution, spread to medial surface of thighs	Adult	Adult (> 20 mL)

Adapted from Tanner, J. M., *Growth and Adolescence*, 2nd edn, Oxford, Eng., 1962, Blackwell Scientific Publications. William A. Daniel Jnr, *Adolescents in Health and Disease*, The C. V. Mosby Co., Saint Louis, 1977 (used with permission).

History and examination

The interview

Establishing a comfortable and trusting relationship requires genuine interest, a non-judgmental attitude, empathy and honesty towards the young person. The key features of a successful adolescent interview can be summarised as follows:

- Begin the appointment on time.
- Begin by seeing the adolescent alone—this avoids the appearance of alignment with parents and invites a more mature response.
- Define the basis of confidentiality—reasonable exclusions are proposed self-destructive or dangerous behaviour.
- Respond openly to the adolescent's initial reactions—this can help to defuse hostility.
- Clarify the reasons for the consultation and fully explore the chief complaint—the young person's view may be at variance to that of parents and/or others.
- Be relaxed, open, flexible and unhurried in approaching the patient. Use an interactive rather than interrogative style of questions.
- Answer questions simply and honestly—listen quietly for the hidden, tangential ways in which young people frequently convey their concerns.
- Respect the teenager's concerns and point of view.

The history

In addition to a thorough medical history (including dietary habits, physical activity and menstrual history in girls) the Adolescent Risk Profile Assessment (the 'HEADSS' examination—developed by the Children's Hospital, Los Angeles) is a useful psychosocial history-taking tool:

- Home
- Education/employment
- Activities (peer group related)
- Drugs
- Sexuality
- Suicide/depression.

The physical examination

Precautions should be taken to protect the patient's modesty and privacy. Permission should be requested and obtained before proceeding with a physical examination. Ongoing dialogue and reassurance will lessen anxiety. Take the opportunity to provide information about developmental/health matters. A pelvic examination is not routinely indicated but may be necessary in the following situations: sexual activity; severe menstrual abnormalities; undiagnosed complaints related to the lower abdominal or vaginal area; if requested by the teenager and it is indicated. Ensure the young person and the family are aware of and agree to the need for pelvic examination. Follow the hospital guidelines on indications and practice for pelvic examination in prepubertal and pubertal girls.

Problems of growth and physical development

Delayed puberty/short stature

Both are relatively frequent complaints, more often in boys than in girls. More than 90% of cases are due to constitutional delay, a diagnosis of exclusion. Short stature is defined as height < 3rd percentile. Delayed puberty (2% of adolescent population) is defined as:

- absence of pubertal development by the age of 13 years (girls), or 14 years (boys)
  or
- failure of the progression of puberty over a 2-year period.

Consult Endocrinology with regard to these problems.

Precocious puberty

This is defined as development of pubertal signs before the age of 8 years in girls or 9.5 years in boys. Endocrine referral is necessary.

Breast problems

Benign masses are common in adolescent females:

- benign fibroadenomas—firm, usually painless lesions that persist
- fibrocystic lesions—often multiple; tenderness varies with the menstrual cycle.

Gynaecomastia

Gynaecomastia is a common finding in the early adolescent male:

- Benign adolescent hypertrophy is by far the most common. There is breast tissue immediately beneath the areola. It is usually tender and may measure up to 5–6 cm in diameter. It requires reassurance and tends to resolve spontaneously.
- Gynaecomastia without evidence of endocrine disorder resembles early normal female breast development. All other primary and secondary sexual characteristics are consistent with normal male adolescence. Surgical management is warranted rarely, if psychological distress is great.
- Gynaecomastia with evidence of endocrine disorder/drug ingestion/chromosomal disorder, such as Klinefelter's syndrome, is rare.

Menstrual disorders of adolescence

Menstrual disorders require a reassuring and gentle approach, and an understanding of basic menstrual physiology.

Following menarche (usually at age 12 or 13), the menstrual cycles are often irregular (anovulatory) for some 1–2 years.

Common pubescent menstrual problems include failure to menstruate, excessive or irregular menstrual bleeding and painful menstrual periods:

- *amenorrhoea* (absent menses):
  - *secondary amenorrhoea*—the most common abnormality in adolescents (usually hypothalamic/pituitary abnormalities; exclude pregnancy, think of eating disorders)
  - *primary amenorrhoea* (no menarche before 16 years of age)— rare; undernutrition and strenuous physical exercise delay menarche (check for congenital abnormalities, such as an imperforate hymen). Assess secondary sexual characteristics. Arrange gynaecological ± endocrine referral.
- *repeated heavy menstrual bleeding*—uncommon; usually due to anovulation; requires detailed investigation (at an appropriate gynaecological service); the addition of a progestational agent such as Primolut may be needed.
- *dysmenorrhoea*—very common; can be severe and disabling; detailed investigation is not usually indicated; usually due to

281

elevated uterine prostaglandin production; reassurance and simple methods are generally sufficient; otherwise a prostaglandin inhibitor such as mefenamic acid (Ponstan) should be prescribed. This can be used in conjunction with paracetamol or codeine.

- *polycystic ovary syndrome*—presents with oligomenorrhoea or amenorrhoea, anovulation or infertility, hirsutism or acne. Refer to adolescent gynaecology.

Nutritional problems

Teenagers are susceptible to a range of diet-related health problems. Eating behaviours in adolescents are affected by external factors (such as peers, media and culture) as well as internal factors (such as mood and personality traits). More than half of all adolescents report abnormal eating behaviours.

Adolescent obesity

- This is the most common chronic condition affecting adolescents. It results from an energy intake in excess of expenditure. Both child and adolescent obesity are becoming increasingly common.
- Obesity is variously defined by:
  - BMI > 95th percentile (check on a BMI-for-age percentile chart)
  - weight percentile more than 2 SD above the height percentile.
- Risk factors:
  - genetic predisposition
  - high calorie food for meals and snacks
  - more sedentary lifestyle and increased TV hours
  - psychosocial factors within the individual and family.
- Underlying organic aetiology is rare; consider this when there is:
  - early onset
  - short stature
  - developmental delay
  - abnormal physical findings.
- Management:
  - both individual and community strategies
  - individual and family assessment with ongoing therapy as indicated

- realistic evaluation and interaction regarding balancing diet, exercise and healthy lifestyle factors
- weight maintenance while growth proceeds
- peer group activities to enhance self-esteem, and provide support and encouragement
- no routine medications.

Anorexia nervosa

- This is the third most common chronic illness of adolescents after obesity and asthma.
- It affects 1:200 female adolescents between 15 and 19 years.
- Females > males, in a ratio of approximately 20:1.
- It is characterised by:
  - a decrease in weight of 15% of ideal body weight (IBW) or failure to gain the equivalent amount of weight; resistance to weight gain
  - preoccupation with foods and fat avoidance
  - distortion of body image; drive for thinness
  - secondary amenorrhoea for more than 3 months or primary amenorrhoea—pubertal arrest.
- Other features may include:
  - calorie purging by increased physical activity, vomiting and restriction of food
  - anxiety
  - obsessive-compulsive traits.
- Admission to hospital becomes necessary when weight loss leads to medical complications such as hypothermia, bradycardia, hypotension, electrolyte or ECG changes.
- Consult Adolescent Medicine and/or Psychological Medicine.
- Management is complex. It requires the integration of skills from a multi-disciplinary team. The hospital program includes refeeding (oral or nasogastric), psychiatric assessment, individual, family and nutritional counselling, physical rehabilitation, schooling and involvement in the arts program.

Bulimia nervosa

- This occurs typically in older adolescents, associated with mood disturbance (depression).
- It is characterised by repeated cycles of bingeing and feelings of guilt relieved by purging (usually with laxatives or vomiting),

which occur three or more times a week for 3 or more months.
- Body image, menstrual disturbance and weight loss tend to be far less severe than with anorexia nervosa.
- Treatment is usually successful on an out-patient basis with medical monitoring, counselling and the use of SSRI (selective serotonin reuptake inhibitor) medications as indicated.

Orthopaedic problems

A number of important conditions occur almost exclusively in adolescents.

Adolescent scoliosis

- About 2–3 per 1000 adolescent girls will develop idiopathic scoliosis of sufficient severity to require treatment. Scoliosis is much less common in boys.
- The best screening test is the forward bending test which increases the prominence of any rib humps (the patient bends forward at the waist, the trunk parallel to the floor, with legs straight and arms dangling with fingers and palms together); school screening is done widely, although not universal.
- Early referral to a specialist orthopaedic surgeon with experience in the condition, prior to the growth spurt, is needed.

Adolescent kyphosis

- This is also known as adolescent round back, Scheuermann's disease and vertebral epiphysitis.
- Clinical manifestations include a round deformity of the back and, in over half of patients, persistent pain localised in the involved area; X-ray findings confirm the diagnosis.

Osgood-Schlatter disease

- This occurs predominantly in active adolescent males.
- There is a painful enlargement of the tibial tuberosity at the insertion of the patella tendon (usually unilateral).
- Treatment consists of physiotherapy directed at hamstring stretching and quadriceps rehabilitation. A short period of rest may be helpful.
- Parental reassurance is very important.
- Similar conditions may affect the patella itself.

Slipped capital femoral epiphysis

- The femoral head slips on the femoral metaphysis; chronic and gradual in 80% of cases.
- It is more prevalent in males than in females (2:1 to 4:1), and often associated with obesity and delayed skeletal maturation.
- Symptoms include hip or knee pain (from obturator nerve referral) or a limp; signs include an externally rotated gait, decreased flexion, adduction and internal rotation of the hip.
- X-ray changes and bone scan findings (increased uptake at involved epiphyseal plate) are characteristic. Ultrasound examination can be helpful.
- Acute orthopaedic referral is required, as surgery is the only reliable treatment.

Chronic illness and disability

Approximately 1 in 10 adolescents have a significant medical condition or physical abnormality requiring ongoing care or support. A chronic disease provides many obstacles to growing up with impact being related to the developmental stage:

- early—distortion of body image; isolation from peers
- mid—enforced dependency; decreased acceptance by peers
- late—impaired relationships with special friends; concerns about marriage and family effects upon education and vocational goals.

Chronic illness can delay physical, emotional, social and psychosexual development; continued dependency and increased social isolation may add to coping difficulties.

Strong family support can make young people resilient to even profound physical and psychosocial disability and illness.

Key issues in management

- A chronically ill teenager has the same developmental needs as all other teenagers.
- Encourage self-management and self-reliance; encourage development of creativity and other skills.
- Limit intrusive medical examinations or procedures as far as possible.
- Provide and discuss honest and comprehensive information about

the condition and its consequences; do not focus only on negative consequences.

- Parents may need help to reduce over-anxiety, over-attention, and over-protection.
- The dying adolescent will generally be aware of the seriousness of the situation; avoid the conspiracy of silence. Provide opportunities for individual and family support. Encourage involvement in management decisions.
- To *improve adherence to treatment* (compliance):
  - Explore general issues (use 'HEADSS').
  - Explore beliefs and expectations around the illness.
  - Give verbal and written information and education.
  - Give clear explanations of the outcome and benefits of therapy.
  - Simplify the treatment regimen and integrate it into daily activities.
  - Involve the young person in decision-making and control, for example appointment making.
  - Frequently monitor progress, encourage and motivate.
  - Know when to seek help; individual or family counselling in preparation for transition to adult status can be motivating.

The transition from paediatric to adult physician care is a process to be considered and started early:

- From about 12 years the young person can be seen alone first, with parents joining the consultation later so that both the young person and family become used to evolving independence.
- The time of transfer is individualised according to the patient's and family's educational and medical needs with flexibility around the 15–19 year age group.
- A transitional clinic with a paediatrician, adult physician and allied health professionals all present has been found to be effective, with emphasis on promotion of self-management skills and provision of resources for the transition. Parent and patient groups can be incorporated into the clinic and facilitate the process.

Depression and suicidality

- Certain groups are more vulnerable.
- Suicidal behaviour is increasing, particularly in males aged 15–19 years.
- The use of methods other than the ingestion of drugs increases the risk of successful suicide.

High-risk groups

- Current suicidal ideation—always take seriously
- One or more previous suicide attempts, particularly a recent one
- Depression
- Antisocial behaviour—fighting/stealing/truancy
- Suicide of a close peer or family member
- Frequent use of drugs or alcohol
- Male sex
- Mismatch between the young person and his/her environment

Precipitating events

These include:

- sudden alienation from parents
- rejection by a peer (usually a highly valued relationship)
- significant and often public failure (usually academic or athletic)
- family disruption or dissolution
- history of suicide in a friend or relative.

Signs of depression

It is important to recognise signs of depression:

- *sad and tearful* and not bouncing back; loss of interest, deteriorating school work, a distancing from family and friends
- *physically unwell* with symptoms (headaches, general malaise) and excessive tiredness
- *sleep disturbance*
- *uncharacteristic behaviour* such as hyperactivity, disruptive, antisocial acts such as stealing.

With all troubled adolescents, ask explicit direct questions about suicidal thoughts and plans, and seek psychiatric advice. *Following all suicide attempts, urgent formal psychiatric assessment is essential.*

Adolescent sexuality and sexual health

Sexuality is a sensitive issue for most people, but can be particularly difficult to broach with an adolescent. About half of all adolescents have had sexual intercourse by the end of high school (Year 12). Not all adolescents are heterosexual—up to 10% of adolescents experience same-sex attraction. Creating a sufficiently trusting relationship with the adolescent patient so that they feel safe to reveal information without fear of judgment or stigmatisation is the key to promoting sexual health. A comprehensive coverage of these subjects is beyond the scope of this book.

Contraception

Condoms

- Condom use should always be encouraged in penetrative sexual relationships.
- Invite the adolescent to ask how to use condoms properly; remind them about storage (away from heat and light), using water-based lubricant, putting them on and taking them off properly.
- The female condom is now available.

Hormonal contraception

- Most forms of hormonal contraception are effective and safe for use in the adolescent population.

The combined oral contraceptive pill (COCP)

- The COCP can be prescribed legally to a young woman of any age for contraception, with her informed consent. It is best to start with a low dose (for example 30 micrograms ethinyl estradiol, 150 micrograms levonorgestrel) monophasic or triphasic regimen.
- The ultra low dose pill (20 and 100 micrograms, respectively) has the same efficacy as the low dose pill, but slightly less margin for error. First-time pill users should be cautious.
- All adolescents starting on the COCP for contraception should be adequately counselled about its use, particularly what to do if pills are missed.

Long-acting injectable progestogen
- These are efficacious and safe but require Guardianship Tribunal approval for women under 16 years of age, due to the semi-irreversible nature of the contraception.

Progestogen implants
- These are very efficacious, reversible, safe and available as a pharmaceutical benefit. Doctors require special training in their use.

Oral progestogen-only pill
- This is not generally recommended for adolescent women because of a narrower margin for error (missed pills, lower efficacy).

Sexually transmitted diseases

- Sexually active adolescents are at greater risk of acquiring sexually transmitted diseases (STDs) than their adult counterparts for both biological and psychosocial reasons. Table 20.3 lists the relative frequency of adolescent STDs.
- Most people with an STD are asymptomatic, yet the sequelae, particularly for women, can be devastating.
- Having one STD increases the likelihood of harbouring another and the diagnosis of one STD should prompt a full screen (Table 20.4).
- Prevention is an important part of management (always consider vaccination, safer sex education opportunities, encouraging partners to be screened and treated).
- Risks for different STDs vary according to sexual orientation, sexual practices and the gender of sexual partners.
- Single dose treatment is often preferable to increase compliance, and the possibility of pregnancy should always be considered when prescribing.

An adolescent who is sexually active and at risk of having an STD and/or requests an STD screen should have the tests in Table 20.4 done.

Management of sexually transmitted diseases

Discussion of the management of patients with sexually transmitted diseases is beyond the scope of this book. Refer to *National*

Management Guidelines for Sexually Transmissible Infections, published by the Australasian College of Sexual Health Physicians, 2002.

Table 20.3 Relative frequency of adolescent STDs

What is common	What is less common
Human papilloma virus	*Trichomonas vaginalis*
Chlamydia trachomatis	Syphilis
Nonspecific urethritis	HIV
Herpes simplex virus	Gonorrhoea in heterosexuals
Gonorrhoea in homosexual males	

Table 20.4 STD screening in asymptomatic adolescents

Females	Males
Endocervical swab for *Chlamydia* culture/PCR	First catch urine for *Chlamydia* PCR
Endocervical swab for gonorrhoea culture	Urethral swab for gonorrhoea culture
High vaginal swab for *Candida*, clue cells, *Trichomonas*	Testicular examination
Papanicalou smear if due (in an adolescent with multiple partners or changing partners, this should be done every year)	
First catch urine for *Chlamydia* if pelvic examination refused or difficult	

Blood tests

Syphilis serology

Hepatitis B serology (prevaccination; vaccination should be routinely recommended)

Hepatitis C Ab if there is a history of injecting drug use or blood transfusion pre-1990

HIV only if indicated/requested following careful history and pretest counselling

Hepatitis A Ab if gay male, Aboriginal

Depending on the sexual practices of both females and males: anal swabs, throat swabs

The symptomatic adolescent

- Many adolescents present with physical symptoms such as recurrent abdominal pain, chest pain, headache and fatigue, which are not attributable to an identified organic disorder.
- Abnormal illness behaviour (or somatisation) should be suspected in those situations where there a discrepancy between the symptomatic complaints, the physical findings and medical investigations (usually all negative).
- As well as a detailed history:
  - Enquire about the time of onset with regard to family, school and peers.
  - Explore the origin of the symptom—borrowing or perpetuation of symptoms is not uncommon.
  - Accept the reality of the symptom and keep an open mind on diagnosis, indicating, however, the need to explore psychosocial issues as part of assessment in an individual and family context.
  - Resist the pressure to provide a diagnosis using excessive and inappropriate investigations.
  - Arrange a family interview as the young person's 'being sick' may mask or reflect family distress or dysfunction.

21

Oncological emergencies

This section includes:

- cancer in childhood
- making the diagnosis
- emergencies at diagnosis
- emergencies during therapy
- pain and symptom control
- immunisation and children with cancer
- long-term follow-up.

Cancer in childhood

- 600–700 children aged 0–15 years develop cancer each year in Australia.
- *Leukaemia* is the most common malignancy of childhood. Current therapy cures about 75% of children with acute lymphoblastic leukaemia (ALL) and up to 50% of those with non-lymphoblastic leukaemia.
- *Other childhood cancers* include cerebral tumours, non-Hodgkin's lymphoma, Wilms' tumour, neuroblastoma, rhabdomyosarcoma, osteogenic sarcoma and Ewing's tumour, germ cell tumour, and retinoblastoma. Cure rates for solid tumours vary between 20% and 95%, with an average of 65%.
- Survival rates are highest if treatment is supervised by a tertiary level paediatric oncology unit. *Prompt referral of newly diagnosed children is essential.*
  - Do not administer chemotherapy (including corticosteroids) prior to initial referral as this may impede accurate diagnosis, hamper treatment planning and worsen prognosis.
  - In exceptional circumstances, emergency treatment may be necessary prior to referral, following discussion with and directed by a paediatric oncologist.

Making the diagnosis

- Early diagnosis simplifies therapy and may reduce early morbidity.
- Always consider leukaemia or other types of cancer in any sick child.
- Cardinal symptoms of cancer in children are:
  - persistent fever/recurrent fever without cause
  - persistent pain (particularly bone pain and headache)
  - a mass
  - purpura
  - pallor
  - strabismus or other eye changes
  - changes in co-ordination or behaviour.
- A full blood count will usually be abnormal at diagnosis in a child with untreated acute leukaemia, commonly revealing two or more of the following: anaemia, neutropenia, thrombocytopenia, circulating abnormal blast cells.
- Other symptoms which should raise the possibility of cancer as a diagnosis are:
  - persistent limp (which may be an indication of leukaemia or bone tumours)
  - progressive weight loss
  - localised joint pain and swelling with fever, mimicking osteomyelitis or arthritis
  - subacute onset of upper airway obstruction (upper mediastinal mass) which may mimic asthma.

Emergencies at diagnosis

Severe anaemia

- Haemoglobin of less than 70 g/L, at diagnosis, in acute leukaemia, may result in life-threatening high-output cardiac failure.
- Transfusion with packed red blood cells must be given promptly in this situation (provided the white cell count is less than $50 \times 10^9/L$).
- Blood transfusions must be group-compatible and cross-matched prior to transfusion.
- CMV-negative blood products should be requested.

Fever and neutropenia in acute leukaemia

- Fever may indicate bacterial septicaemia and can occur prior to diagnosis as well as during treatment.
- Such infection is life-threatening, and necessitates prompt broad-spectrum antibiotic therapy following blood culture (and other appropriate cultures).
- Where the child has not yet arrived at a paediatric oncology unit, urgently seek advice on the choice of antimicrobials from a paediatric oncologist.

Severe thrombocytopenia in acute leukaemia

- A platelet count less than 20×10^9/L can be associated with life-threatening bleeding (for example, cerebral haemorrhage), especially if platelet transfusion is delayed.
- Platelet transfusion must be group-compatible.
- CMV-negative blood products should be requested.

Transfusion of packed red blood cells and/or platelets should be undertaken promptly, and prior to referral to the paediatric oncology unit, in children with severe anaemia or thrombocytopenia. Such transfusions do not hinder the diagnosis of the underlying leukaemia, and may be life-saving. (Premedication with steroids is contraindicated.)

Other presentations which require urgent intervention at the time of diagnosis

- *Acute-onset weakness in lower limbs or bowel/bladder dysfunction*: These symptoms could indicate spinal cord compression and require urgent tertiary referral for investigation and treatment.
- *Acute thoracic inlet obstruction*: Respiratory difficulty, especially when supine, with or without cough, wheeze and upper mediastinal mass on chest X-ray and with or without distension of veins in the neck or arms, can be due to malignancy (especially lymphoma). Do not anaesthetise the child! Do not arrange biopsy! Seek advice urgently!
- *Very high circulating blast cell count*: Counts greater than 500×10^9/L at diagnosis are associated with blood vessel sludging, due to high blood viscosity, and hence cerebrovascular accidents. The risk is greater when thrombocytopenia is also present. Seek advice urgently. Management prior to referral may need to include

platelet transfusions, additional intravenous fluids and, in exceptional circumstances, exchange transfusion.

Emergencies during therapy

Children with cancer receive programs of carefully planned multidisciplinary therapy which may extend for 2 years or more from the time of diagnosis. This therapy commonly includes chemotherapy administered according to strictly monitored national or international protocols. Radiotherapy and surgery are also often used.

Infection relating to immunosuppression—from the underlying disease or its treatment—is the major source of emergencies during treatment. Other causes of emergencies include bleeding, raised intracranial pressure, electrolyte abnormalities and drug side-effects.

Febrile neutropenia

- Fever (body temperature 38°C or higher) associated with neutropenia from chemotherapy-induced bone marrow depression will inevitably occur during treatment.
- In this situation, the diagnosis must be presumed to be septicaemia until proven otherwise, and appropriate broad-spectrum antibiotics must be commenced urgently after appropriate 'septic work-up'.
- Children with febrile neutropenia are normally treated in the paediatric oncology unit.
- Where transfer is not possible, consult the paediatric oncologist urgently for advice.

Infectious diseases

- Measles and varicella may be life-threatening in patients who are receiving chemotherapy and who are immunosuppressed.
- The risk of exposure to patients with measles, chickenpox or herpes zoster should be lessened by the isolation of susceptible children in emergency departments, and by the education of the family, childcare and school personnel.
- If non-immune children with cancer are exposed to measles or VZV, they should be given passive protection with normal human immunoglobulin 0.5 mL/kg to maximum 15 mL for measles, or VZIG 2 mL 0–5 years old, 4 mL 6–12 years old, 6 mL > 12 years old for varicella.

Pain and symptom control

Severe pain occurs in up to 50% of children with cancer. It can usually be adequately treated with either non-opioid or opioid analgesics (see Chapter 6). Children are particularly distressed by painful procedures (blood collection, lumbar puncture and so on). The best general principle is to prevent procedural pain, as far as possible, from the beginning of therapy.

Vomiting is commonly associated with chemotherapy but otherwise may be present as a nonspecific symptom (see Chapter 6).

Aspirin should be avoided in children receiving chemotherapy as it inhibits platelet aggregation. Paracetamol can be used for pain and/or fever.

See Chapter 33 for *palliative care, dying* and *death*.

Immunisation and children with cancer

Children being treated for cancer, even those in remission, should *not* receive live vaccines (for example Sabin polio vaccine, MMR, BCG) until at least 6 months after chemotherapy has finished. Inactivated vaccines are not dangerous to the recipient but are usually less effective. Household contacts may receive MMR but not oral polio vaccine.

Long-term follow-up

Routine follow-up and surveillance for possible recurrence or after-effects of treatment continue indefinitely after the completion of planned treatment. Recurrences of the underlying cancer will rarely occur later than 5 years after completing the original treatment. The quality of life for long-term survivors of childhood cancer is usually very good.

Growth, puberty, fertility, intellectual function and psychological wellbeing may all be affected as a result of therapy for childhood cancer. Formal follow-up of all survivors of childhood cancer should continue into adult life. It is recommended that patients beyond the immediate post-treatment phase be referred to a paediatric oncology late-effects clinic, staffed by healthcare personnel with experience in the detection and management of the late sequelae of therapy.

22

Abuse of children

This chapter includes:

- child abuse: your reporting responsibility
- Child Protection Unit (CPU) of the Children's Hospital at Westmead
- physical abuse
- sexual abuse
- emotional abuse and neglect.

Child abuse: your reporting responsibility

Children can be abused physically, sexually and emotionally and/or have their needs neglected by their parents or caretakers. It is important to be aware of children who are at risk of abuse or neglect and know how to respond appropriately. It is mandatory for all doctors in New South Wales to report all forms of abuse or suspected abuse, and all staff of New South Wales public hospitals have a departmental directive to report abuse. Healthcare workers who fail to comply with this obligation may be guilty of an offence, with maximum penalties exceeding $22 000.

Child Protection Unit (CPU) of the Children's Hospital at Westmead

The CPU should be contacted early for consultation if you suspect a child has been abused. Contact the social worker on call for child protection (extension 52434 at the Children's Hospital at Westmead, or via the switchboard). The unit can provide consultation, assessment, medical examination, notification and ongoing therapeutic intervention. A doctor and social worker are on call

24 hours a day, 7 days a week to respond to urgent referrals. For in-patients, referral to the CPU should be made after discussion with the consultant caring for the child.

Admission policy for in-patients

Children with injuries or other problems that appear likely or possibly due to abuse are admitted under the general physician, general surgeon or subspecialty surgeon on call, as appropriate to the medical problem. The CPU is involved early, via consultation.

Interaction with other services

The CPU works within Interagency Guidelines for Child Protection Intervention in close co-operation with the Department of Community Services (DoCS). Although the CPU will often accept responsibility to make a report to DoCS, it is the duty of all Department of Health staff to act on their concerns when child abuse is suspected, and it is the prerogative of any staff member to make a report on the basis of their genuine concerns. Substantiation or proof of abuse is not required. The paramount consideration is the safety and welfare of the child.

What is a report?

A report is information provided to DoCS about a child whom they have reasonable grounds to suspect is at risk of harm, in this case by a person working in the delivery of healthcare to children. Children under the age of 16 years, young persons (aged 16–17 years) and unborn children may all have a report made about them.

Making a report to DoCS

A healthcare worker who has reasonable grounds to suspect that a child has suffered abuse or is at risk of harm should make a report to the DoCS Helpline on 13 36 27.

You will need to supply:

- your name, position and the name of your Area Health Service
- your grounds for concern for the child.
  After a verbal report has been made, you should then either:
- fill out the form for reporting to the DoCS Helpline and place a copy of this in the patient's health record
  or
- document the report in the patient's health record on a separate page under the heading 'Report to DoCS'.

The DoCS Helpline operates 24 hours a day, 7 days a week. DoCS is required by law to make its own assessment of whether the child or young person is at risk of harm.

If the situation is life-threatening, notify the police on 000.

Notification details

- Name and description of the child/young person
- Current whereabouts of the child/young person
- Whether the risk of harm relates to a staff member of the hospital or another organisation
- Reasons for concern about the risk of harm
- When the child was last seen
- Information about parents/caregiver
- Name and address of alleged perpetrator (if known)
- Aboriginality
- Child's views about the report being made
- Whether an interpreter is needed

Making a notification or furnishing information will not be held to constitute a breach of professional etiquette or ethics or to be a departure from acceptable standards of professional conduct. The worker will not be liable for defamation proceedings and the notification will not constitute a ground for civil action for malicious prosecution.

For more detailed information on the role NSW Health plays in child protection, refer to the manual *NSW Health Frontline Procedures for the Protection of Children and Young People*.

Physical abuse

You should consider the possibility of physical abuse when a child presents with injuries along with:

- a history inconsistent with the physical findings, or that is vague, bizarre or variable
- an unexplained delay between the injury and presentation for medical attention
- multiple injuries or bruises, particularly bruising around the face, trunk or in areas not often injured in normal play
- bruises with a pattern indicating the objects used, for example flex cords, shoe imprints, sticks or evidence of finger marks on the face, arms or body where the child has been gripped tightly

- fractures which are not consistent with the child's developmental stage, are of varying ages and sites and for which there is no adequate explanation. Metaphyseal 'corner' fractures and periosteal reactions are strongly associated with physical abuse, as are posterior rib fractures
- burns in a distribution inconsistent with the history given, cigarette burns
- severe head injury without an associated history of major trauma, especially in infants
- retinal haemorrhages
- a history of repeated injuries.

Additional features in the overall situation may include:

- recurrent presentations to the Emergency Department with minor complaints (may be 'pleas for help')
- social isolation
- a history of involvement with multiple agencies, none of whom has been able to help the family
- domestic violence
- presentation of the child as 'bad', management problems with the child and inappropriate emotional reactions to the child
- admission by parents of fears that they may injure the child
- physical or mental health issues for the parent affecting their ability to care for the child
- the parent appearing affected by drugs or alcohol.

Remember, most significant physical abuse occurs in a context of significant emotional abuse and/or neglect. Remember also that most of this information will not be apparent and will not be volunteered unless it is actively sought by direct questioning.

Management

It is essential when dealing with suspected child abuse to avoid confrontation, accusation and repeated interrogation. At the same time it is important to remain honest about your concerns and what action you are planning. Very often, the abuser has experienced an emotionally or physically abusive childhood themselves and is mistrustful of authority. This does not condone their actions but may help you to understand them better.

In situations where concerns arise that a child has been abused or is at risk of abuse, the following actions are recommended:

Patients of the Children's Hospital at Westmead

- Document the history and injuries precisely and provide emergency medical treatment as needed.
- Document any relevant observations that would justify concerns, such as inappropriate behaviour or comments by the parents, statements or behaviour by the child, observations of the parent–child interaction.
- Discuss your concerns with the consultant caring for the child if the child is an in-patient.
- Inform the parents of your concerns about the child's injuries, and the need for further assessment by the CPU.
- Refer to the Child Protection Unit (CPU) social worker on call who will liaise with the CPU medical officer or consultant paediatrician on call.
- Form an initial case plan in consultation with the CPU.
- An assessment of the child and family may be made by the CPU.
- CPU will make a report to the Department of Community Services (DoCS) if abuse is suspected. The parents will be informed of this.
- Department of Community Services may contact the police to investigate in cases where there have been significant physical injuries.

If the parents threaten to remove the child from the hospital against medical advice, do not attempt to restrain them yourself. Call Security and discuss with the CPU. The CPU will contact DoCS immediately to discuss appropriate action.

Further appropriate tests may include:

- medical photography: photographs should include the name of the child, an identifying view of the whole child, a view of the injuries with an associated identifying feature of the child, for example the face, and the date on which the photographs are taken. It is helpful to use a tape measure next to the injuries so that sizes can be determined and a Kodak colour chart so that colours can be accurately processed. Where possible, these photographs should be taken by the hospital's clinical photographer.
- FBC, film, coagulation studies, platelet aggregation studies
- skeletal survey (X-ray): periosteal lifting, metaphyseal and other fractures may not be apparent until calcification occurs (2–3 weeks)

- nuclear bone scan: detects more recent injuries and soft tissue injuries
- CT scan of head
- an ophthalmology examination in all head injury cases or where a shaken baby is suspected
- EUC, liver function tests, serum amylase, urine microscopy for RBC to detect covert abdominal trauma
- CT scan of abdomen: persistent tachycardia in a semicomatose child with no clear history of injury suggests occult blood loss and is an indication for abdominal CT scan.

A protection planning meeting is held to arrange continuing management of the child and family. This will involve members of the house staff who initially referred the case, nursing staff, the Child Protection Unit, the Department of Community Services and other community services who may have been involved with the family, e.g. Drug and Alcohol, Community Health.

Patients outside the Children's Hospital at Westmead

Where concerns arise about children seen outside the Children's Hospital at Westmead, a report should be made to the DoCS Helpline. The parents should be informed of the grounds as well as the mandate for the report. DoCS will investigate and refer the child for documentation of injuries if necessary. The doctor who sees the child should take a precise history, use diagrams to document the injuries, note the colour, tenderness, size and pattern of injuries and arrange for clinical photography to be done.

Sexual abuse

Repeated studies of young people indicate that approximately 33% of girls and 10% of boys will experience some form of significant sexual abuse by the age of 18 years. Most abusers are known to the child, usually a family member. Stranger assault is not as common. Sexual abuse is often a frightening, confusing or overwhelming experience for the young child, who may be reluctant to disclose to strangers, particularly if the first disclosure has caused considerable family emotional turmoil. It is best to listen to the child and to let them tell their story with a minimum of interruptions and no direct questioning.

Indicators of child sexual abuse include:

- a child giving a story of sexual interference, particularly if this is consistent and contains peripheral details which are confirmed by the parent
- sexual activity between children which involves coercion and a power imbalance
- age-inappropriate behaviour, persistent sexualised behaviour
- recurrent vaginal discharge
- inadequately explained genital and perianal trauma or bleeding
- self-destructive behaviours, drug dependency, suicide attempts, self-mutilation
- eating disorders (anorexia, bulimia)
- persistent running away from home
- reluctance to leave hospital
- multiple unexplained medical ailments, psychosomatic symptoms
- unexplained emotional disturbance, depression
- sexually transmitted infections, pregnancy.

Sexual abuse may also be occurring in children with physical or emotional abuse.

If a child discloses abuse what should I say?

- Tell them that you believe them.
- It is not their fault no matter what the circumstances.
- You know other children to whom this has happened; it is not just them.
- You will try to stop it happening.
- Adults sometimes do wrong things.
- They were right to tell.
- Do not make any promises that cannot be kept, particularly about keeping information secret.
- Try to remain calm.
- Listen to the child's story.
- Make the child comfortable while you organise things.
- Explain to the child what you are going to do to arrange help.
- Avoid confronting the suspected offender.

Management

In cases of sexual abuse, taking the history and carrying out the physical examination must be done with great sensitivity, with privacy and in an atmosphere of calm reassurance. Medical examinations should not be carried out by an inexperienced person. Medical training in this area is available through specialist Child Protection Centres.

Patients of the Children's Hospital at Westmead

- Discuss your concerns with the consultant caring for the child and make a referral to the CPU.
- In the case of a medical emergency, for example haemorrhage, the child's medical needs take priority and emergency treatment should be provided in consultation with the CPU doctor on call.
- The CPU will notify DoCS who may conduct an investigation.
- The child will be seen by a CPU doctor.
- In a specialist unit such as the CPU the following are undertaken:
  - The history and medical examination are documented in a 'Child Sexual Assault Protocol'.
  - A forensic specimen kit may be collected.
  - Pregnancy prophylaxis and screening/treatment for sexually transmitted infection are provided if indicated.
- A witness, usually a female member of staff, must be present at the examination. Internal examinations are rarely necessary, but if needed it is often preferable to perform them under anaesthesia.
- Families may need crisis counselling immediately post-disclosure. This may take place over 6 to 8 weeks. Longer term therapy may be required, particularly as there is a high incidence of intergenerational abuse and this incident may revive memories in other family members.

Sexual assault

- Where sexual assault has occurred or is suspected, the CPU social worker on call should be contacted promptly.
- The child should first be interviewed by DoCS and/or specially trained police officers (the Joint Investigation and Response Team).
- The police are often involved in sexual assault cases as this is a criminal offence.
- The child and non-offending parent(s) are then seen at a Child Sexual Assault Centre such as the Child Protection Unit for assessment, crisis counselling and medical examination if indicated.

- Forensic medical evidence can be collected up to 7 days following an assault.

Emotional abuse and neglect

Failure to meet the physical and emotional needs of the child will lead to failure of his or her emotional development, particularly of a healthy attachment to the parent, the development of self-esteem and the capacity to trust and love others. Abuse in these areas often is manifested as clinging attachment, rejection of the parents, behavioural problems, and psychosocial or developmental delay. These have serious repercussions in later life and again are frequently inter-generational. They are equally as important as physical and sexual abuse but often harder to define.

Indicators of neglect and emotional abuse

- Non-organic failure to thrive
- Delayed developmental milestones
- Unhygienic living conditions
- Delay in seeking medical attention, including incomplete immunisation
- Leaving children without adequate supervision
- Scavenging or stealing food by the child
- Extended stays at school, public places or others' homes
- Self-comforting behaviour
- Extreme longing for adult affection
- A flat and superficial way of relating
- Unwillingness to leave the clinic or ward on discharge
  Other features in the situation may include:
- verbal abuse, such as yelling or screaming at the child as the main means of communication, belittling, constant threats and lack of encouragement
- an unavailable parent—drug and alcohol addiction, the 'too busy' parent, frequent changes in partners, chaotic parental lifestyle, maternal depression, psychosis.

Management

- Referrals should be made to the CPU social worker on call. For in-patients, this should be after discussion with the consultant caring for the child.

- The CPU medical officer and social worker will assess the case and liaise with the Department of Community Services and other services with whom the family may have been in contact.
- Psychosocial, developmental and paediatric assessments may be arranged to determine the needs of the child.
- Case conference and regular review of these families is important, with links between the medical and CPU staff.

In addition to the use of community resources, the CPU provides counselling for parents and children. It is important to deal with the parents' emotional needs to be able to help the child in the long term.

23

Important skin conditions

This chapter includes:

- scabies
- impetigo
- staphylococcal scalded skin syndrome
- tinea
- warts
- atopic dermatitis
- seborrhoeic dermatitis
- molluscum contagiosum
- herpes simplex virus infection
- haemangiomas
- common napkin rash.

Scabies

Clinical features

- Severe itch which is worse at night
- Rash which may be manifested as blisters, burrows, excoriated papules, impetigo or patches of eczema at the sites of mite infestation. These include wrists, elbows, anterior axillary folds, between fingers, palms and soles in babies, nipples and penis. A 'secondary rash' with punctate, excoriated papules may be present on the anterior trunk.
- The rash is often present in contacts because the infestation is caught by close physical contact.

Management

- Treat the patient and all close contacts.
- The preferred treatment for this condition is Lyclear (5% permethrin). Its safety in infants under 2 months old is not established. In the very young infant the treatment of choice is precipitated sulfur.

Treatment using Lyclear

- Apply to cool, dry skin.
- Apply it all over from the neck down. This must include between the fingers, between the toes, in the groin, and all over the back.
- Leave on for 24 hours.
- Repeat the application 1 week later in the same way.

Treatment using precipitated sulfur

- The preparation is 10% sulfur in white soft paraffin.
- This is applied all over, including face and scalp (avoid the area just around eyes).
- It is applied 4 times a day for 2 consecutive days.
- The treatment should be repeated in 1 week.
- It should be noted that recurrence quite often occurs following this treatment and that re-treatment with Lyclear may be required later.

Impetigo

Impetigo is a bacterial infection caused by *Staphylococcus aureus* or pyogenic streptococci. It occurs in two forms, crusted and bullous.

Crusted

This may be caused by staphylococci and/or streptococci. In staphylococcal disease, the typical lesion is a golden crust covering a shallow ulcer with an oozing base. The child is otherwise well and asymptomatic. The lesions of streptococcal impetigo are deeper ulcers with collections of pus in the early stages and later a firm, adherent crust. The child may be febrile and the lesions are often painful. Lesions may be superimposed on other skin diseases such as insect bites, head lice, scabies or eczema.

Management

- Look for underlying disease.
- Swab lesion.
- Give oral antibiotics. *Note*: Over 40% of staphylococci in the community are resistant to erythromycin, so cephalosporins or flucloxacillin are often required.
- Give saline baths.

- If streptococcal, remember the possibility of poststreptococcal glomerulonephritis.

Bullous

This is caused by staphylococcal strains which produce epidermolytic toxin. Small blisters appear and enlarge quickly and rupture, producing large denuded areas which are glazed in appearance and dry quickly. The lesions are not itchy and rarely tender. The child is systemically well.

Management

- Swab lesion.
- Give oral antibiotics.
- Give saline baths.

Staphylococcal scalded skin syndrome

This condition is caused by systemic spread of an epidermolytic toxin produced by certain strains of staphylococci. The primary infection may be umbilical, conjunctival, nasopharyngeal or in a wound. The child is febrile with signs of systemic toxicity. The skin is bright red, often all over, and extremely tender. The child prefers not to be held. There is superficial blistering with sheeting off of skin, leaving the appearance of a scald. The process often begins in the genital and perioral areas and may become widespread.

Management

- Admit if severe.
- Swab any obvious source of infection and/or posterior nasopharynx. *Do not* swab denuded areas, as these are sterile.
- Give flucloxacillin—orally if possible as insertion/strapping of an intravenous cannula is painful; however, intravenous administration is often required.
- Nurse with minimal handling on non-stick sheeting.
- When skin starts to improve and dry out, use bath oils and emollients.

Note: Fluid loss is rarely a problem except in neonates.

Differential diagnosis

- Stevens-Johnson syndrome—in this condition, the blisters are deeper and often haemorrhagic. There is mucosal involvement (*not* seen in staphylococcal skin syndrome). The skin is not red all over and is less acutely tender.
- Burns

Tinea

Tinea is a fungal infection of the skin, hair and nails. Classical features include itch, definite edge, tendency to clear in the centre and scale. Tinea may involve the scalp, general body skin or nails (very rare in children).

Scalp

Clinical features

- Signs of inflammation such as scale, erythema, oozing or pustulation
- Short broken-off hairs, all of which are the same length in an individual case (0.5–2 mm)
- Itch, not pain

  Note: Inflammation and broken hairs = tinea

Differential diagnosis

- *Alopecia areata*: Complete hair loss, area smooth and bald, no inflammation
- *Trichotillomania*: Hairs broken off at different lengths, scalp not inflamed, history of hair twisting or pulling

General body skin

Clinical features

- Scaly, itchy lesions which are usually dry, have a definite edge and have a tendency to clear in the centre. There are often small papules or pustules within the lesion.
- Asymmetrical distribution

Differential diagnosis

- Discoid eczema: Often weeping and usually very symmetrically distributed, particularly on extensor aspects of limbs

- Psoriasis: Silvery scale when scratched. There may be scalp and nail involvement.

Management of tinea

- Scrape for microscopy and culture.
- Topical antifungals, such as Canesten (clotrimazole 1%) and Ecostatin (econazole nitrate 1%), have a place for early, localised, skin lesions.
- For widespread or resistant disease and all cases of scalp and nail tinea, use Griseofulvin orally. Griseofulvin should be given after meals, preferably with milk.

Dosage guide

- 0–1 years: 125 mg/day
- 1–3 years: 125 mg b.d.
- 3 years-puberty: 125 mg t.d.s.
- After puberty: 500 mg/day

Duration of therapy

- Scalp: 3 months
- Other areas: 2 months

Warts

Common warts

These are ordinary warts, as seen on hands, knees and so on. They have a tendency to disappear spontaneously.

Management

- Daily apply salicylic and lactic acid mixture (a common preparation is 15% salicylic acid, 15% lactic acid in equal parts of collodion and acetone). Then cover the wart with sticking plaster.
- If there is no improvement *and* warts are worrying the child, consider referral for liquid nitrogen.
- For multiple refractory warts, oral cimetidine, 40 mg/kg once daily, has been successful, usually within 5–8 weeks.

Plantar warts

Plantar warts occur on the soles of the feet. Predisposing factors include hyperhidrosis and orthopaedic abnormalities producing pressure points.

Management

This may involve two approaches:

- weekly, apply Upton's paste under plaster
- daily, paint with 20% solution of formalin and pare weekly.

Note: Cautery or excision of a wart on the sole may result in a painful scar and in general is *not* advisable.

Atopic dermatitis

Atopic dermatitis can begin at any age, but 75% show the first sign by 6 months. Fifty per cent will be clear by puberty and most of the remainder will be clear by 30 years. Involvement *may* be lifelong, however, so the term 'infantile eczema' should be abandoned.

Clinical features

- The skin is dry, with patches of weeping eczema, lichenified skin and evidence of scratching.
- The characteristic distribution is face to 1 year of age, extensor aspects of legs at crawling stage, and flexural at a later age.
- Associated features include asthma and hayfever in both patient and relatives.

Management

- Avoid the term 'infantile eczema'.
- Explain that the skin will need care for many years, possibly indefinitely.
- Avoid wool, nylon, sand, perfumed and medicated products.
- Use bath oil over the long term.
- Use all over b.d. of emollient, such as 10% glycerine in sorbolene cream, in the long term. If this stings, use Eucerin ointment.
- *Topical steroids*: In general, ointments are preferable to creams. Never use topical steroids stronger than hydrocortisone on the face. Elsewhere fluorinated steroids, such as Aristocort 0.02%,

can be used for short periods, t.d.s. Always cease steroids when eczema settles.
- Use nocturnal sedation if necessary, for example Vallergan syrup.
- Give oral antibiotics after a swab if secondary bacterial infection develops.

Seborrhoeic dermatitis

Seborrhoeic dermatitis is a condition of infancy and adult life. It does not occur in children. If it occurs at the 'wrong age', think of drugs (especially antiepileptics), psoriasis or malignant histiocytic disorders.

Clinical features
- Red background with greasy, yellow scale; usually not pruritic
- Characteristic distribution in the scalp, centre of face, behind ears, neck fold, axillae and groin

Management
- *Scalp*: Sulfur 2% and salicylic acid 2% in aqueous cream—apply nocte and wash out mane
- *Flexural areas*: 1% hydrocortisone, with an antimonilial agent
- *Face*: 1% hydrocortisone cream

Molluscum contagiosum

This is a poxvirus infection, which is rare under 1 year of age, and occurs particularly in the 2–5 year age group. The spread of lesions is enhanced in warm water and outbreaks occur among children who swim together or share baths or spas. Further spread of mollusca in the individual is also encouraged by being in warm water.

The typical lesion is spherical and pearly white with a central umbilication 1–5 mm in diameter. Lesions occur on any part of the skin surface with common sites being the axillae and sides of the trunk, the lower abdomen and anogenital area. A secondary eczema often occurs around lesions.

Each lesion lasts for only weeks and if the child is kept out of heated pools and spas and has showers rather than baths at home the proliferation is curbed and the numbers of lesions usually decreases quickly. If these measures are rigidly adhered to, treatment is rarely required. The most definitive treatment is de-roofing of the lesion with a large cutting-edged needle and wiping out the contents. This can be done with nitrous oxide sedation.

Herpes simplex virus infection

Primary herpetic gingivostomatitis

Clinical features

- Ulceration of the tongue, gums, lips and anterior buccal mucosa
- Severe systemic toxicity, with fever
- Lymphadenopathy
- Swelling of soft tissues of face and neck which can be extreme and resemble cellulitis

Management

- Ensure adequate fluid intake. A drip is often required.
- Clean the child's mouth with large cotton wool swabs, with water only.
- IV aciclovir is indicated only if the infection is severe, for example if IV fluids are needed or if the child has eczema.

Disseminated herpes in the atopic ('eczema herpeticum')

Clinical features

- Evanescent, umbilicated vesicles and pustules with a tendency to coalesce, then form punctate erosions
- Usually limited to face, neck and upper chest
- Often severe systemic toxicity

Management

- Confirm HSV by immunofluorescence of skin lesion swab.
- Cease all topical eczema therapy.
- Use saline packs or dressings.
- If severe, give IV aciclovir (5 mg/kg/dose, 8-hourly).

Haemangiomas

Clinical features

These may be superficial or deep or combined lesions:

- *Superficial lesions* usually appear in the first weeks of life as areas of pallor followed by telangiectatic patches. They then grow rapidly into lobulated, well-demarcated, bright red tumours (strawberry naevi). Rapid growth continues over the first 4–5 months; the growth rate then slows and further growth after 6 months is unusual. After a stationary phase, signs of involution appear with the appearance of grey areas which enlarge and coalesce. The tumour becomes softer and less bulky and in 90% of cases disappears by 9 years of age.
- Deeper haemangiomas may occur alone or beneath a superficial lesion. They also usually appear after birth and undergo a growth phase which, however, may be less striking than that of the more superficial lesions. The overlying skin is normal or bluish in colour, or may be surmounted by a superficial haemangioma. As they resolve, they soften and shrink over, and complete disappearance occurs in many cases; occasionally some redundant tissue remains.

Complications

- Ulceration may occur during the rapid growth phase of superficial haemangiomas. Some scarring is inevitable.
- Ulceration of lesions on eyelids, lips or ala nasae can lead to full thickness tissue loss.
- Haemangiomas may encroach on vital structures:
  - the eye—leading to amblyopia
  - the mouth or nose—interference with feeding
  - the larynx—a marker for this is a fast-growing, extensive lower face or neck haemangioma, particularly when there is accompanying intraoral involvement. Arrange lateral airways X-ray, and *urgent* ENT consultation if there is stridor.
- Giant haemangiomas may cause high-output heart failure.

Management

- Simple observation and reassurance while awaiting natural resolution is the ideal approach for most haemangiomas.

- Indications for active intervention, using oral corticosteroids, are an alarming growth rate, threatening ulceration in areas where serious complications could ensue, interference with vital structures and severe bleeding. These patients should be referred urgently to a dermatologist. Early treatment is essential.

Common napkin rash

- All napkin rashes result from a combination of moisture, candidiasis and dermatitis (seborrhoeic, or irritant from urine and faeces).
- Miliaria (sweat duct occlusion) is a common feature.
- Treat with a combination cream: 1% hydrocortisone, with an antimonilial agent. A silicone or zinc barrier cream may be added.
- Treatment includes frequent nappy changes; superabsorbent disposable napkins are preferable to cloth napkins.

Infections presenting as a 'napkin rash'

- *Herpes simplex virus*: 4–6 mm erosions coalescing to produce geographic lesions, with pain, swelling and lymphadenopathy; severe cases require IV aciclovir
- *Enterovirus exanthems*: Often associated with blisters and/or erosions on hands and feet and in the mouth
- *Chickenpox*: Especially where there is a pre-existing napkin rash
- *Kawasaki syndrome*: A red, peeling eruption: look for other signs
- *Impetigo*: Staphylococcal, streptococcal
- *Scalded skin syndrome*: See above
- *Streptococcal*: Perianal disease or vulvitis—treat with 10 days of full dose penicillin and topical mupirocin (Bactroban)

Other causes of napkin rash

- *Psoriasis*: A characteristic well-marginated bright-red rash covering most of the napkin area. Treat with hydrocortisone/antimonilial agent; expect recurrences.
- *Erosive*: Associated with severe diarrhoea. Often perianal. Orabase paste may be useful treatment.
- *Gluteal granulomas*: A peculiar form of napkin rash with purplish nodules on top of pre-existing napkin rash. Responds slowly to standard therapy.

- *Fixed drug eruption*
- *Zinc deficiency*

An infant with napkin eruption which is atypical, unusually severe or unresponsive to standard treatment should be referred.

24

Ocular emergencies

This chapter includes:

- equipment necessary to examine the eye
- trauma
- acute red eye
- preseptal and orbital cellulitis
- relative ocular emergencies.

Equipment necessary to examine the eye

Ocular emergencies are infrequent. The initial treatment is crucial as it will often determine the outcome for the eye. The necessary equipment is:

- a good light source
- magnification—2 × binocular loupe
- an ophthalmoscope
- fluorescein in the form of fluoristrips
- sterile disposable hypodermic needles, cotton tip applicators, epilation forceps, eye speculum, Desmarres' retractors, Eye Stream solution, local anaesthetic eyedrops, eyepads and micropore strapping.

Trauma

Foreign bodies

Conjunctival foreign bodies

- The foreign body is often located on the tarsal conjunctiva of the upper eyelid.
- Remember to evert the upper eyelid; this is done by grasping the

lashes and pulling them down and then everting the eyelid over a cotton tip applicator held at the upper margin of the tarsal plate.
- Attempt to irrigate the foreign body off the conjunctiva with Eye Stream.
- If irrigation is unsuccessful, wipe the foreign body off with a moistened cotton tip applicator.
- Insert antibiotic eye ointment.

Corneal foreign bodies

- These are extremely irritable and painful.
- Instil a local anaesthetic eyedrop into the eye.
- Attempt to wash the foreign body off with Eye Stream or wipe it off with a moistened cotton tip applicator.
- If unsuccessful, attempt to remove the foreign body with a sterile hypodermic needle.
- Approach from the temporal aspect of the cornea; this way there is minimal risk of injury if the child suddenly moves forwards.
- Extra care should be taken if the foreign body is in the visual axis.
- Removal may need to be done under general anaesthesia.
- Insert antibiotic eye ointment and pad the eye.
- Continue treatment with the antibiotic eye ointment until the cornea is completely healed.

Intraocular foreign bodies

- These are extremely rare in children.
- Suspect in a child who has been watching someone use a hammer on metal where the child complains of a sore eye or blurred vision.
- Arrange for plain X-ray or CT of the eye and orbit.
- A child with an intraocular foreign body requires hospitalisation for definitive treatment.

Corneal abrasion

- This generally results from trauma to the cornea from injuries such as a scratch from a twig or a fingernail.
- There is profuse epiphora and photophobia.
- To examine the eye instil an anaesthetic eyedrop.
- Fluorescein is helpful in determining the extent of the abrasion.
- Treat with instillation of antibiotic eye ointment or drops.
- If the eye is very painful a cycloplegic eyedrop (cyclopentolate 1% or homatropine 2%) should be instilled.

- The eye is padded firmly to prevent eyelid movement under the pad.
- The child is followed daily until the abrasion has healed.

Burns
Thermal

- A thermal burn may affect either the eye itself or the eyelids. Thermal burns occur in isolation, such as contact between the eye and a lit cigarette, or may be associated with extensive burns of the body.
- Instil an anaesthetic eyedrop and fluorescein.
- Treat thermal burns on the cornea as for corneal abrasions.
- Treat burns to the eyelid as for other facial skin burns.

Chemical

- Acid burns generally cause only superficial ulceration of the cornea.
- Alkali burns are much more serious because of the ability of the alkali to penetrate the cornea.
- With any chemical burn, first aid treatments consist of profusely irrigating the eye; tap water may be used.
- When the child is seen in Emergency, instil local anaesthetic eyedrops and further irrigate the eye with Eye Stream or saline to neutralise any chemical.
- Particles of lime, if present, must be removed as soon as possible.
- Remember to evert the eyelids as particles are frequently found on the tarsal conjunctiva and in the fornices.
- Instil a cycloplegic eyedrop and antibiotic eye ointment.
- Firmly pad the eye and refer the child for ophthalmological assessment.

Superglue

- Problems are generally caused by accidentally touching the eyes with the glue on the fingers.
- Reassure the parents that it will not harm the eye (superglue is used in the treatment of corneal wounds).
- If the eyelids and eyelashes are stuck together they can be left alone. They spontaneously open in 2 to 3 days. The eyelashes can be cut off to allow eyelid opening if desired or if both eyes are stuck closed.
- The cornea and conjunctiva should be examined and stained with

fluoroscein as soon as is practical. Any corneal abrasion should be treated as above.

Eyelid lacerations

- Penetrating injury of the eye or brain must be excluded.
- The most serious are those involving the eyelid margin.
- Dog bite injuries frequently are associated with a laceration of the medial end of the lower eyelid, involving the lower lacrimal canaliculus.
- Give tetanus toxoid and systemic antibiotics.
- Instil antibiotic eyedrops.
- Admit the child so that the eyelid laceration can be repaired under general anaesthesia.
- Careful repair under magnification is essential to avoid notching of the eyelid and also to achieve repair of the canaliculus if it has been torn in the accident.

Lacerations of the eyeball

Conjunctiva

- This is usually not serious and the conjunctiva will heal quickly with the use of antibiotic eyedrops.
- More extensive lacerations may require suturing under general anaesthesia.

Cornea and sclera

- Lacerations of the outer coat of the eyeball (penetrating eye injury) may lead to damage to intraocular structures and extrusion of intraocular contents.
- Instil antibiotic eyedrops into the eye.
- Do not apply any pressure to the eyelids.
- Apply a sterile eye pad and eye shield.
- Commence systemic antibiotics.
- Admit the child for definitive treatment under general anaesthesia.

Blunt ocular trauma

Hyphaema

- Haemorrhage into the anterior chamber after trauma may range from a barely perceptible deposit inferiorly to complete obscuration of the iris.

321

- A secondary haemorrhage may occur several days after the original injury and may be associated with raised intraocular pressure.
- Admit the child to hospital.
- Give bedrest, with sedation if necessary. Allow toilet privileges.
- Pad the injured eye.
- Treat associated corneal or conjunctival injury.
- The problem generally resolves within 3 to 4 days.
- Long-term follow up is necessary, due to the risk of retinal detachment or glaucoma.
- Some children with small hyphaema may be considered for ambulatory treatment.

Lens damage

- Trauma may cause subluxation of the lens or even cataract formation.
- Refer the child for ophthalmological assessment.

Vitreous haemorrhage

- Partial or complete vitreous haemorrhage may occur from trauma.
- It is diagnosed by the presence of a dull or absent red reflex of the pupil.
- Vitreous haemorrhage may accompany hyphaema.
- There is no emergency treatment. Refer the child for ophthalmological assessment as soon as possible.

Retinal detachment

- Retinal detachment may be a consequence of blunt trauma.
- It is diagnosed by ophthalmoscopy.
- Refer the child to an ophthalmologist for assessment and treatment.

Blowout fracture of the orbit

- This should be suspected if the child presents with a 'black eye'.
- Restricted movement of the eyeball together with diplopia suggests a blowout fracture of the orbit with entrapment of soft tissue.
- Feel the orbit margin.
- Check infraorbital nerve integrity by checking the skin sensation of the cheek.

- The diagnosis can be confirmed by radiological investigation (CT scan) of the orbit.
- Definitive treatment is usually delayed until approximately 2 weeks after the injury when the swelling has settled and the damage can be fully assessed.

Non-accidental injury (NAI)

- Ocular signs are frequently present in the child with non-accidental injury (shaken baby syndrome).
- Examine the fundi with an ophthalmoscope if NAI is suspected, looking for widespread retinal haemorrhages.
- Unexplained subconjunctival or eyelid haemorrhages should also raise suspicion of NAI.
- Arrange for ophthalmological consultation and retinal photography (if available) to document retinal damage.

Acute red eye

Acute glaucoma

- This is extremely rare in childhood but may occur in association with a subluxated lens that causes pupil block.
- It may occur with Marfan's syndrome, homocystinuria or Weill Marchesani syndrome.
- Glaucoma is associated with pain and blurred vision.
- Admit the child for ophthalmological treatment.

Acute iritis

- This causes pain, photophobia and blurred vision in one eye.
- It is associated with ciliary flush (conjunctival injection is more marked about the limbus).
- There is a sluggish, small/irregular pupil.
- Treat by dilating the pupil with atropine 1% eyedrops and instil steroid eyedrops.
- The cause of the iritis should be investigated; the most common association in a child is ANA-positive juvenile chronic arthritis. This form of iritis usually presents with a white eye.

Conjunctivitis

- There is diffuse redness of the conjunctiva and tarsal plates with associated discharge.

- In severe neonatal conjunctivitis, suspect the possibility of gono-coccus or *Chlamydia*. Remember to treat the parents.
- A conjunctival swab for smear culture and sensitivity is indicated in neonates and also in other cases of severe conjunctivitis.
- Treatment consists of appropriate antibiotic eyedrops and ointment.
- Neonates with severe conjunctivitis require hospitalisation for treatment.
- Viral conjunctivitis may be unilateral and is generally not associated with any discharge from the eye. The eyes tend to be watery.

Keratitis

- The eye is injected and there is associated epiphora, photophobia and pain.
- Keratitis may result from trauma, but the possibility of being due to herpes simplex infection must always be suspected.
- Instil an anaesthetic eyedrop and fluorescein.
- Examine the eye with a bright light and look for any disruption of the corneal epithelium.
- Herpes simplex keratitis shows a typical branching corneal ulceration.
- Herpes simplex keratitis is treated with aciclovir eye ointment which is applied 4-hourly; a cycloplegic eyedrop is also instilled if there is extreme discomfort.
- After the initial treatment, refer the child for ophthalmological follow-up.
- Steroid eyedrops must be avoided in the patient with herpes simplex keratitis.
- If keratitis is due to a corneal ulcer the treatment is as previously described (see 'Corneal abrasion' on p. 319).

Preseptal and orbital cellulitis

- Preseptal and orbital cellulitis may occur in a child with associated upper respiratory tract infection.
- These conditions may also occur with conjunctivitis, dacryocystitis, meibomian cysts and sinusitis.
- Frequently, there is no history or signs of any underlying cause.
- In preseptal cellulitis there is usually diffuse swelling and redness of the eyelids with or without pyrexia.

- Admit the child with preseptal cellulitis to hospital and commence intravenous cefotaxime and flucloxacillin—see Chapter 10.
- Preseptal cellulitis generally responds within 48 hours.
- If there is a failure to respond within 48 hours, then arrange a CT scan of orbits and sinuses.
- The child with orbital cellulitis may become extremely unwell.
- Orbital cellulitis is associated with proptosis, chemosis and restriction of the eye movement.
- The child with orbital cellulitis is admitted and commenced on intravenous cefotaxime and flucloxacillin—see Chapter 10.
- Urgent CT scan of orbits and sinuses is indicated as there are generally underlying sinus disease and subperiosteal abscess.
- If sinusitis is diagnosed consult an ENT surgeon about the need to drain the sinus.

Relative ocular emergencies

Leukocoria (white pupil)

When a child is seen with leukocoria the clinician must differentiate between the following:

- cataract
- retinoblastoma
- pseudoglioma.

  Refer to an ophthalmologist as soon as possible.

Strabismus

- Strabismus can be a manifestation of underlying ocular or intracranial disease.
- Children do not grow out of strabismus.
- The child with strabismus should be referred for ophthalmological assessment and treatment as soon as possible.
- Children in the first 3–4 months of life may have intermittent strabismus, which is transient and harmless.

Unilateral proptosis

- Proptosis is a rare problem in children.
- Unilateral proptosis that comes on rapidly and is painless should excite suspicion of an orbital tumour, especially a rhabdomyosarcoma.

- The child should be referred to an ophthalmologist as soon as possible for assessment.

Postoperative problems

- Children may present with problems following strabismus, ptosis and intraocular or other surgery.
- Many instances relate to normal healing processes and no more than reassurance is necessary.
- Some instances represent infection or other complications.
- Discuss these problems with an ophthalmologist.

25

Common ENT conditions

This chapter includes:
- nasal discharge
- inhaled foreign body (bronchial)
- ingested foreign body
- tonsillitis
- acute otitis media
- discharging ears
- glue ear
- epistaxis
- laceration of the oral cavity.

Nasal discharge
- Most nasal discharge is due to the common cold.
- In colds, discharge is clear initially, then normally becomes mucopurulent. This is not an indication for antibiotics.
- Allergic rhinitis is more likely to cause a blocked nose, but may cause chronic nasal discharge, often with nasal itch and sneezing.
- Persistent unilateral nasal discharge, often foul-smelling, may be due to a foreign body. This can often be removed under direct vision using nitrous oxide analgesia.

Inhaled foreign body (bronchial)
- A bronchial foreign body often presents with a history of chronic cough, or sudden onset of wheeze, or a choking, cyanotic episode.
- Chest auscultation may reveal unilateral wheeze and/or reduced air entry over one lung field.
- Chest X-ray may show hyperinflation of one lung or lung segment or a radio-opaque foreign body in the airway.
- Contact the ENT surgeon urgently, and keep the child 'nil by mouth' for rigid laryngobronchoscopy.

Ingested foreign body

- An ingested foreign body may lodge high in the oesophagus, causing drooling, inability to swallow and/or airway obstruction. In the lower oesophagus a foreign body may cause vomiting.
- Chest X-ray may show a radio-opaque foreign body with a pocket of air above. Look for air in the mediastinum, indicating oesophageal perforation.
- Keep the child 'nil by mouth' and notify the ENT surgeon. Rigid oesophagoscopy is likely to be required.

Tonsillitis

- Group A streptococcal tonsillitis is uncommon under the age of 5 and very rare under 3 years of age.
- In preschool children, exudative tonsillitis is usually viral due to adenovirus (which often causes high fever and sometimes also conjunctivitis), EBV or HSV.
- In school-age children about 25% of tonsillitis is due to group A streptococcus.
- Ideally, a positive culture should be obtained before starting treatment.
- Where empiric therapy is desirable, use penicillin V, not ampicillin (because of the risk of rash with EBV).
- Peritonsillar abscess (quinsy) is a rare complication of tonsillitis in childhood. It causes trismus (spasm of the jaw muscles) and swelling of the soft palate. It requires drainage by ENT as well as intravenous antibiotics.

Acute otitis media

- Almost half of all episodes of acute otitis media are viral and will resolve with or without antibiotics.
- It is often worth waiting for a day or two before giving antibiotics to a child with red eardrums as many resolve spontaneously.
- The commonest bacterial causes are *S. pneumoniae*, *H. influenzae*, and *Branhamella catarrhalis*.
- Empiric antibiotic therapy is usually with amoxycillin.
- Poor response to amoxycillin may be due to beta-lactamase-

producing organisms; second-line drugs are amoxycillin–clavulanate and cotrimoxazole.

- Myringotomy should be considered where there is a bulging drum with severe pain.
- Acute mastoiditis is a complication of acute otitis media and causes fever, swelling and redness behind a protruding pinna. This requires admission and a cortical mastoidectomy.

Discharging ears

- Ear discharge may arise from otitis media through a perforated eardrum or a grommet. This is usually profuse and painless. Arrange a swab and treat with oral and topical antibiotics, based on the swab result.
- This condition is common in remote communities and is often chronic.
- Painful scanty ear discharge with swelling of the ear canal or pinna is due to otitis externa. Treat with aural toilet and antibiotic ear drops. When severe, intravenous antibiotics may be necessary.

Glue ear

- This is the commonest cause of childhood hearing impairment and speech delay.
- It affects 15–30% of children aged 3–10 years.
- The diagnosis is confirmed with a hearing test and tympanometry.
- Medical treatment is the initial treatment of choice:
  - antibiotics for 10–30 days (amoxycillin first, then, if unsuccessful, amoxycillin–clavulanate or cotrimoxazole)
  - Eustachian tube exercises (such as blowing up balloons)
  - treatment of any nasal or nasopharyngeal disease
  - steroids—advocated, with antibiotics, by some authorities.
- Surgical treatment (grommet insertion) is indicated for failed medical treatment with ongoing hearing loss or other serious problems. Grommet insertion can often be done as an outpatient, elective procedure.

Epistaxis

- Bleeding is usually from a venous plexus at the front of the nasal septum known as Little's area.

- Mild cases often respond to firm pressure to the tip of the nose, along with an ice-pack to the forehead, for 10 minutes. Sit the child forward and ask him or her to breathe through the mouth.
- More persistent bleeding may need cauterisation of the bleeding vessel with a silver nitrate stick or nasal packing by ENT.
- Check the blood pressure, clotting studies and FBC and establish intravenous access when persistent bleeding is present. Consult ENT for persistent, recurrent or posterior nasal bleeding.

Laceration of the oral cavity

- This may occur when a child falls with an object, like a ruler, in the mouth.
- There is usually bleeding and a laceration of the hard or soft palate.
- Keep the child 'nil by mouth' during assessment as suturing may be required.
- Most lacerations are small, stop bleeding spontaneously and require no treatment.
- Arrange a lateral soft-tissue X-ray, looking for retropharyngeal air, which would indicate a posterior pharyngeal tear.
  See also Chapter 26.

26

Dental and oro-facial emergencies

This chapter includes:
- trauma
- infection
- other dental problems
- usual eruption times for the primary and permanent dentition.

Trauma

This chapter is a guide for initial management of oro-facial conditions likely to be seen by medical staff as emergencies.

Trauma and infection are the most common reasons for children presenting to an emergency department with an oro-facial problem. The trauma usually involves the face and in particular the mouth, while infections are either bacterial (usually involving decayed teeth) or viral (associated with soft tissues).

Traumatic incidents

Most traumatic incidents involving the hard and soft tissues of the mouth will require a dental consultation. Having the dental officer on call talk directly with the patient's caregivers can be reassuring and may be all that is required for a minimal injury. When the accident is of greater concern, such as significant oral bleeding has occurred or there is displacement of teeth, the dental officer on call will need to examine the patient.

Trauma to teeth and jaws

Traumatic injuries to the face and jaws should be assessed and treated as early as possible to avoid long-term oro-facial sequelae, such as disturbed jaw growth, loss or malposition of primary and permanent teeth and soft tissue, and the need for extensive restorative dentistry.

Soft tissue lacerations

- All soft tissue lacerations, especially gingival tissues, should be assessed for degloving and for the need to reposition and suture.
- Where teeth are significantly displaced there will be associated displacement and laceration of soft tissue. It is very important for long-term periodontal and gingival health of the traumatised teeth that displaced soft tissues are adequately repositioned and sutured. Alveolar bone should never be left exposed.
- Check that mucosal lacerations do not extend through to the skin layer. Such full thickness lacerations can often be disguised by swelling of the perioral tissues.

Suspected fracture of the mandible and maxilla

- Tetanus prophylaxis and antibiotics (penicillin, metronidazole) should always be given for a compound fracture into the mouth or skin. The key points in recognition of a facial fracture are pain, facial swelling, stepping (of bone border), limited jaw opening, palatal or sublingual haematoma, and altered occlusion.
- The paediatric dentist and/or maxillo-facial surgeon on call should be involved in the management of these children from the time of presentation.
- Admission will be required.
- Initial radiographic examination should include orthopanto-mography (OPG), plain films and, where indicated, CT scan.
- Make sure to check whether a child can bite together evenly. Allow for the front teeth not touching due to pre-existing distortion from a dummy or finger sucking habits. Obtain a dental opinion if in doubt.

Tooth fractures

- Crown fractures usually involve enamel and dentine. Fractures of the crown can also involve exposure of the 'nerve'. This is usually seen as a pink or bleeding area in the centre of the fracture. The root of the tooth and the alveolar bone can also be fractured, often with minimal damage to the crown of the tooth.
- Once the extent of the crown and/or root fractures has been

established (including 'nerve' involvement), appropriate treatment can be planned.

- It is important to locate any missing tooth fragments. These may lodge in the lungs or in soft tissue lacerations. Consider a chest X-ray.
- Assess tetanus prophylaxis status and the need for antibiotics.
- Arrange a dental consultation as soon as possible. All that may be necessary is to discuss the case with the dental staff on call who can provide appropriate advice and follow-up care.
- Early (same day) placement of a temporary restoration by a dentist to seal and protect exposed dentine significantly reduces the potential for 'nerve' death.

Luxated and avulsed primary incisor teeth (children age 0–6 years)

- Teeth can be displaced in any direction (luxation) or dislodged totally from their socket (avulsion). These injuries are usually associated with alveolar fractures—fracture of the bone housing the teeth but not including basal bone. A dental consultation needs to be arranged as soon as possible. Discuss the degree of displacement and/or fracture, and soft tissue damage with the on-call dentist.
- Appropriate treatment may include extraction of one or more teeth and suturing of soft tissues.
- If a primary tooth is avulsed, do not replant it. Such teeth are not reimplanted because of the risk of damaging the underlying permanent tooth.

Luxated and avulsed permanent incisor teeth

- Ideally, teeth should be repositioned/reimplanted in the socket immediately. Handle the tooth gently by the crown only and not by the root surface. The tooth must be kept moist if it is being examined. Soak gauze in saline and gently hold the tooth with the gauze while examining it.
- If it is not possible to reimplant the tooth it must be stored in tissue culture medium, or milk, or wrapped in plastic wrap. This is an interim measure only and urgent dental management is required to minimise the risk of tooth loss. *Note*: Tissue culture medium is kept refrigerated in the Emergency Department.

- Teeth reimplanted within 30 minutes, with appropriate interim storage, have the best long-term results.
- Order appropriate radiographs: OPG, lateral cephalogram and chest X-rays.
- Once the tooth has been reimplanted, splinting and stabilisation by the dentist on call will be required, along with treatment of soft tissue lacerations.
- A temporary splint can be constructed from aluminium foil moulded around the tooth.
- Urgent dental follow-up should be arranged. Follow-up is essential because root canal therapy (endodontics) will most likely be undertaken within a week or two of the injury.

Infection

Infection with facial swelling

When a child presents with a facial swelling, raised temperature and general malaise, admission to the hospital is usually required, for full assessment as well as intravenous fluids and antibiotics (penicillin and metronidazole).

Infection without facial swelling

For children with oral infection without obvious facial swelling but with a raised temperature and/or general malaise (for example, a primary herpes infection) a dental consultation may be required. The child is unlikely to need admission to the hospital unless severely dehydrated or medically compromised.

Other dental problems

The following problems may present as emergencies, but require careful triaging to accurately determine the true emergency nature of the situation:

- lost fillings or artificial crown (if associated with significant pain)
- damaged orthodontic appliances. If damaged orthodontic wires are traumatising oral mucosa they can be treated easily by using a haemostat to 'tuck' the offending piece of wire back in to the tooth bracket, or using wire cutters to remove the offending wire. Alternatively there is some sticky 'red wax' available at triage to

mould over the offending piece of wire and give adequate relief to traumatised mucosa.

Such situations as a superficially chipped tooth or minor lacerations not needing suturing can best be treated with warm saline rinses and the use of a chlorhexidine gluconate 0.2% rinse.

All patients should be advised to contact their usual dental provider for an appointment at the earliest opportunity.

Oral bleeding

- Always wear gloves.
- If possible, irrigate the child's mouth with water or saline.
- Remove loose blood clots using gauze or tweezers.
- Identify the source of bleeding, such as a soft tissue laceration or tooth socket.
- A bleeding tooth socket is frequently associated with the extraction of a tooth that had presented with untreated infection.
- A persistently bleeding tooth socket can often signal a haematological disorder. Local haemostatic measures are still the first line of treatment.

Bleeding from a tooth socket

- Firmly compress the alveolar bone between finger and thumb.
- Apply pressure to the bleeding gum (not the adjacent teeth) for 20 minutes using a tightly folded gauze pad. In cases where the child is uncooperative, a parent must be encouraged to hold the gauze pack in place for the appropriate time. It is not necessary to pack anything into the socket.
- Sedation/analgesia (for example, IM pethidine) may be required and this should be given immediately if indicated.
- Topical thrombin may be placed on the pack.
- Antibiotics should be given if infection is present. This is usually indicated by a history of pain, abscess and/or sinus formation prior to the onset of bleeding. Penicillin is the drug of first choice.
- Dental consultation is usually required if bleeding continues.

Intermittent facial and/or dental pain

Children who present with facial and/or dental pain (for example, after eating) and who are otherwise well usually require analgesia and appropriate dental follow-up (private or public). Spontaneous dental pain is indicative of irreversible inflammation of the dental pulp (the nerve). Children who also suffer from serious medical conditions (cardiac, haematological, oncological) require acute dental care.

Table 26.1 Usual eruption times for the primary and permanent dentition

Primary (or deciduous) teeth (total 20)	Age (months)
Central/lateral incisors	6–12
Cuspids	16–20
First molars	12–16
Second molars	20–30

Permanent teeth (total 32)	Age (years)
Central/lateral incisors	6–10
Cuspids	10–12
First bicuspid	10–12
Second bicuspid	11–12
First molars	6–7
Second molars	11–13
Third molars	17–21

There is wide variation in eruption times, particularly of the deciduous teeth. At 1 year an infant has six to eight teeth, at 18 months 12 teeth, and at 2–3 years 20 teeth. If there are no teeth erupted by 12 months, dental consultation should be sought.

The first permanent teeth to erupt are the lower, first molars followed by central incisors.

Fluoride supplementation

See Chapter 4.

27

Acute poisoning and envenomation

This chapter includes:

- accidental ingestion of drugs and chemicals
- poison removal methods
- supportive treatment
- snake and spider bite.

Accidental ingestion of drugs and chemicals

Consult the Poisons Information Centre (13 11 26) on all except obviously trivial poisonings.

Some general points

- Most accidental ingestions of drugs and chemicals by children are harmless, though severe poisoning and occasionally death still occur. Therefore do not delay assessment and any appropriate treatment.
- Poisoning in young children has been greatly reduced by child-resistant packaging and scheduling changes.
- The likelihood of serious poisoning can usually be predicted if the amount of drug or chemical missing can be accurately assessed.
- Guidelines which included uncritical use of ipecac-induced emesis or gastric lavage are now outmoded; these often led to unnecessary, unpleasant and dangerous treatment. Poison removal methods are now advised much more selectively.

General principles of management

- *First, do no harm!*
- Assess the situation:

- Identify the suspected poison, likely dose and time of ingestion as accurately as possible.
- Assess general appearance, vital signs and obvious abnormalities.
- Respiratory or circulatory support, if needed, takes precedence over other measures.
- *Consult the Poisons Information Centre* in all cases, unless you are certain the poisoning is trivial. You should now have a plan of action.
- Remove the poison, if possible and if appropriate:
  - Attempts at poison removal are carried out only when a significant risk of poisoning is considered likely—that is, in only a small proportion of childhood accidental ingestions.
- Provide supportive therapy.

Poison removal methods

Activated charcoal

- Adsorption of the ingested poisons with activated charcoal is the preferred method of poison removal, in most instances. It should be given within 30 minutes of ingestion, but may still be advised at an hour or later.
- It is useful for most drugs and organic chemicals, but is not useful with alcohols, strong acids or alkalis, or with metallic salts, such as those of iron and lithium.
- Give 1 g/kg, up to 50 g, in a slurry made with water.
- Children will often refuse to drink charcoal slurries; they are then given via a nasogastric tube.
- The nasogastric tube should be a size above the 'feeding-tube' gauge.
- With liquid poisons, such as paracetamol syrup, aspiration of the tube prior to charcoal administration may be useful.
- Emesis follows the use of charcoal about 5–20% of the time; lung damage from aspiration of charcoal and gastric contents is a significant hazard.
- Unconscious children can be given activated charcoal. However, they require airway protection.
- Activated charcoal is used selectively—only where significant poisoning is a possibility, and where the benefits of activated charcoal are assessed as outweighing potential disadvantages.

- In some severe poisonings, repeat doses of activated charcoal may be advised by the Poisons Centre, up to 1 g/kg 4-hourly.

Gastric lavage

- Gastric lavage will occasionally be advised by the Poisons Centre.
- It is usually considered only for poisons not adsorbed by activated charcoal, though it may occasionally be advised prior to activated charcoal use when potentially fatal poisoning is considered likely.
- Gastric lavage beyond 1 hour after ingestion is much less likely to be beneficial, and should be used only if advised by a toxicologist.
- Airway protection (tracheal intubation by an anaesthetist, with full resuscitation facilities present) will be required with a drowsy or unconscious child, and with most small children generally.
- It should not be used following ingestion of caustics or petroleum distillates (kerosene, turpentine and so on).

Whole bowel lavage

- This is occasionally advised for potentially very severe poisoning, for example with iron tablets.
- Iso-osmolar polyethylene glycol (ColonLYTELY, Glycoprep) is given orally or by nasogastric tube, 15–25 mL/kg/h until rectal effluent is clear (usually about 4 hours).

Outmoded techniques

- Syrup of ipecac has no place in hospital management. If it has any use at all, this may be for emergency induction of vomiting, for poison removal, in very isolated areas, and only after consultation with the Poisons Centre.
- Catharsis using magnesium sulfate or other osmotic agents has no place in poison removal.

Systemic removal methods

Peritoneal dialysis, haemodialysis, forced diuresis and exchange transfusion are very rarely, if ever, necessary for poisoned children. The Poisons Centre will advise on these if necessary.

Use of a pharmacological antagonist or chelating agent

Pharmacological antagonists (for example naloxone, for opioid poisoning) and chelating agents (for example DMSA, for lead poisoning) are useful in only a small proportion of poisonings. However, they will be advised by the Poisons Centre if they are likely to be useful.

Supportive treatment

- In severe established poisoning, survival will often depend upon the quality of supportive care.
- Respiratory and circulatory support, once necessary, take precedence over all other management measures.
- Where arrhythmias are a potential problem, use cardiac monitoring.
- Use pulse oximetry in very unwell children.
- Inotropes may be necessary for depressed myocardial function.
- Fluid requirements may vary widely.
- Control convulsions, hypothermia and hyperthermia.
- Emotional support for the family and careful follow-up are essential.

Ask for laboratory assistance

- A drug screen done on urine gives the opportunity of diagnosing or proving commoner drug ingestions; such tests may be ordered as urgent investigations, where clinically warranted, or the urine stored appropriately for subsequent testing.
- Specific assays are often useful in determining severity, and sometimes in guiding therapy, for instance with paracetamol, ethanol, iron, lithium, salicylate and theophylline poisoning.

Snake and spider bite

Important information relevant to Australian snake and spider bite

- Many bitten children develop no symptoms, because no venom has been injected.
- The creature is not always seen—tentatively believe a child who claims to have been bitten.
- Venoms of different snakes are antigenically distinctive, but with most:
  - there are often only minor or absent local effects
  - neurotoxicity (progressive paralysis) and/or coagulopathy are the most serious systemic effects.

- The CSL Venom Detection Kit (VDK) when used with a swab from the bite site (for the best yield) or with urine (less often useful) often gives positive identification of the snake. No VDK is available for spider bites.
- Red-bellied black snakes and death adders are often correctly identified by non-experts; for all others a recognised professional herpetologist is needed, especially where such identification will determine the choice of antivenom used in treatment.
- Any bite from a large black or dark-coloured spider must be considered potentially dangerous, as distinguishing funnel-webs (*Atrax* or *Hadronyche*) from non-venomous species requires expert training.
- Funnel-web spider bites cause severe local pain; systemic symptoms (abdominal pain, dyspnoea, perioral numbness, sweating, salivation) indicate the need for immediate evaluation and treatment.
- Red-back spider bites cause severe local pain and relatively gradual progression of symptoms; when seen the spider is usually correctly identified.

First aid principles

- Apply a pressure bandage over the bite site, then the limb; if crepe bandages or other material for this are unavailable, use a broad (not tight) tourniquet around the proximal limb.
- Immobilise the limb by splinting; carry the victim to help.
- *Do not* wash or clean the bite site, *do not* cut or incise the bitten area, *do not* try to suck the venom from the wound, *do not* use a tight tourniquet or constrictive bandage, *do not* try to catch the snake.

Management principles

- *Delay systemic venom absorption*: Apply compression bandage; immobilise.
- *Transfer to hospital*: When appropriate personnel and antivenom are available, remove first-aid measures.
- *Maintain circulation and respiration* and use other supportive measures as appropriate, but do not delay specific therapy (antivenom—see below) when needed.
- *Consult the Poisons Information Centre* who will arrange for a consultant to discuss management with you directly.

341

- *Arrange bite site swab and urine testing* with the CSL Venom Detection Kit (VDK).
- *Arrange baseline tests*, including clotting studies.
- *Give antivenom* if the victim has clinical and/or laboratory evidence of significant envenomation. Choice of antivenom is based on results of the CSL VDK, or on accurate snake or spider identification, or on the basis of accurate knowledge of all possible snake types in the area.
- *Anaphylaxis* is always a potential hazard when antivenoms are given. Have adrenaline 1:1000 drawn up and ready to use.
- The dose of antivenom is whatever is required to reverse the effects of the venom, such as paralysis or coagulopathy. If in doubt consult.

28

Preanaesthetic preparation

This chapter includes:

- consent for operation and anaesthesia
- preoperative assessment.

Consent for operation and anaesthesia

- Consent must be obtained from a parent or legal guardian or, when appropriate, from the Department of Community Services.
- A signed form is usual. Occasionally, in urgent circumstances, verbal consent may be acceptable after discussion with the parents by telephone.
- In an emergency, when parents are unavailable, the chief executive or executive director of the hospital may give consent.

Preoperative assessment

Medical assessment

Medical assessment by an anaesthetist is routinely made preoperatively:

- Any underlying medical condition is noted; assessment is made for anaesthetic fitness, with particular reference to the cardiovascular and respiratory systems.
- During this consultation, the anaesthetist attempts to develop rapport with the child and family, to allay anxiety, to explain anaesthetic procedures and to discuss the risks relevant to anaesthesia.
- Postoperative pain management is also explained.
- Loose teeth are noted and recorded.
- A history of previous anaesthesia is sought, and any problems, such as significant nausea and vomiting, noted.

Premedication

Premedication is prescribed when indicated. Drugs chosen for this have one or more of the following effects:

- anxiolysis
- analgesia
- antisialagogue action (antisalivatory)
- vagolysis—to prevent bradycardia and reduction in cardiac output during deep halothane induction, particularly in the very young whose cardiac output is heart-rate dependent. Venous access in a child with chubby hands and feet may be difficult and emergency administration of atropine may be delayed. For this reason atropine before induction (either IM or orally) is helpful (maximum of 20 micrograms/kg)
- antiemetic action
- reduction in gastric acidity
- promotion of gastric emptying
- bronchodilatation
- topical anaesthetic action
- SBE prophylaxis.

Premedicant drugs may be given orally, parenterally, by inhalation or topically, for example EMLA, amethocaine creams.

Intercurrent infection

In the assessment, certain infections are of special relevance. Active upper respiratory tract infection generally contraindicates elective surgery because respiratory tract irritability is increased, with coughing and laryngeal spasm more likely to occur during induction of anaesthesia, resulting in increased risk of hypoxia.

In an otherwise well child with minimal respiratory tract symptoms, the anaesthetist may decide to proceed with anaesthesia for elective surgery but each case has to be assessed individually.

Oral herpes simplex virus active infection may contraindicate anaesthesia for elective surgery because of the risk of dissemination of the virus.

Dental caries may complicate intraoral manipulations. It may be advisable to postpone elective surgery pending dental treatment.

Previous steroid medication

- Steroid therapy may suppress adrenal function and the patient may not respond appropriately to the stress of surgery and anaesthesia.
- Supplemental steroid is usually given if there is a history of at least 1 week of steroid therapy within the last 6 months.

Current medications

These must be documented because of the potential for interaction with drugs administered during anaesthesia.

Hypersensitivities and allergies

An allergic history must be elicited and documented. Besides drug allergies, hypersensitivity to adhesive tape and latex (in surgical gloves and IV injection ports) is also relevant.

Preoperative fasting

- No solid food, cow's milk or formula should be given for at least 6 hours before anaesthesia.
- Clear fluids, for example non-residue drinks such as cordial, fizzy drink and apple juice (not orange juice), are allowed up to 2 hours before anaesthesia.
- It is important that babies be given oral fluids up till the minimum fast period prior to anaesthesia.
- Breastfed babies may continue feeds until 4 hours before anaesthesia. Some may require intravenous fluids preoperatively if hypoglycaemia is a significant risk.
- Fluid and electrolyte imbalance should be corrected before anaesthesia, for example when associated with intestinal obstruction.
- For children with diabetes mellitus see also Chapter 15.

29

Sedation for procedures

This chapter includes:

- general considerations
- patient selection
- essential equipment
- care guidelines
- sedative agents in common use
- antagonist drugs.

General considerations

Although many children tolerate diagnostic and therapeutic procedures awake, the provision of general anaesthesia or sedation with or without analgesia is increasingly seen as a standard of care, especially for invasive procedures. For some children, general anaesthesia is necessary (for example, for those who are developmentally delayed or who have complex medical conditions) and needs to be booked on a general anaesthesia list. In selected cases, sedation by non-anaesthetists can be a safe and flexible alternative. The guidelines below aim to enhance the safety of procedural sedation.

The aims of procedural sedation

- Minimise physical discomfort or pain.
- Control behaviour, particularly movement.
- Minimise psychological disturbance.

  These aims must never compromise patient safety.

When procedural sedation fails

- All sedation regimes have a failure rate.
- Should sedation fail, the child should be rescheduled for an appropriate general anaesthesia list.

Degrees of sedation

Four degrees of sedation, defined below, cover the continuum from minimal sedation to anaesthesia. At the Children's Hospital at Westmead, only minimal sedation and conscious sedation can be administered by non-anaesthetists. Deep sedation, when required or when inadvertently obtained, requires the involvement of anaesthetists.

1 *Minimal sedation (anxiolysis)*: a drug-induced state in which patients respond normally to verbal commands. Although cognitive function and co-ordination may be impaired, ventilatory and cardiovascular functions are unaffected.

2 *Conscious sedation*: a medically controlled state of depressed consciousness that (a) allows protective reflexes to be maintained; (b) retains the patient's ability to maintain a patent airway independently and continuously, and (c) permits appropriate responses by the patient to physical stimulation or verbal commands, such as 'open your eyes'.

3 *Deep sedation*: a medically controlled state of depressed consciousness or unconsciousness from which the patient is not easily aroused. It may be accompanied by a partial or complete loss of protective reflexes, and includes the inability to maintain a patent airway independently and respond purposefully to physical stimulation or verbal command.

4 *Anaesthesia*: a medically controlled state of depressed consciousness accompanied by loss of protective reflexes, including the inability to maintain a patent airway independently and respond purposefully to physical stimulation or verbal command.

The sedation period

This is the time between administration of a sedative regimen and that time when the patient recovers to the point where he or she meets specified discharge criteria. During this time, cognitive function and co-ordination may be impaired and the child may be at risk of partial or complete loss of protective airway reflexes. It is therefore very important to adhere to the monitoring and care guidelines set out below.

Common settings where sedation may be required

- *Medical Imaging Department*: For MRI and CT scans, urodynamic studies and nuclear scans

- *Out-patient clinics*: For change of gastrostomy buttons, removal of sutures and so on
- *Neurophysiology Department*: For nerve conduction studies, EEGs
- *Cardiology Department*: For transthoracic ECHO or ECG
- *Wards*: For difficult intravenous cannulation, dressing changes, drain removal, liver and renal biopsies, auditory evoked brainstem responses

Nominated responsible staff member

Whenever procedural sedation is employed, a nominated staff member must take responsibility for the care of the child during the sedation period. This staff member must have the skills and training to observe the patient's vital signs, airway patency, adequacy of ventilation and level of sedation. He or she must be able to commence resuscitation procedures and know who to call for additional help.

Medical staff who prescribe sedative agents should be familiar with the pharmacology of the sedative agents being used, their adverse effects profile and the use of appropriate antagonist agents. For the duration of the sedation period, a medical staff member who possesses skills in resuscitation (administration of oxygen, insertion of IV line, use of bag and face mask to support ventilation) must be available. In many instances, the hospital resuscitation team will provide this support.

Patient selection

Factors that must be taken into account before prescribing sedation

- Patient's age, weight, developmental stage and medical condition
- Duration of procedure and degree of stimulation/pain
- Degree of immobility required
- Concurrent medication—especially other drugs that may act synergistically with sedatives, for example opioid analgesics, antiepileptics, antidepressants
- Context—in-patient or out-patient; previous response to sedation

Remember, non-pharmacological techniques, good psychological preparation and parent education and involvement may obviate or reduce the need for drug sedation. A parent information leaflet ('fact sheet') is available and should be used where appropriate.

Contraindications for sedation by non-anaesthetists

Sedation by non-anaesthetists is contraindicated in the following situations:

- premature infants with a postnatal age of less than 12 weeks
- any child or infant with:
  - raised intracranial pressure
  - vomiting, bowel obstruction
  - altered state of consciousness
  - gastro-oesophageal reflux
  - snoring, stridor or sleep apnoea
  - pneumonia or an O_2 requirement
  - history of difficult airway
  - hypovolaemia or sepsis
  - craniofacial abnormality or neck swellings.

Essential equipment

For every procedural sedation, the following equipment *must* be available:

- standard hospital resuscitation trolley
- functioning suction apparatus
- oxygen supply with appropriate patient delivery system (masks/tubing and/or breathing circuits)
- pulse oximeter—pulse oximetry is mandatory for all but the most minor sedative regimens
- naloxone and flumazenil
- an emergency call system to summon extra help.

For some procedures, an ECG monitor and blood pressure monitor are also required.

Care guidelines

Fasting

- Patients should be fasted from solids and liquids for 2 hours prior to any sedative regime. This includes bottle- and breastmilk, jelly and clear fluids.
- *Note*: When deeper levels of sedation/analgesia are required (for instance when oral sedatives are to be used in combination with

nitrous oxide), patients should be fasted from solids, jelly and milk for 4 hours prior to the procedure. Clear fluids may continue up to 2 hours prior to sedation.

- Always liase with an endocrinologist before prescribing a sedative and/or fasting a child with diabetes mellitus. See Chapter 15.

Consent

Informed consent must be obtained for both the procedure and the sedation.

Staffing

A minimum of two clinical staff members should be present for the care of a child during a procedure. One member is to be responsible for continuous observation of the patient's vital signs, airway patency, adequacy of ventilation and level of sedation.

- Staff responsible for the administration of sedative drugs must be confident and competent in their use, must be able to initiate resuscitation procedures and must know when to call for additional help.

Observation requirements

- Monitor and document the patient's temperature, heart rate and respiratory rate hourly until discharge criteria are met.
- Continuous pulse oximetry should be used for the same amount of time.

General care

- Sedated patients should be placed in the left lateral position until they are awake.
- Oxygen, suction, pharyngeal airway and a self-inflating bag must accompany the patient until discharge criteria are met.

Transport protocol

- In the sedation period (between sedative administration and the time when discharge criteria are met) portable oxygen and suction must accompany the patient during transport.
- Oxygen saturation must be monitored during transport.
- The patient should be accompanied by a confident and competent staff member who must be continuously responsible for

observation of the patient's vital signs, airway patency, ventilation and level of sedation, and be able to initiate resuscitation procedures and know how to call for additional help.

Discharge criteria (for outpatients)

- Cardiovascular function and airway patency are satisfactory and stable.
- The patient is easily rousable, and protective reflexes are intact.
- The patient can talk (if age-appropriate).
- The patient can sit up unaided (if age-appropriate).
- The child has returned to his/her presedation level of responsiveness.
- The state of hydration is adequate.
- There is no respiratory distress.
- There is no more than minimal pain.
- There is no significant nausea, vomiting and dizziness.

Discharge criteria (for return to general ward/general nursing care)

- Cardiovascular function and airway patency are satisfactory and stable.
- The patient is rousable, and protective reflexes are intact.
- There is no respiratory distress.
- Pain is adequately controlled.

Antagonist drugs

Naloxone

Dose

- 5 micrograms/kg/dose IV over 1–2 minutes for opioid-induced respiratory depression
- Can be repeated every 2–3 minutes
- Maximum dose 2 mg

Caution: Because the duration of action of naloxone is shorter than that of the typical opioids it reverses, any child requiring naloxone must be observed carefully for the return of opioid-induced side-effects.

Flumazenil

Dose

- 5 micrograms/kg/dose given IV for benzodiazepine-induced oversedation
- Can be repeated every 1–2 minutes
- Maximum dose 40 micrograms/kg or 2 mg

Caution: Resedation may occur; flumazenil may increase the risk of seizures in predisposed patients.

Benztropine

Dose

- 10 micrograms/kg/dose given IV or IM for dyskinesia and dystonia induced by droperidol or metoclopramide
- Can be repeated after 15 minutes

Table 29.1 Sedative agents in common use

Formulation	Dose	Administration	Side-effects	Used for
Chloral hydrate				
Syrup 1 g/10 mL i.e. 100 mg/mL	> 3 months: 50 mg/kg = (0.5 mL/kg) (oral/rectal) Max. 1 g	Give slowly or dilute with water to improve palatability and avoid gastric irritation. Give orally 30 minutes before procedure; for rectal use dilute 1:1 with olive oil and give via soft feeding tube.	Nausea, vomiting, gastric irritation, diarrhoea, delirium, disorientation, ataxia, paradoxical excitement, respiratory depression, airway obstruction, ketonuria, leucopoenia, rash.	*Not for infants < 3 months or ex-prems* Used for CT and MRI scans, nuclear medicine studies, brain stem auditory evoked responses, Dexa scans, EEGs, applying gallows traction. Used in dosage 20 mg/kg with pethidine 1.5 mg/kg IM for removal of sutures following cleft lip surgery.
Midazolam				
Syrup 1 mg/mL Parenteral solution, 5 mg/mL	0.5 mg/kg (oral/buccal) 0.2 mg/kg (nasal)	Give oral solution 30 min before procedure. Apply injection solution to buccal mucosa, or as drops into nostrils, 15–20 min before procedure.	Ataxia (supervise well to prevent falls); coma, apnoea, respiratory depression, airway obstruction, low BP, excitement, confusion. *Note:* Synergistic action with opioids.	Echocardiography (using nasal). In combination with nitrous oxide and topical anaesthetic cream for lumbar puncture, bone marrow aspiration, IV cannulation, skin biopsy, removal of central lines, etc.
Ketamine				
Parenteral preparations 50 mg/mL and 100 mg/mL	3–10 mg/kg oral (lower dose for analgesia only; higher doses may induce dissociative anaesthesia)	Use 100 mg/mL solution mixed with apple juice. Give orally 30 minutes before procedure.	Hallucinations and emergence phenomenon, raised intracranial pressure, seizure activity, hypertension, tachycardia, nausea, vomiting, salivation, bronchorrhoea.	Can be used in combination with midazolam (0.5 mg/kg orally), both given 20–30 min before the procedure.

continues . . .

Table 29.1 Sedative agents in common use (*continued*)

Formulation	Dose	Administration	Side-effects	Used for
Nitrous oxide				
100% gas	Inspired concentration 30–70%, with oxygen	Only by accredited nursing and anaesthesia staff, under the supervision of the Pain and Palliative Care team. Check the hospital's *Policy and Procedure Manual*.	Nausea and vomiting; symptoms related to gas expansion, therefore *contraindicated with pneumothorax, bowel obstruction, recent craniotomy.*	Botulinum toxin injection, urodynamic studies, abdominal paracentesis, gastrostomy tube changes, venous cannulation including long-line insertion, dressing and plaster cast changes, minor laceration repairs, lumbar puncture. Used in conjunction with morphine (0.5 mg/kg oral) and midazolam (0.3–0.5 mg/kg oral) and paracetamol for burns baths. Also used in combination with codeine (1 mg/kg oral) and paracetamol for gastrostomy button changes.

Check the latest specific guidelines in the ward policy and procedure manual and/or the hospital intranet.

30

Management of burns

This section includes:

- first aid measures
- management of the shock phase
- replacement of losses of water, electrolytes and protein
- monitoring of the shock phase
- local treatment of the burn wound
- general aspects of management
- skin grafting procedures.

First aid measures

- *Remove the source of heat* by:
  - smothering the flames (rolling the patient on the ground, preferably in a blanket or coat) and extinguishing them with water
  - removing charred clothing or clothes soaked with hot fluid.
- *Cool the surface of the skin* by applying cold water at 8–25°C (not ice or iced water) as soon as possible for 60–90 minutes to the affected part only.
- *Cover the burn* with a clean cloth or plastic film 'cling wrap'.
- *Analgesia*: Apply cold fluid, or for burns > 5% give intravenous morphine in small increments.

Only small burns confined to one extremity, or a very small patch on the trunk, are suitable for out-patient management. Admission is required for all children with burns of > 5% body surface area, suspected inhalation injury or suspected non-accidental injury, and most children with burns of hands, face, feet or perineum.

Management of the shock phase

Initial assessment

- Remove all clothing, jewellery and any previous dressings.
- Record accurate bare weight.
- Record and assess the extent of the burn:
  - *Area*: Use a chart of the body outline and record the area as accurately as possible using visible landmarks (such as the umbilicus, nipples and skin creases). The rule of nines is a good guide (head and neck 9%; arms each 9%; legs each $2 \times 9\%$; trunk anterior and posterior surface each $2 \times 9\%$). In infants the head is larger: $2 \times 9\%$ at the expense of the legs, each 14%. To calculate the proportions in children over 1 year, take 1% off the head for each year of life and add it to the legs (for example for a 4-year-old, the head = $18 - 4 = 14\%$, the legs are each $14 + 2 = 16\%$).
  - *Depth*: The initial assessment of depth is unreliable: never predict depth to parents. For the purpose of fluid replacement, mild superficial erythema can be ignored. Areas that are pink and blanch with pressure and have a pinprick sensation are usually superficial; dark red, mottled or pale waxy areas are deep.

Respiratory tract injury

- This results from inhalation of hot gases (thermal injury) and/or smoke (chemical damage).
- The clinical signs are hoarseness, stridor, cough, visible redness of pharynx, overt respiratory distress or hypoxia.
- All children with major burns should have humidified O_2.
- If the child is thought to have respiratory burns consider ICU admission.
- Consider intubation as airway obstruction can progress rapidly.

Carbon monoxide poisoning

- This may occur in children burnt in confined spaces.
- The clinical signs are loss of consciousness, confusion or disorientation.
- Give O_2 at high flow rates.
- Arrange a carboxyhaemoglobulin level.
- Consider for hyperbaric O_2.

Analgesia

- Give analgesia by IV injection (IM or subcutaneous morphine has a slow and unreliable absorption). Burns are very painful. Early use of analgesia makes subsequent procedures such as IV cannula insertion, bathing and dressings easier for everyone. When the patient is stable, consider continuous morphine infusion. Nitrous oxide inhalation is useful when children over 1 year old are bathing.

Fluid replacement

- Damaged capillaries leak protein-rich fluid, seen as exudate on the surface or oedema. It starts immediately after the burn. Oedema increases most rapidly for 8 hours, stops increasing by 48 hours, and is largely reabsorbed over the subsequent 5 days. Loss from the surface of the burn continues until it is healed.
- Progressive hypovolaemia, shock and death can occur unless this fluid is replaced.
- IV replacement is necessary in all burns > 10% in children and sometimes in smaller burns, especially in babies.

Antibacterial measures

- Use topical silver sulfadiazine with chlorhexidine from the start after the initial cleaning of the burn and after discussion with the Burns Unit.
- Tetanus prophylaxis: DTPa (ADT if child is > 8 years) or tetanus toxoid is given IM unless the last booster was given < 10 years previously.
- Routine use of antibiotics is not indicated.
- Swabs of the burn and throat are taken.

Replacement of losses of water, electrolytes and protein

Delivery

An intravenous infusion must be set up, preferably situated in an area free from burns. In major burns, two large IV cannulae are needed.

Calculations

The procedure employed at this hospital as a guide to rehydration is as follows.

The first 24 hours

- Start with 3 mL/kg/% burn as Hartmann's solution.
- Give 50% in the first 8 hours after the burn injury.
- Give the next 50% in the next 16 hours.
- In addition, give maintenance fluids for children less than 40 kg.
- Adjust fluid input to achieve a urine output of 1 mL/kg/h (the acceptable range is 0.5–2 mL/kg/h).
- Commence feeds via a nasogastric tube as soon as possible.

Example

A 16 kg, 3-year-old child with a 25% body surface area burn, occurring at 5 p.m., arrives in the Emergency Department at 7 p.m.

Resuscitation fluid for 24 hours = $16 \times 25 \times 3$
$$= 1200 \text{ mL}$$

50% of this to be given in the first 8 hours after the burn = 600 mL

Maintenance fluid for 24 hours = $16 \times 80 = 1280$ mL

Maintenance fluid for 8 hours = 426 mL

To complete this fluid by 8 hours after the burn (5 p.m. + 8 hours = 1 a.m.), i.e. 6 hours after starting IV, give Hartmann's solution 100 mL/h plus maintenance fluid 70 mL/h as IV N/2 or oral milk, or combination of both.

Reassess frequently; adjust Hartmann's to give urinary output 16 mL/h.

The second 24 hours

- Give 0.3 to 0.5 mL/kg/% as colloid (Albumex; that is, 4% albumin).
- In addition, give maintenance fluids.
- Give additional Hartmann's if it is needed to maintain urinary output.
- Maintenance fluids should be given as nasogastric feeds, or if

necessary 4% dextrose and N/4 saline, or 2.5% dextrose and N/2 saline.

- Increased requirements are needed in situations such as delayed resuscitation, inhalation burns, previous dehydration and in the very young child.
- Decreased requirements occur with pre-existing cardiac disease.
- If the patient is not responding to crystalloid therapy, then colloid can be commenced in the second 12 hours.

The formulae are a guide only. Patients require repeated reassessment and fluids should be increased without hesitation if, for example, the urinary output falls. In the presence of anuria reassessment should be by an experienced person. Overhydration can be harmful; if urine output is > 2 mL/kg/h, fluids should be slowed.

Monitoring of the shock phase

Clinical observations

- Anxiety and restlessness are early signs of hypovolaemia and hypoxaemia.
- Use skin colour and temperature to assess peripheral circulation.
- Temperature, pulse and BP charts are useful in showing changes over a few hours, but can be influenced by other factors.

Urinary output

- Urine output is the most useful guide to the adequacy of tissue perfusion. An indwelling catheter is needed for all patients with > 20% BSA burn, for perineal burns or if the clinical course indicates.
- Aim for 1 mL/kg/h: 0.5–2 mL/kg/h is acceptable.

Central venous pressure monitoring

Consider for burns in excess of 25% BSA.

Laboratory studies

- Haemoglobin, haematocrit and serum electrolytes are measured on admission (they usually reflect haemoconcentration). Repeat as clinically indicated.
- With extensive burns, repeat serum electrolytes frequently in the first few days.

Blood transfusion

Blood transfusion is occasionally required with extensive severe burns where there has been red cell destruction.

Electrolyte supplements

- K^+ supplements are frequently necessary, but should never be given when there is oliguria or impaired renal function.
- Hyponatraemia can occur, usually on day 2 or 3.

Limb ischaemia

- Circumferential burns to limbs can cause distal ischaemia (oedema within a tube of rigid skin). Assess the colour, temperature, capillary return, sensation and movement. Use Doppler to assess blood flow. Elevation of the limb is important.
- Circumferential or near-circumferential trunk burns can restrict ventilation. Escharotomies to relieve pressure are occasionally necessary and should be done by the surgeon.

Local treatment of the burn wound

Local therapy of burns is aimed at obtaining wound healing as rapidly as possible.

- Topical silver sulphadiazine (with 0.1% chlorhexidine) is one treatment, but more advanced dressings are presently being trialled. Discuss with the Burns Unit. Gentamicin should not be used topically because of the selection of gentamicin-resistant *Pseudomonas aeruginosa*.
- Following resuscitation and analgesia, local care is given. Wash the area with dilute Hibitane. Initially, dressings may be done in bed but progress to a full bath in dilute Hibitane as soon as possible. Leave intact blisters alone and trim away loose keratin. Apply the dressing to the burnt area and bandage it in place.
- Dressings are repeated daily until the healing is almost complete or grafting is required.
- Swabs of burn surface (after the bath) are sent for culture twice weekly. Rising fever, vomiting, drowsiness or convulsions may be due to sepsis. If sepsis is suspected, take blood cultures and treat the patient with antibiotics if the clinical situation demands or if

cultures are positive in a patient with evidence of local or general sepsis.

- Semipermeable occlusive dressings (Omiderm, Duoderm, Comfeel or Cutinova) can be used when it is possible to predict that the burn will not need grafting.

General aspects of management

Nutrition

- A hypermetabolic state leads to an increase in nutritional requirements.
- All patients in the Burns Unit are seen by the dietitian.
- Children with minor burns may require only supplements to milk, juices and ordinary meals.
- Children with major burns require tube feeds (usually nocturnal). Traumacal or Isocal is used for children over 6 months of age, and a supplemented infant formula is used under 6 months of age. Start feeds as soon as the patient is admitted. Zinc supplements are also given.

Physiotherapy

- Limitation of joint movement occurs acutely due to pain and after healing as a result of scar contracture.
- It is essential to maintain mobility of joints, particularly when scar contracture is likely to occur.
- Commence active and passive movements of involved joints early (supervised by a trained physiotherapist).
- Splinting of involved joints may be employed.

Occupational therapy

This is an essential adjunct to treatment as a means of providing stimulation for the child and in preventing psychological regression.

Emotional aspects

- Burns invariably produce emotional problems in both the child and the family. Care of these emotional problems is just as important to the long-term outcome of the burn as the physical treatment.
- The social worker bears the primary responsibility for detecting major emotional problems. The social worker is usually involved

in the initial assessment of the possibility of the child being at risk.
- The nursing staff are involved in supporting the family to allow anger and guilt to be expressed.
- The physiotherapist and occupational therapist will often have different insights into the family's emotional problems.
- Keep explanations clear and simple as the parents of a child who has just been burnt are in a state of emotional turmoil.

Scar problems

- All scar tissue contracts. Many patients require long-term management with physiotherapy and sometimes surgery. Scarring is unlikely if the burn heals in < 10 days and is almost invariable if healing takes > 21 days.
- Many scars hypertrophy—keloid is severe hypertrophy. Continuous surface compression lessens the amount of hypertrophy and helps to control itching.
- Compression is best provided by a two-way stretch garment which is custom-made for the individual patient. Measurement for the garment is complex and in the Children's Hospital at Westmead is done by the physiotherapist to the Burns Unit. The garments are worn night and day except in the bath and are replaced every 2–3 months.
- Compression is used until scars become pale and inactive, usually 9 to 18 months. Other surface applications may also be used.

Skin grafting procedures

- Full thickness burns always require skin grafting. Deep partial thickness burns are frequently best treated with grafting. The timing and method of grafting will be decided by the surgeon.
- It is usual to carry out autografting when it is clear that full thickness injury has occurred.

31

General surgery

> **This chapter includes:**
>
> - penile problems
> - scrotal problems
> - hernias
> - abdominal pain
> - vomiting
> - delayed passage of meconium
> - congenital gut evisceration
> - diaphragmatic hernia
> - fever in the postoperative period.

As a general principle, be aware of both common and life-threatening conditions. Obtain a relevant history and perform an appropriate examination. Before performing tests, ask 'Can I wait and re-examine?' in well patients presenting early, or 'Should I talk to a surgeon?' in instances where the patient is seriously ill. Talk before tests.

See Chapter 7 for fluid and electrolyte therapy in surgical conditions.

Penile problems

A generation ago, circumcision of newborn boys was almost routine in Australia. Routine circumcision is no longer recommended, and only about 10% of boys are now circumcised. Parents of young boys now need to be taught that the normal foreskin does not require any special care during infancy or childhood. No attempt should be made to forcefully retract it—this can result in trauma and subsequent phimosis.

In a newborn baby boy, the foreskin is fused to the glans. The opening in the foreskin is usually just large enough to visualise the end of the glans. This is termed 'physiological phimosis'. It is normal. Over time adhesions between the foreskin and glans resolve. By 5 years of age the foreskin is retractable in 80% of boys, and by puberty this will be close to 100%. Residual adhesions only rarely require treatment. As the foreskin separates, desquamated epithelium ('infant smegma') may be visible between the two layers—it is harmless and should be ignored. It will spontaneously discharge.

After puberty, boys should be instructed to retract their foreskin gently in the bath or shower each day and clean the glans with water. It is important they replace the foreskin after cleaning: if left retracted, paraphimosis may develop.

Phimosis

This is a narrowing at the end of the foreskin so that it cannot be withdrawn. Remember that at birth the foreskin is completely adherent to the glans, and becomes progressively retractable with age.

- If you can retract the foreskin sufficiently to see the urethral meatus, then there is no obstruction. If the opening of the foreskin is surrounded by thickened, white scar tissue, this is pathological phimosis.
- If the child can pass urine without difficulty, use a steroid cream (such as half-strength betamethasone) applied to the foreskin three times a day for 6 weeks.
- If the child cannot pass urine or has pain when urinating, then talk to a surgeon about immediate treatment.
- If the parents wish the child to be circumcised, then this is a reasonable first-line treatment after phimosis has developed.

Balanitis

Redness of the foreskin is common and rarely requires treatment. If there is redness, swelling and a purulent discharge, this is posthitis and treatment is required. The discharge should be cultured and the condition treated with a combination of a topical antifungal and a topical antibiotic cream plus an oral antibiotic (for example, a cephalosporin). Pathological phimosis should be excluded.

If there is a combination of balanitis and phimosis, sometimes a dorsal slit is required to treat the infection. Consult a surgeon.

Balanitis xerotica obliterans (BXO)

BXO is a sterile inflammation of the foreskin. It is also known as lichen sclerosus et atrophicus. It mimics balanitis, but does not respond to antibiotics. The foreskin becomes thickened and white. The treatment is circumcision, and possibly also steroid creams.

Paraphimosis

In this condition, the retracted foreskin cannot be returned to its normal position, covering the glans. The problem usually arises because the foreskin has been retracted and left behind the glans. The foreskin becomes swollen and difficult to reduce.

- Treatment usually requires surgical referral. It is only the rare co-operative child who allows you to gently compress the oedema and reduce the paraphimosis without an anaesthetic.
- Circumcision is not usually required after treatment of paraphimosis. The child just needs to learn to reduce his foreskin after retraction.

Scrotal problems

Acute scrotum

- Any boy with a red, swollen scrotum should be referred urgently to a children's hospital, with a call to the triage desk to alert the Emergency Department so that the child does not sit in the waiting area. The child should be fasted.
- With a torsion of the testis, time is critical. After 12 hours very few testes can be saved.
- Do not be misled by lack of pain. Most children over 10 years have classic severe pain, with pallor and vomiting, but young children, age 2–4 years, may not complain of pain. Do not presume a diagnosis of epididymo-orchitis or torsion of the testicular appendix without surgical consultation.
- Adolescent testicular torsion may present with referred loin or abdominal rather than groin or testicular pain.
- Ultrasound and nuclear scans should not be ordered unless considered necessary by the surgeon. Generally, these tests waste valuable time and can be misleading.
- The surgeon will usually explore the scrotum as it is difficult to exclude testicular torsion on history and examination.

365

Hydroceles

These are usually present in the first year of life, are painless, can be large, have a 'bluish appearance' and transilluminate brilliantly. Textbooks say that hydroceles are scrotal swellings that the examiner can easily get above. In practice, this is not always so, as the swelling can extend up towards the deep inguinal ring.

- *History*: The key features are that there is no pain, the infant is feeding normally and behaves normally.
- *Examination*: The key features are that the swelling is not red or tender and you can get above the swelling, or the top part at least seems smaller.
- *Management*: If in doubt discuss with a surgeon. Do not order an ultrasound. The surgeon will recommend repair if hydroceles are still present at 2 years, but 90% resolve spontaneously.
- Hydroceles first appearing past the age of 12 months require a different approach—consult a surgeon.

Undescended testes
Newborn to 6 months

- If you cannot clearly feel a smooth 1–2 mL volume testis on each side refer the patient to a surgeon. Remember that a 'thickening' can be gubernaculum tissue and the testes may be undescended or absent.
- Every infant with bilateral undescended testes should be examined for the possibility of ambiguous genitalia, especially if the penis is abnormal. If in doubt, consult.
- Some testes can descend in the first few months after birth, so if a testis can be felt in the groin, it is reasonable for you to review the patient at 6 months, before referring.
- Tests such as ultrasound, CT scans and endocrine are usually unnecessary. They should be reserved for specialist use.

Over 6 months

- Take a history, and review the boy's 'Blue Book': were the testes recorded as being present at birth?
- Examine the child supine and in the squat position. The squat position overcomes the cremasteric reflex and the testes should be easily felt in the scrotum. Tests are not indicated.
- If the testes cannot be milked into the scrotum in the supine

position and are not in the scrotum in the squat position, then refer the patient to a paediatric surgeon.

- The current preference is to operate on undescended testes at 12 months of age, so refer early once you are satisfied that the testes are undescended. If the testes are not in the scrotum by 6 months, they are not going to descend.

Hernias

Inguinal hernia

- The younger the child, the more difficult it is to make a confident diagnosis of inguinal hernia and the more likely it is for a hernia to become irreducible.
- *History*: The most common presentation is of a lump coming and going in the groin. Get the parent to point to make sure it is above the inguinal ligament.
- *Examination*: The hernia may be apparent, but examination is often normal. A thickened spermatic cord can be a clue to a hernia. Check carefully that the parents are not feeling a lymph node or an undescended testis.
- *Tests*: Nil. Do not request ultrasound or CT scan.
- *Management*: This depends on age.
  - *Less than 3 months*: Ring the paediatric surgeon and try to have the child reviewed that day. Surgery is as soon as practicable.
  - *3–6 months*: Ring the surgeon's secretary so the child is seen at the next rooms or clinic. Surgery is usually within 6 weeks.
  - *Over 6 months*: Refer to the surgeon's clinic; surgery is usually within 3 months.

Irreducible inguinal hernia—boys

- The parents often notice a swelling when changing the nappy. The child is often irritable, not wanting to feed and if there is a prolonged, complete bowel obstruction, there is bile-stained vomiting.
- On examination, there is a tender swelling in the groin that you cannot get above. Sometimes you can feel the testis separately below but often it is not easily felt.
- *Management*: Refer to the surgeon urgently. The longer the hernia remains incarcerated and the younger the child, the more likely there is to be damage to the testis or bowel. The surgeon is

most often able to reduce the hernia by gentle pressure, and operate the next day. Manual reduction requires experience and should be done in a hospital with strict nursing protocols to detect quickly any infant who deteriorates, in the unlikely event that perforated bowel is reduced back into the abdomen.

- Do not use morphine, especially in infants under 3 months of age, as an aid to attempt to reduce an inguinal hernia. It can depress respiration unexpectedly.
- Gallows traction is ineffective.

Irreducible inguinal hernia—girls

- Often the ovary comes out into the hernia sac, and while it is technically irreducible it is not an emergency, unless it is also twisted. The girl is characteristically 3–6 months old and a smooth, mobile, ovoid structure can be moved about but not reduced.
- *Management*: If not tender, refer to the next clinic. If tender, swollen and red, refer urgently to the surgeon as there may have been secondary torsion of the ovary.

Umbilical hernia

- This is common in newborns, resolves without treatment in over 90% of cases and almost never results in intestinal obstruction during childhood.
- Therefore, even if the hernia appears large (due to the skin being lifted up), carefully feel the size of the abdominal wall defect. If it is less than 1 cm, reassure the parents that the hernia has a 90% chance of resolution and review the child when aged 2½ years; if the hernia is still present, refer to a paediatric surgeon who will operate when the child is about the age of 3 years.

Abdominal pain

The key variables are age and the characteristics of the pain.

- *In infants*:
  - Examine the inguinal regions for hernias.
  - Culture the urine to exclude urinary tract infection.
  - Always consider the possibility of intussusception.
- *In older children*: Always consider appendicitis as a possible diagnosis.

Intussusception

Clinical features

- The peak incidence is between 2 months and 2 years, but it can occur at any age.
- The pain is colicky, with quiescent periods, often with marked pallor.
- Vomiting is clear early, bile-stained after 12–24 hours.
- There may be a palpable sausage-shaped mass, or fullness with some tenderness.
- There may be red currant stools—it is always important to do a rectal examination, as this sign may otherwise be missed.
- Intussusception can be a great mimicker, so always consider it as a differential diagnosis in children with vomiting with a provisional diagnosis of 'head injury' or 'meningitis'; and in any obtunded child, especially with 'gastroenteritis'. Take a careful history of the pain (and vomiting) and perform a full examination, including a rectal examination. If this does not suggest an intussusception and the child is relatively well, with no pallor and no tachycardia, observe and re-examine. If the child is unwell, discuss with a surgeon.

Treatment

- Urgent fluid resuscitation is needed occasionally if the child is in hypovolaemic shock. Placing a venous cannula should be achieved quickly, so that there is no delay in getting on with the enema reduction.
- The treatment is urgent enema reduction (with air or barium). If this is not effective, then open surgical manual reduction or resection is required.

Appendicitis

- This can occur at any age.
- Under the age of 5 years, it often mimics gastroenteritis, presenting with diarrhoea, and can progress quickly to perforation and peritonitis.
- The key to diagnosis remains a good history and a thorough examination.
- If a child with abdominal pain (and possibly appendicitis) is well, with no tachycardia, minimal fever and no signs of peritonism,

then review the next day, ideally by the same doctor, is a reasonable plan of management.

- If the child is unwell, even if the diagnosis is unclear, seek a surgical opinion.
- Graded compression ultrasound and spiral CT are being increasingly used as diagnostic tests for appendicitis. However, these are best used as an adjunct, after surgical consultation, for a small subgroup of patients. Do not order these tests before a surgical consultation.

Other causes of abdominal pain

- *Meckel's diverticulum* can cause abdominal pain at any age, but is commonest at about 2 years of age. It is more common for Meckel's diverticulum to present with painless PR bleeding than with abdominal pain.
- *Adhesions*: Think of these if there has been any previous surgery.
- *Inflammatory bowel disease*: There will often be a long history of poor weight gain, diarrhoea and systemic features.
- *Gallstones*: These are being seen with increasing frequency in children. The pain is not as classical as in adults but is usually associated with meals. An ultrasound is the best investigation.
- *Psychogenic*: While not immediately dangerous, this can be very destructive socially unless handled carefully. Children with psychogenic pain often see multiple doctors, have many investigations and can miss a lot of school. The best approach is comprehensive, unhurried consultation with a consultant, perhaps an ultrasound and friendly reassurance in a relaxed environment in normal working hours. Referral to Psychological Medicine may occasionally be needed.
- *Gynaecological*: Ovarian dysfunction is an important differential diagnosis. Remember that any female who has started her periods can be pregnant.

Vomiting

The principal variables are age and colour of the vomit.

Newborn, with mucousy clear froth

Oesophageal atresia is the major condition to diagnose (or exclude).

- Polyhydramnios will often have been present antenatally.

- The diagnosis can be made, as follows:
  - A 10 FG feeding tube will stop at about 10 cm from the lips.
  - An abdominal X-ray will show a gasless abdomen if there is no fistula.
- Refer urgently to the surgeons.
- Do not attempt to feed.
- Leave a 10 FG tube to be gently aspirated every 15 minutes, or more frequently if the newborn is mucousy.
- The best nursing/transport position is supine.

Newborn to 2 days with bilious vomiting

Atresia or *Hirschsprung's disease* are the serious surgical conditions to consider, but consider medical conditions, such as sepsis, in your differential diagnosis.

- A plain abdominal X-ray will help pick the level of the atresia, if present.
- Abdominal distension will usually be present.
- Early referral to a neonatal unit is wise.

Infant with milk vomiting

Pyloric stenosis is the major condition of concern.

- If small amounts of milk are 'vomited' from birth, especially if with effortless regurgitation as opposed to vomiting, consider as gastro-oesophageal reflux and manage expectantly. See Chapter 16.
- If there is sudden or progressive onset of increasing volumes that then become forceful (projectile), consider pyloric stenosis to be a likely diagnosis:
  - 20% have a positive family history.
  - Pyloric stenosis may present early, without weight loss and with normal electrolytes.
  - Do a careful examination, feeling with your left index finger from the left side. If the child will not lie still, try a dummy to suck or a small feed (test feed).
  - If you cannot feel a tumour and the infant is well (no weight loss) and passing urine at least every 12 hours, you can safely review the infant the next day.
  - If the child is unwell, seek a surgical opinion.
  - While an ultrasound can diagnose the thickened muscle, it

should be used only if the surgeon has trouble feeling the swelling (10% of cases).

Infant with bilious vomiting

Malrotation is the major condition requiring diagnosis or exclusion.

- Malrotation usually presents in the first 4 weeks of life but can present at any age.
- Any infant who has a green vomit (even if small) has *malrotation* and *potential volvulus* until proven otherwise. This is a major surgical emergency. Any delay increases the risk of necrosis of the small intestine, and therefore death.
- Any infant with green vomiting and bowel obstruction requires *urgent surgical referral*.
- In less urgent situations, for instance if there has been an episode of acute vomiting which has settled, malrotation can be excluded by a contrast meal and follow-through done by an expert paediatric radiologist. This must be done even if the bilious vomiting is of small volume and transient.

Delayed passage of meconium

- Any delay beyond 24 hours in the passage of a normal amount of meconium raises the possibility of Hirschsprung's disease. The child should be referred to a paediatric surgeon for consideration of a rectal biopsy.
- Other features consistent with this condition include abdominal distension and bile-stained vomiting. These latter features may also be due to sepsis or other serious conditions. When the child is present, transfer to a tertiary neonatal unit and surgical consultation are both required urgently.

Congenital gut evisceration

- Do not put wet gauze on the defect because this will rapidly cool the infant.
- Instead, insert a nasogastric tube and wrap the bowel in plastic cling-film, such as 'Gladwrap'.
- Check the blood sugar (exomphalos and low blood sugar in a large baby with horizontal ear creases suggest the possibility of Beckwith's syndrome).

Hypoglycaemia should be urgently treated with 10% dextrose infusion to prevent fits and brain damage.

Diaphragmatic hernia

- Think of diaphragmatic hernia if there is a scaphoid abdomen and shift of the cardiac impulse. The chest X-ray shows loops of bowel in the chest.
- In severely affected infants the need to intubate and assist ventilation is obvious.

In less severely affected infants there is time to discuss management and transfer. A nasogastric tube is required to decompress the stomach. Bagging with a mask is contraindicated as it may inflate the gut, exacerbating the respiratory distress.

Fever in the postoperative period

This may be due to infection, or to non-infective causes.

- Early postoperative fever may be caused by surgical trauma, pulmonary atelectasis, bacteraemia, septicaemia or an intercurrent illness.
- Wound infection, intra-abdominal abscesses and anastomotic leaks usually become apparent 4–7 days postoperatively, often with fever as an important symptom.

Investigation and further management

- History and clinical examination, including IV sites and surgical wounds
- Investigations:
  - Swab any purulent discharge.
  - Urine microscopy and culture; blood culture
  - FBC, EUC
  - Chest X-ray if clinically indicated
- Inform the surgical team; decide on other diagnostic tests in discussion with them.
- If the child appears septic or has proven infection, antibiotics will be required; discuss the choice of antibiotics with the surgical team.
- Do not delay antibiotic treatment in an unwell child with possible bacteraemia or septicaemia.

32

Trauma and orthopaedics

This chapter includes:

- severe trauma—early management
- fractures
- lacerations
- acute-onset limp.

See also:

- head injury (Chapter 17)
- non-accidental injury (Chapter 22)
- resuscitation (Chapter 3)
- osteomyelitis (Chapter 11)
- septic arthritis (Chapter 11)
- adolescent orthopaedic problems (Chapter 20).

Severe trauma—early management

Early management

The approach to the severely injured child requires a combination of rapid assessment looking for life-threatening injuries with early management of the injuries found. The types of injuries which, if untreated, will result in the rapid demise of children include airway obstruction, haemo/pneumothorax, ruptured liver or spleen, pelvic fractures and intracranial haematoma.

The Trauma Team must be called immediately to all high-risk cases (high-energy mechanisms of injury and patients who already have altered vital signs or obvious major trauma). The surgical registrar is the team leader. All team members have tasks assigned (see the *Hospital Trauma Manual*).

The following plan, promoted by the Royal Australasian College of Surgeons, should be used to structure your assessment and resuscitation.

Primary survey (ABCDE)

This is your initial quick assessment of the patient looking for life-threatening conditions such as airway obstruction. Treat problems as you find them.

Airway with cervical spine control

- Clear the airway and administer oxygen.
- Be aware of the possibility of cervical spine injury—no airway manoeuvres must move the neck, so as to prevent the development or exacerbation of cervical spinal cord injury. Children are more likely than adults to have spinal cord damage without X-ray evidence of spine fracture.
- Even in the presence of facial fractures and lacerations, remember simple measures to improve airway obstruction and oxygenation such as suction, Guedel airway, and bag and mask ventilation before proceeding to intubation.

Breathing

Look for signs of respiratory distress, tachypnoea, an obstructed pattern of chest wall movement, cyanosis or agitation suggesting hypoxia, reduced breath sounds or altered percussion note, and tracheal deviation suggesting tension pneumothorax. Tension pneumothorax requires immediate needling of the chest (anterior, midclavicular line, second interspace). The flail segment of the chest cage will benefit from splinting and assisted ventilation using positive pressure. Cover an open pneumothorax. Remember that respiratory distress may be due to aspiration of the stomach contents.

Circulation

Do external haemostasis for lacerations. Identify shock—children are able to maintain a normal BP in the face of a larger percentage loss of blood volume than adults, but will rapidly deteriorate subsequently, so give volume for tachycardia, poor perfusion, decreased capillary refill, and altered level of consciousness not due to head injury even in the absence of frank hypotension. Treat shock with rapid administration of 20 mL/kg of normal saline or Hartmann's solution, repeated if signs of shock persist. Ongoing signs of shock warrant urgent blood transfusion.

Disability

Assess neurological disability rapidly by assessing pupillary size and reaction and making a gross assessment of level of consciousness (*AVPU*: *A*wake, needing *V*erbal stimulation to get a response, responding only to *P*ainful stimuli, or *U*nresponsive).

Exposure

Uncover the child to permit examination (remembering to keep him or her in a warm environment and to re-cover as soon as possible).

Resuscitation

- Attach ECG and pulse oximeter. Give oxygen.
- Catheterise the bladder and stomach. Children are prone to air-swallowing and acute gastric dilatation. Use an orogastric rather than a nasogastric tube if a base-of-skull fracture is suspected.
- Establish IV access if this has not already been done (preferably with two large bore cannulae). Possible access sites are the long saphenous vein, external jugular, cubital at the elbow, and intraosseous.
- Take blood for cross-match and do the tests listed below.

Secondary survey

This is a more thorough assessment to discover less severe injuries and severe, but previously occult, injuries.

- *Look, listen and feel.* Perform a 'top-to-toe' examination. Remember to feel the fontanelle in babies. Look for retinal haemorrhages by fundoscopy. Feel the clavicles and examine the back. Palpate the rib cage and pelvic girdle for stability. Look for bruises and marks such as seat belt, fist or tyre marks. Don't forget to examine the orifices: nose, ears, mouth (and perineum by the surgical registrar). Look for signs of child abuse. Pancreatic, duodenal and lumbar spine injuries may be present but not obvious on initial examination.
  - Take a more thorough *history*, especially about the mechanism of the injury.
  - Ask for a history of drug or other *allergy*.
  - Organise *lab tests*: Hb, electrolytes, creatinine, cross-match, Dextrostix, amylase.
  - 'Trauma series' *X-rays*: lateral cervical spine, chest and ?pelvis.

- Consider *other tests* depending on the findings, for example CT head. Diagnostic peritoneal lavage (DPL) is not usually performed in children, abdominal CT being preferred.
- *Definitive care*:
  - Splinting of fractures and vascular access, securing of catheters
  - Surgery as needed
  - Stabilisation and transfer to the paediatric intensive care unit after consultation

Trauma is the commonest killer of children after the first year of life. An efficient systematic approach to a severely injured child's assessment and initial management will minimise mortality.

Fractures

Both upper and lower limb fractures are common in children. 'Greenstick', buckle and epiphyseal fractures are all more likely in children than in adults. A good account of how the injury occurred is essential in understanding the type and extent of the injury.

- Pain and swelling suggest a fracture; fractures are more common than sprain injuries in children. Do not diagnose a sprain without negative X-rays.
- Immobilise, splint, cover open wounds with sterile dressing, give analgesia, then X-ray.
- X-rays should normally include the joint above to the joint below; contralateral X-rays are useful with subtle bone injuries, especially around the elbow.
- Always provide adequate analgesia. Use morphine or pethidine, IV or IM, for other than minor injuries.
- Always consider the possibility of nerve damage and vascular compromise at or below the fracture site.
- Open injuries almost always require surgical exploration. This decision rests with the surgeon.
- Consult the orthopaedic service without delay:
  - for any displaced fracture
  - if there is an associated open injury—give antibiotic cover immediately
  - if there is any evidence of nerve damage or vascular compromise
  - for any fracture through the joint
  - for any displaced growth plate fracture.

- Consider the possibility of non-accidental injury:
  - in children aged less than 2 years
  - for spiral or other unusual fractures
  - where there are unexplained injuries elsewhere
  - where the history doesn't 'fit' the injury
  - when presentation is delayed.

Management of fractures

- *Clavicle*: Use a broad arm sling and review at 10–14 days. Fracture displacement matters only if the overlying skin is threatened.
- *Supracondylar humerus*:
  - Undisplaced and minimal swelling: collar and cuff, 3–4 weeks.
  - Displaced or swollen: immediately refer to the orthopaedic surgeon; anaesthetic and internal fixation may be required.
- *Lateral condyle humerus*: This is an important fracture to recognise—2 mm of displacement requires internal fixation.
- *Distal radius only* (ulna intact):
  - Greenstick and undisplaced fractures: plaster of Paris; initially just a backslab to allow for swelling; allow thumb and fingers free movement.
  - Displaced fractures: immediately refer to an orthopaedic surgeon.
- *Radius and ulna*: Both require a long arm backslab above the elbow. This controls elbow flexion and forearm rotation. Immobilise in neutral rotation (thumb points to ceiling).
- *Metacarpal bones*:
  - Undisplaced: crepe bandage, then review at 10–14 days.
  - Displaced: requires orthopaedic referral.
- *Femur*:
  - Remember analgesia.
  - Consider femoral nerve block if a skilled person is available. This is ideal.
  - With gross trauma, especially in older children and adolescents, anticipate shock (place IV line, replace volume, cross-match blood).
  - The type of traction will be chosen by the orthopaedic surgeon. Keep the patient fasted.
- *Tibia and fibula*:
  - These require a long leg plaster backslab. Admission to hospital is recommended if there is gross swelling.
  - Displaced: requires orthopaedic referral.

- *Ankle*:
  - Fractures are near or through growth plates. Orthopaedic referral is required.
- *Metatarsal bones*: If the patient is unable to weight bear, backslab and review in 10 days.
- *Fingers and toes*:
  - Undisplaced—strap to adjacent fingers or toes.
  - Avulsion fractures near joints—splint the digit in extension and review at 10 days.

Immobilisation

A good backslab is the mainstay of acute orthopaedic care. Use two slabs for even better immobilisation. Make sure the limb is well padded at the prominences, and that padding does not impinge on circulation, and wrap with a crepe bandage firmly but not tightly. When immobilising the forearm, the plaster should come only to the metacarpal heads dorsally, and to the distal palmar crease on the volar side. If the hand needs to be immobilised, the wrist should be extended 30 degrees, the metacarpophalangeal joints bent to nearly 90 degrees, and the interphalangeal joints should be in full extension. This is the 'safe' position for the hand.

Lacerations

Skin lacerations are very common in children and often require no more treatment than local antisepsis. The aim is a good functional and cosmetic result with the least pain and distress to the child. Delay in treatment promotes infection, poor healing and scarring.

The laceration

- *How did it occur?* Assess the likelihood of embedded foreign material, or nerve, tendon or visceral injury. If in doubt seek surgical consultation.
- *Is the skin blood supply at risk?* This is indicated by poor skin perfusion. Do not use local anaesthetics with added adrenaline. Nerves run next to vessels—do not grab blindly with clamps. Seek surgical consultation if in doubt.
- *Are special areas involved?* Lacerations involving lips, crossing the vermilion border, eyelids, eyebrows and scalp margins require surgical expertise for best results. Consult.

- *Does it really need closure?* Short, shallow lacerations often do not require closure. Tongue and oral mucosa tears require closure only where there are gross gaps or bleeding. Puncture wounds should not normally be sutured.
- *Are there multiple lacerations?* In this situation, or if there are mucosal lacerations requiring repair or if the child is extremely distressed and/or uncooperative, consider general anaesthetic.

Handling the child before and during treatment

- Give simple, truthful and age-appropriate information to the child. Then get on with it!
- Give the child and the parents some part in the procedure to perform, if possible. Tell the child what you are doing at each stage.
- The need for a patient, kind, confident and expeditious approach from all professionals involved cannot be overestimated.

Sedation and analgesia

- See Chapter 29 for information on sedation.
- Local anaesthesia is the most important measure to reduce pain and distress when wounds must be sutured.

According to the circumstances, infiltrate the wound with local anaesthetic (1% xylocaine infusion, up to 0.5 mL/kg, 5–10 minutes before starting the procedure); use a long thin needle and infiltrate through the wound margins where possible.

Topical anaesthesia, using local anaesthetic solutions or gels, is being developed. Where available, its use will be governed by local policies and procedures.

Closure methods

These include adhesive strips, suturing and tissue glues. The choice will be determined by the type of laceration and the experience of the doctor.

- *Suturing*: The aim is to achieve close approximation of the wound edges; this can be done with one or two layers of suture material. Surgical consultation is essential whenever there is significant bleeding or the possibility of tendon or nerve injury.
- *Tissue glue (cyanoacrylates)*: These are useful for lacerations up to 3 cm in length. Tissue glue should not be used near the eyes or

on mucosal surfaces or where wound edges are under tension. It should not be used for deep, infected or puncture wounds where bleeding does not stop with pressure.

- It is applied with the edges of the wounds held together so glue does not get into the wound. Take care not to adhere instruments or your own fingers to the patient. If a poor result is apparent, immediate removal and re-gluing can be done.
- Thin separate sterile strips can be used to keep the wound edges in the correct position while other parts of the wound are glued.

Tetanus prophylaxis

- If the child has been fully immunised in the past 10 years, no booster or other antitetanus measures are needed.
- If the immunisation status is uncertain, or incomplete:
  - For clean, minor wounds, give tetanus toxoid, then subsequently complete the course of immunisation.
  - For tetanus-prone wounds, give tetanus toxoid (as above) as well as tetanus immunoglobulin.
  - See *The Australian Immunisation Handbook* (NHMRC) if tetanus toxoid and/or tetanus immunoglobulin is necessary.
- Always take the opportunity to review all of the child's immunisations and give catch-up immunisations, if needed.

Acute-onset limp

Acute or sub-acute onset of limp is common in children. It is usually due to pain and only rarely due to muscle weakness or neuropathy. Causes are numerous; only the common and/or serious conditions are listed in Table 32.1.

- The history is very important. Take into account only witnessed trauma that caused the child pain at the time. Most children have had a minor fall in the previous few days, including those with osteomyelitis and leukaemia.
- Careful physical examination is necessary, including observation of the gait, and checking for limited movement.
- Carry out investigations based on likely causes (Table 32.1).

Table 32.1 Common causes of limp in children

Cause	Consider when	Tests
Acute		
Fracture	Pain, swelling, history of injury	X-ray (2 views, plus normal side)
Sprain, soft tissue injury	Pain, swelling, history of injury; make this diagnosis only after considering all other possibilities	Exclude fracture by X-ray if necessary
Irritable hip (transient synovitis)	Recent viral infection, lack of trauma, especially in 3–8-year-old children	FBC, ESR, exclude other causes
Infection (including joints and spine)	Lack of history of trauma	FBC, ESR, consider ultrasound and/or bone scan
Sickle cell crisis	Any child with sickle cell disease	FBC
Sub-acute or acute		
Juvenile rheumatoid arthritis	Fever, multiple joint involvement, morning stiffness	FBC, ESR, ANA if suspicion high
Leukaemia, or solid malignant tumour	Pallor, easy bruising	FBC, marrow biopsy if any doubts
Perthes' disease	Longer history of limp, intermittent, well otherwise	AP pelvis, frog lateral views of hips
Slipped femoral epiphysis	Teenage child, limb in external rotation	AP pelvis, frog lateral views of hips

33

Dying and death

This section incudes:

- palliative medicine
- limiting life-sustaining treatment
- procedures following death of a child
- principles of bereavement care
- looking after yourself.

Palliative medicine

Palliative medicine is the study and management of patients with active, progressive, far-advanced disease for whom the prognosis is limited and the focus of care is quality of life. As such, the domains of concern are the physical, psychological and spiritual wellbeing of the child and the family.

Concepts of death

There are large variations in the rate of acquiring a mature concept of death, which reflect individual children's experience and environment.

Pre-school-age children

In early childhood, children have usually heard the word 'death' and may have some sense of its meaning as a departure or an absence, but no understanding of its universality or irreversibility. Due to their ability to enter into the world of the imagination, younger children may believe their thoughts are sufficient to cause events such as the death of a sibling.

School-age children

Younger children may still associate bad thoughts and deeds with the cause of the death, and may feel intense responsibility and guilt.

However, older children have more developed cognitive abilities and may well respond to logical explanations. By 9 or 10 years of age, most children have an adult concept of death as being inevitable, universal and irreversible.

- *Adolescents* facing impending death may express anger by being medically non-compliant, or by isolating themselves from their peers. Adolescents are best supported by realising their needs as children while recognising their developing skills as adults.

Pain and other symptom management

- *Pain*: See Chapter 6 for the general principles of pain management.
- *Seizures*: See Chapter 17 for the general principles of seizure management.

Gastrointestinal symptoms

Mouth problems

Debility and lowered immunity can lead to problems with mouth care. Adequate local hydration and meticulous cleaning are the keys to preventing mouth sores. Dry mouth is often not due to dehydration but rather to poor oral hygiene.

Nausea and vomiting

The aetiology of these symptoms should be determined, as therapies directed at the underlying cause may be more effective than simply prescribing antiemetics. Raised intracranial pressure, gastritis, partial or complete bowel obstruction and so on are common causes of this symptom in the dying child. Phenothiazines, lorazepam or dexamethasone may be effective in treating nausea and vomiting, when traditional antiemetics have failed.

Constipation

Inactivity, opioids, and poor oral intake predispose a dying child to constipation. Other causes may be related to complications of the underlying illness itself (for example bowel obstruction, involvement of the sacral nerve roots). Treatment is usually with both a stool softener and a stimulant.

Cardiorespiratory symptoms

Cardiorespiratory symptoms are common in dying children. The cause of cardiorespiratory deterioration must be determined accurately in order to implement effective therapy. The combination of morphine and benzodiazepines can often alleviate the distress and anxiety associated with terminal dyspnoea.

Sleep disturbance

Sleep disturbances are common in children, but more especially in the dying child. The aetiology is complex and related potentially to the underlying condition and associated symptoms, and to the anxiety and fear of impending death.

Emotional support is the mainstay of treatment. A low dose of amitriptyline, unless contraindicated, may be helpful.

Skin

Skin problems are common in the dying child. Children who are most susceptible to the development of pressure ulcers include those who have decreased sensation, are immobile and remain in one position, are malnourished, have skin that is frequently wet from urine, stool or sweat, or have fragile, easily damaged skin. Consideration must be given to changing their position frequently and to the use of appropriate mattresses.

Limiting life-sustaining treatment

Cardiopulmonary resuscitation (CPR) covers a number of treatments, including, at times, tracheal intubation, external cardiac massage and the use of inotropes. CPR will often be inappropriate where the diagnosis and prognosis are known and where active 'curative' treatment is no longer being given.

- It is *not* appropriate to write 'not for resuscitation' in the clinical notes, or to display this on the bedhead.
- Once the physician or surgeon in charge decides to limit some or all CPR treatment options, this will be discussed with the parents or guardians, and when appropriate with the child, and with nursing and other medical staff.
- The treatment plan will then be documented in the clinical record, specifically:

- what treatment will continue to be given
- what CPR options will not be used. The plan, for instance, may specify suctioning of the airway and oxygen administration, but indicate that assisted ventilation and cardiac compression will not be done.
- The treatment plan may be changed, when necessary, by the physician or surgeon in charge, and for hospitalised children should be rewritten in the clinical notes at least once each week.

Procedures following death of a child

Essential *communications* and *decisions* are outlined in the *Purple Folder* available in every ward of the Children's Hospital at Westmead. This also contains all necessary forms for the three common categories:

- deaths referred to the coroner
- other deaths, no autopsy
- other deaths, with hospital autopsy.

It is necessary to do the following:

- Certify that death has occurred.
- Notify the physician or surgeon in charge:
  - Decide if it is a coroner's case.
  - Decide about requesting an autopsy (non-coroner's cases).
- Notify the next of kin and explain the procedures to follow.
- After discussion with the family, nursing staff may notify the social worker, chaplain and other family.
- Notify the local doctor and other consultants involved.
- For coroner's cases:
  - Leave all drips, tubes, and so on, in situ.
  - Contact the police; complete the required forms in triplicate.
  - Follow required procedures for identifying the body to police.
  - Give the police officer the required copies of the forms.
- For non-coroner's cases, complete the relevant certificates including the Cremation Certificate.
- Check you have omitted nothing, by consulting the Purple Folder (or your own hospital's procedures manual).
- Arrange family follow-up.

Principles of bereavement care

The loss of a child is one of the most painful experiences for parents, and siblings are often the forgotten mourners. The dying and death of a child, whether anticipated or sudden, often creates an intense response in the family and professionals involved.

Parents often need some specific guidelines to help themselves and their surviving children—in particular, how to:

- take care of themselves physically, to deal with their feelings of guilt and blame
- allow surviving children their own method of grieving and get help for the surviving children if they need it
- find ways to spend time with their remaining children
- not compare the dead child with the surviving children.

It is the responsibility of healthcare professionals to ensure that parents and family are fully informed, as well as optimally supported and comforted, after the death of a child. Depending on the experience, training, skill and previous relationship with the child and parents, it may be appropriate for a medical practitioner to be the main resource for a family in bereavement. Other professionals at the Children's Hospital at Westmead who may be of great help to a family in bereavement include senior colleagues, social workers and chaplains.

Looking after yourself

Both junior and senior medical staff will be distressed by the death of a child in their care. Telling parents their child is likely to die, telling parents about the unexpected death of a child and discussing the possibility of death with a child or adolescent should produce strong emotions in any physician. At such times, though, it is often of value to the family for the doctor to demonstrate calm, control and strength at the same time as being kind and empathic. Showing how upset you may feel is often better done in the presence of peers or other professionals, rather than with the family.

Medical staff can decide whether to deal with their emotions privately, for instance on their own, or with their family. However, the Children's Hospital at Westmead recognises the need of its staff to deal with death formally—a 'critical incident debriefing' or 'defusing' with as many as possible of the various staff involved in the care of the child may be held within a few days of an unexpected or particularly distressing death. This is facilitated either by a professional from the Children's Hospital at Westmead Employee Assistance Program or by peers specifically trained in this process. Critical incident debriefing is not intended to be therapy, there is no pressure on participants to disclose personal material, and attendance is voluntary.

The goals of debriefing are:

- to acknowledge the impact of the event in order to reduce the likelihood of burnout
- to normalise commonly experienced reactions and educate on how to manage uncomfortable or distressing feelings including where to go for further confidential assistance
- to create, strengthen and maintain effective networks within the team.

In addition, the Director of Clinical and Physician Training (ext. 53635 at Westmead) or the staff counsellor, Employee Assistance Program (ext. 53555 at Westmead), can arrange times for confidential conversation.

34

Growth charts

This chapter includes:

- measurement
- percentile charts.

Measurement

Height, weight and head circumference should be routinely recorded during examination.

Body measurements of healthy children of any age vary greatly. Although the 3rd and 97th percentiles are used as the lower and upper limits of 'normal', for the purpose of determining the need for investigation, most children outside these limits are in fact entirely normal.

Inherited constitutional factors are the most important determinants of growth. Variations may result from underfeeding, overfeeding, emotional deprivation and many diseases.

A series of measurements over months or years is of much greater value than single measurements. In general, growth is a sensitive indicator of the health of a child. From the age of 2 years to adolescence, children tend to grow consistently along one percentile and any deviation from this should be assessed.

Some disparity between height, mass and head circumference percentiles for any particular child is more the rule than the exception.

Standing height

The child is measured without shoes, standing with heels, buttocks and shoulders against a vertical surface. The child is asked to look straight forward, and stretch his or her neck to be as tall as possible.

Supine length

Younger children are measured on a flat surface between vertical boards.

Weight

Weight should be measured without clothing, or (in older children) with minimal underclothing.

Percentile charts

Following advice from National Health and Medical Research Council, the Australian Department of Health has determined that percentile charts from the US National Center for Health Statistics be used for Australian children. The percentiles on these charts are generally similar to the previous National Health and Medical Research Council Charts (1980) except that, above the age of 8 years, American children tend to be taller and heavier, this becoming more marked in the teenage years.

Except where indicated otherwise, all of the following percentile charts are derived from the US National Center for Health Statistics data.

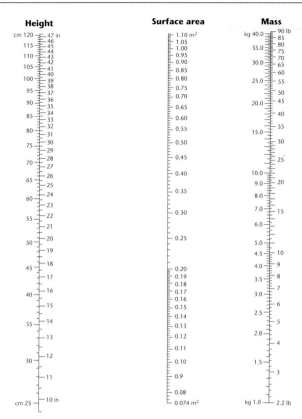

Figure 34.1 Nomogram for calculating the body surface area of children
Source: Reproduced from Documenta Geigy Scientific Tables, 6th edn, by permission of J. R. Geigy S.A., Basle, Switzerland

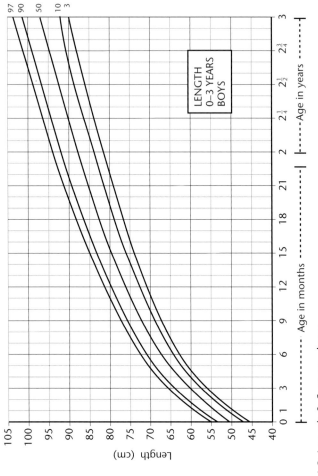

Figure 34.2 Length 0–3 years—boys
Source: Figures 34.2–34.13 come from US National Center for Health Statistics data.

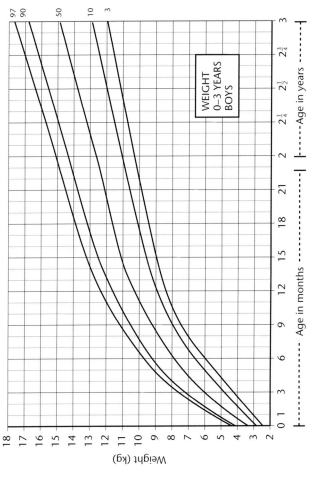

Figure 34.3 Weight 0–3 years—boys

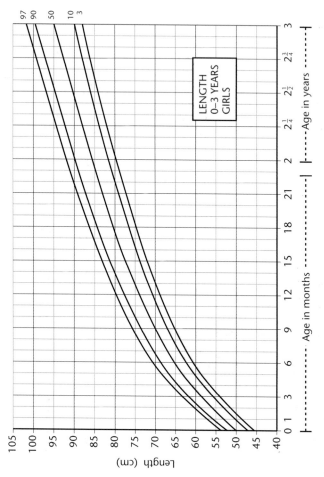

Figure 34.4 Length 0–3 years—girls

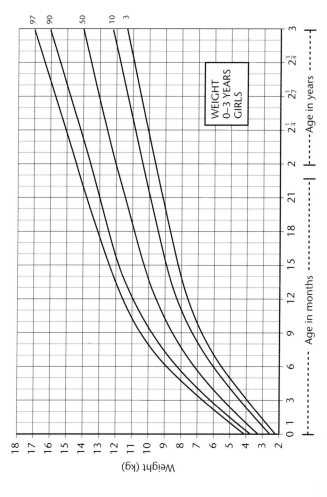

Figure 34.5 Weight 0–3 years—girls

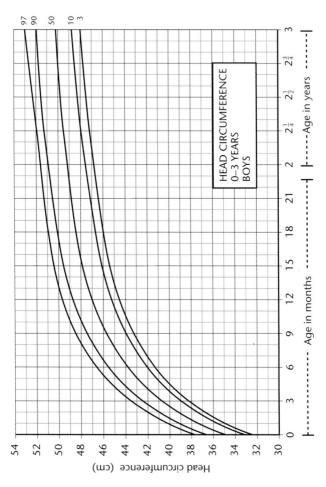

Figure 34.6 Head circumference 0–3 years—boys

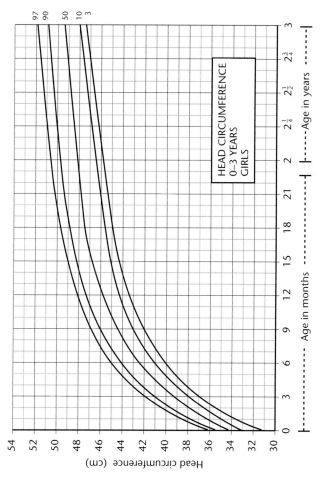

Figure 34.7 Head circumference 0–3 years—girls

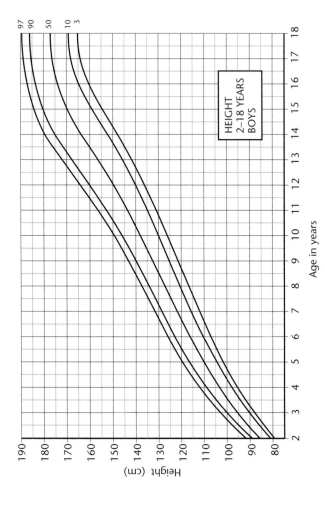

Figure 34.8 Height 2–18 years—boys

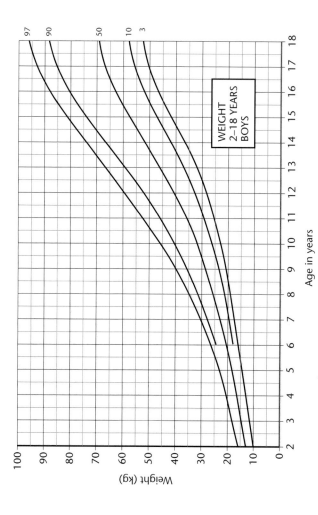

Figure 34.9 Weight 2–18 years—boys

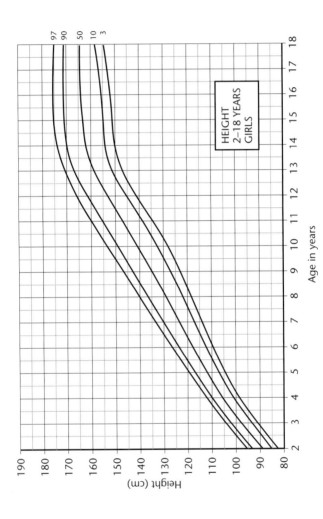

Figure 34.10 Height 2–18 years—girls

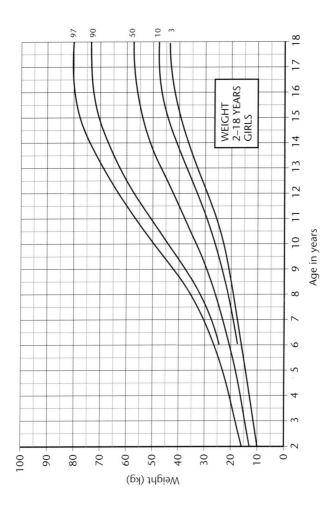

Figure 34.11 Weight 2–18 years—girls

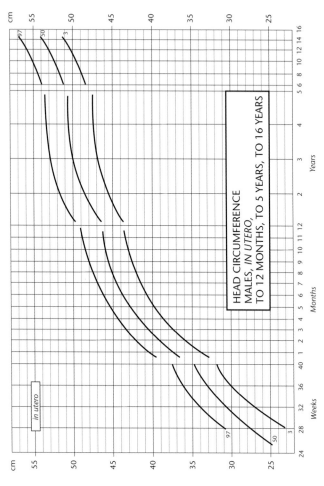

Figure 34.12 Head circumference of males, *in utero*, to 12 months, to 5 years and to 16 years
Source: National Health & Medical Research Council 1980

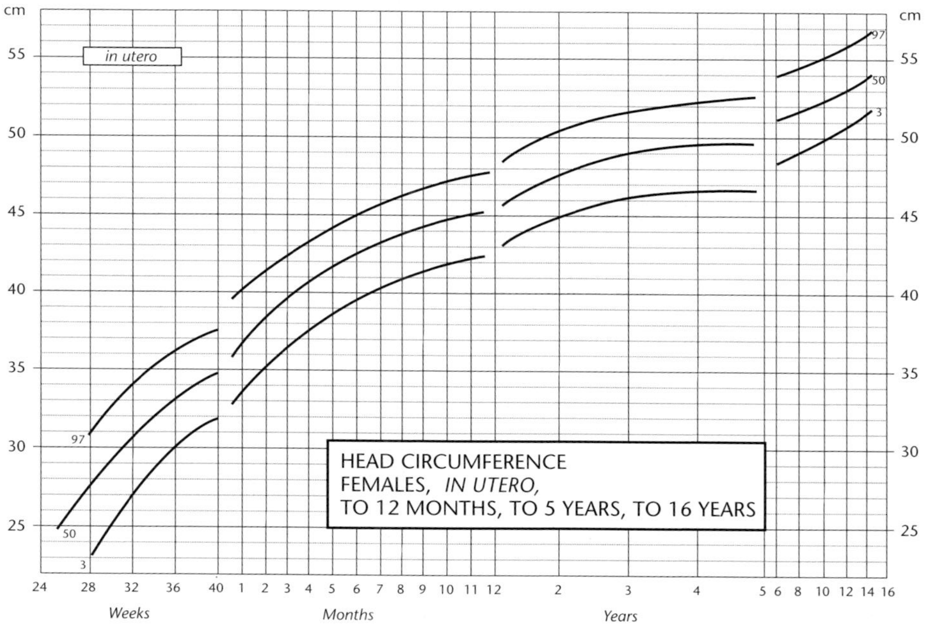

Figure 34.13 Head circumference of females, *in utero*, to 12 months, to 5 years and to 16 years
Source: National Health & Medical Research Council 1980

35

Developmental assessment and screening

This section includes:

- developmental assessment
- health screening in childhood.

Developmental assessment

The examination of any child is not complete until the child's development has been assessed. Some of the major developmental milestones are listed in Table 35.1.

Knowledge of normal development will allow you to recognise patterns which vary from the normal and will also help you to reassure parents when milestones are normal.

Basic equipment required

- Wooden blocks (approximately 2 cm high)
- High-pitched bell and low-pitched rattle
- Fluffy, red woollen ball
- Pencil and paper
- Picture book with simple, coloured pictures
- Small safe objects (such as jellybeans) for testing pincer grasp
- Selection of small, safe, interesting toys

The history

The information obtained will only be as good as the questions you ask. Questions should be concise and precise. You will obtain much of the information about the child's social behaviour as well as information about the child's language from the parents. Remember when asking about language development to distinguish between expressive language (what the child can say) and receptive language (what the child can hear and understand). Receptive language should be well in advance of expressive language.

Timing of the assessment

The developmental assessment is best done at the beginning of the examination when the child is more likely to be co-operative. The child's best performance should be obtained. This will be at a time when the child is not ill, miserable or just woken up. A few moments spent making friends with the child and observing him or her at the beginning of the assessment are well spent.

A useful structure

Table 35.1 divides the milestones into the four areas traditionally used in assessing development: gross motor function; vision and fine motor; social skills and understanding; and hearing and speech.

This helps give some structure to your assessment and helps to avoid forgetting major areas. It is also a useful way to describe the child's development. The order in which the child is tested does not particularly matter as long as all areas are covered. Remember to note what the child does spontaneously during your examination as you can mentally tick this off as an appropriate or inappropriate milestone. As young infants have fairly short attention spans, the developmental assessment should be done quickly as well as efficiently.

Interpreting your findings

Allowances should be made for prematurity, unusual familial patterns (late walkers but otherwise normal) and for fatigue or illness. Some areas of development have more significance than others. The child's alertness, concentration and interest in surroundings are more important than gross motor milestones.

Limitations to developmental assessment

There is a wide range of normal development. The further the child deviates from normal, the more confident you can be that there is likely to be a problem. Advanced intelligence cannot be predicted on the basis of advanced developmental milestones, particularly gross motor milestones. However, if a child shows delays in several areas this raises the possibility of global developmental delay and needs reassessment and further investigation. Specific delays in some areas

Table 35.1 Normal developmental milestones

Age	Gross motor	Vision and fine motor	Social skills and understanding	Hearing and speech
Newborn	Prone: pelvis high, knees under abdomen, turns face to side.	Can fix on a visual object and follow it briefly horizontally.		Variable response to sound.
1 month	Lifts head momentarily when held in ventral suspension.	Follows object through 90°.	Quietens when picked up.	Soft guttural noises when content.
6 weeks	Head lag not complete when pulled to sit.	Hands often open.	Social smiling.	Quiets in response to soft sound 15 cm from ear.
3 months	Prone: lifts chest off bed taking weight on forearms. Only slight head lag when pulled to sit.	Holds rattle placed in hand. Starts to look at own hands.	Pleasurable response to familiar, enjoyable situations (bottle, bath).	Turns head to soft sound at ear level.
6 months	Spontaneously lifts head when supine. Prone: lifts chest on extended arms.	Hand regard goes. Transfers objects between hands. Palmar grasp.	Shows fear of strangers. Can imitate (e.g. cough), laughs.	Visually locates soft sounds at 40–50 cm on ear level.
9 months	Crawls. Stands holding onto support. Sits unsupported for 10 minutes.	Pincer grip developing.	Looks for toy fallen out of sight. Can play peek-a-boo.	Tries to communicate vocally. Localises soft sounds above and below ear at 1 metre.

12 months	Walks alone with one hand held.	Throws objects on floor repeatedly. Less likely to take all objects to mouth.	Knows and turns to own name. Drinks from cup.	Says 2 or 3 words with meaning.
18 months	Jumps using both feet. Walks backwards.	Spontaneous scribble. Tower of three or four blocks.	Points to two or three parts of the body. Indicates toilet needs.	5–20 recognisable words. Understands many more.
2 years	Runs well. Kicks ball without over-balancing.	Copies vertical and circular strokes. Tower of six or seven blocks.	Develops negative behaviour. Fantasy play. Gives first name.	Two- and three-word phrases.
3 years	Rides tricycle. Stands on one foot momentarily.	Copies circle, nine-block tower.	Mainly dry by night. Competent with fork and spoon. Knows own sex. Very imaginative play.	Gives full name. Uses plurals. Three- to five-word sentences.
4 years	Hops on one foot. Stands on one foot for 3–5 seconds.	Copies cross. Draws person with three parts. Matches five primary colours.		Asks many questions. Gives name and address. Names four primary colours.
5 years	Can skip.	Copies square. Draws person with six parts.	Understands rules of play. Washes and dries face and hands.	Speech fluent, good articulation.

with normal development in others raise the question of an isolated defect; for example, delayed speech in a child who is normal in other milestones suggests a hearing loss.

Health screening in childhood

Table 35.2 gives a guide to what should be examined, at various ages beyond the newborn '6-week' check, to permit early detection of problems where such 'screening' has shown to be useful. It has been adapted from guidelines of the National Health and Medical Research Council, 1999.

Note: Immunisation status should be checked at every opportunity, and 'catch-up' vaccination offered.

Table 35.2 Recommended schedule of child health surveillance

	Height	Weight	Head circum-ference	Hearing	Vision	Develop-ment	Congenital heart disease	Congenital hip dislocation	Testes	Scoliosis
4/12	✓	✓	✓	✓	✓	✓	✓	✓	✓	✓
6/12			✓				✓		✓	✓
12/12	✓	✓	✓	✓	✓		✓		✓	✓
18/12			✓			✓	✓	(gait)	✓	✓
2½-			✓				During other exam	(gait)		✓
3½ years										
4–5 years	✓	✓	✓				✓	(gait)		✓
10 years	✓	✓	✓	✓		✓	✓	✓	✓	✓ Females
12 years	✓	✓	✓	✓		✓	✓	✓	✓	
15 years	✓	✓	✓	✓	✓	✓	✓	✓	✓	✓

Source: National Health & Medical Research Council 1999

Appendix: drug dosage guidelines

To reduce errors caused by misinterpretation of your intentions, the following should be observed:

- Don't use abbreviations for *micrograms* or *units*. However, abbreviations can be used for grams (g) and milligrams (mg).
- Liquid medications should be ordered by weight of active ingredients, *not* by volume, for example paracetamol 120 mg, *not* paracetamol mixture 5 mL. Likewise, tablets, capsules and ampoules should be ordered by strength, for example propranolol 40 mg, *not* propranolol 1 tablet.
- The *route* of administration should be clear, for example IM, IV, SC, oral.
- *Decimal prescribing*:
  - Don't write a decimal point without a prefix, for example write 0.5 mg, *not* .5 mg.
  - Don't write a decimal point and zero after a whole number, for example write 2 mg, *not* 2.0 mg.
  - Avoid using a decimal expression when a more recognisable alternative exists, for example write 500 mg rather than 0.5 g, write 50 micrograms rather than 0.05 mg.
- *Prescribing digoxin*: After calculating the dose of digoxin, the prescriber *must* have the dose checked and countersigned by a second medical officer.

The guidelines to paediatric drug doses in Table A.2 are not comprehensive and in part reflect patterns of usage at the Children's Hospital at Westmead.

Every effort has been taken to ensure that drug doses are correct and reflect current recommendations at the time of publication.

The abbreviations used in Table A.2 are:

- IV: Intravenous
- IM: Intramuscular
- SC: Subcutaneous
- O: Oral (also nasogastric or intragastric)
- ET: Endotracheal or intratracheal
- R: Restricted drug at the Children's Hospital at Westmead (seek pharmacy advice before prescribing)
- Cont.: Continuous
- SL: Sublingual

- TR: Therapeutic Range
- SAS: Special Access Scheme.

Note: When a drug is prescribed on a 'per weight' basis, doses for teenagers and obese children may exceed the usual adult dose. Some patients may therefore be at risk of overdose. The maximum patient weight for drug calculations is 40 kg (unless otherwise specified). Calculations for obese patients should be based on lean body mass.

Table A.1 Acceptable abbreviations in prescribing

Route		Dose		Timing	
Oral	O or PO	gram	g	for 1 day	1/7
		milligram	mg	for 1 week	1/52
Sublingual	SL	micrograms	micrograms	twice-daily	b.d.
Nebulised	neb	maximum	max.	morning	mane
Intravenous	IV	millilitre	mL	3 times/day	t.d.s.
Intramuscular	IM	litre	L	4 times/day	q.i.d.
Subcutaneous	SC	millimole	mmol	hourly	hourly
Rectal	PR	one, two	i, ii	4-hourly	4-hourly or 4/24
Topical	top	three, four	iii, iv	at night	nocte
Endotracheal	ET	millilitres/ hour	mL/h	as required	p.r.n.

Table A.2 Guidelines to paediatric doses

Name	Indication	Route	Dose (maximum weight for calculations = 40 kg)	Interval	Dose limit	Notes
Acetazolamide	Epilepsy	O	8–30 mg/kg/day	6–24-hourly	1 g/day	Modify dose in renal failure
	Acute glaucoma, benign intracranial hypertension	O/IV	20–40 mg/kg/day	6-hourly		
	Diuretic	O/IV	5 mg/kg/dose	24–48-hourly		
N-acetylcysteine	Paracetamol overdose	IV infusion	150 mg/kg IV over 15–60 min; followed by 50 mg/kg IV over next 4 hours; then 100 mg/kg IV over subsequent 16 hours	Cont. infusion		Consult Poisons Information Centre prior to administration. Adverse reactions are rate-dependent.
Acetylsalicylic acid (see aspirin)						

Drug	Indication	Route	Dose	Frequency	Maximum dose	Notes
Aciclovir						Restricted (except topical). Maintain adequate hydration. Modify dose in renal failure.
	Neonatal HSV infection:	IV	20 mg/kg/dose	8-hourly		
	Severe HSV infection: encephalitis (postneonatal), ocular, eczema herpeticum, severe mucocutaneous	IV	10 mg/kg/dose	8-hourly	400 mg/dose	
	Less severe HSV infection (mucocutaneous)	O	10 mg/kg/dose 5 times daily		400 mg/dose	
	Severe varicella	IV	10 mg/kg/dose	8-hourly	400 mg/dose	
	Herpes zoster, ophthalmic herpes zoster, varicella	O	10 mg/kg/dose 5 times daily		400 mg/dose	
Activated charcoal (see charcoal)						
Adenosine	Supraventricular tachycardia	IV rapid bolus	0.05 mg/kg–0.25 mg/kg/dose Commence with 0.05 mg/kg and increase in increments of 0.05 mg/kg until control achieved.	Every 2 min	12 mg/dose or total cumulative dose of 30 mg	Administer as a rapid bolus, followed by a rapid saline flush and monitor with continuous ECG strip.

Name	Indication	Route	Dose	Interval	Dose limit	Notes
Adrenaline	Cardiac arrest/resuscitation	IV	Initial: 10 micrograms/kg/dose Subsequent: 10–100 micrograms/kg/dose	Every 3–5 min		10 micrograms/kg = 0.1 mL/kg of 1:10 000 100 micrograms/kg = 0.1 mL/kg of 1:1000 If needed, higher inotropic doses can be infused.
		ET	100 micrograms/kg/dose			
	Inotrope	IV infusion	Dose range: 0.05–1 micrograms/kg/min	Cont. infusion		
	Anaphylaxis	SC/IV/IM	5–10 micrograms/kg/dose	Repeat p.r.n.		
	Croup	Neb.	0.5 mg/kg/dose of 1:1000 (0.5 mL/kg/dose)	Every 30 min p.r.n.	5 mL of 1:1000	
Allopurinol	Hyperuricaemia	O	10–20 mg/kg/day	6–12-hourly	600 mg/day	Modify dose in renal failure. Use urate oxidase if IV route necessary.
	Tumour lysis (oncology)	O	300 mg/m²/day	8-hourly		
Alprostadil (prostaglandin E1)	Maintenance of ductal patency	IV infusion	Initial: 0.05–0.1 micrograms/kg/min. Titrate to response. Maintenance: doses as low as 0.005 micrograms/kg/min may be effective	Cont. infusion		Respiratory depression may occur.

Drug		Route	Dose	Frequency	Max	Notes
Amikacin	t.d.s. regimen	IV/IM	7.5 mg/kg/dose	8-hourly	500 mg/dose	*Restricted:* Modify dose in renal failure. Do not use a single daily dosing regimen for neonates, patients with renal impairment, oncological disease or streptococcal/enterococcal/endocarditis. Levels: See nomogram (daily). Trough: < 10 mg/L (t.d.s.) Peak: 20–30 mg/L (t.d.s.)
	Single daily dosing regimen (see note)	IV/IM	20 mg/kg/dose	24-hourly	1.5 g/day	
Amiloride	K-sparing diuretic	O	0.3–0.5 mg/kg/day	12-hourly	5 mg/dose	
Aminophylline	Asthma	IV	Intermittent bolus: 5 mg/kg/dose	6-hourly		Continuous infusion only in ICU. Monitor levels 6 hours after commencement of infusion: TR 55–110 micromol/L. *Note:* Loading dose may not be needed if taking oral theophylline.
		IV infusion	Load: 10 mg/kg over 60 min then ≤ 9 years: 0.9 mg/kg/h > 9 years: 0.7 mg/kg/h	Cont. infusion		

Name	Indication	Route	Dose	Interval	Dose limit	Notes
Amiodarone	Arrhythmia	IV	Load: 5–10 mg/kg/dose over 1–2 hours	Single dose	15 mg/kg/day	Only administer on Cardiology advice. Monitor liver, thyroid and pulmonary function if long-term therapy anticipated.
		IV infusion	Load as above then 10 mg/kg/day until arrhythmia controlled.	Cont. infusion		Multiple drug interactions.
	Oral maintenance	O	First week: 12 mg/kg/day	8-hourly	600 mg/day	
			Second week: 8 mg/kg/day	12-hourly	400 mg/day	
			Subsequent: 4 mg/kg/day	24-hourly	200 mg/day	
Amitriptyline	Enuresis/neuropathic pain	O	1–1.5 mg/kg/day	24-hourly	200 mg/day	No longer commonly used for depression.
	Depression/conduct disorder	O	1–2.5 mg/kg/day	24-hourly		
Amlodipine	Hypertension	O	0.05–0.3 mg/kg/day	24-hourly	10 mg/day	Commence with a small dose and increase as tolerated.
Amoxycillin	Usual dose	O	7.5–25 mg/kg/dose	8-hourly	1.5 g/day	Ampicillin is used intravenously at CHW.
		IM/IV	10–25 mg/kg/dose	8-hourly	8 g/day	
	Severe infection	IM/IV	50 mg/kg/dose	4- or 6-hourly		
Amoxycillin and clavulanic acid (Augmentin Duo ®)		O	22.5 mg/kg/dose	8-hourly	1.5 g/day	Dose based on amoxycillin. Non Duo Augmentin® prescribed 8-hourly

Drug	Indication	Route	Dose	Frequency	Maximum	Comments
Amphotericin B	Systemic fungal infection	IV	0.5–1 mg/kg/dose	24-hourly	1.5 mg/kg/day or 60 mg/day, whichever is less	Adverse reactions may occur—observe closely during 1st dose. Premedication with corticosteroids, antihistamine and antipyretic may be warranted. Ensure adequate hydration and normal serum Na⁺ prior to administration. Normal saline bolus (10 mL/kg) pre dose may reduce nephrotoxicity. Monitor for hypokalaemia and nephrotoxicity.
	Severe infection (e.g. *Aspergillus*)	IV	1 mg/kg/dose	24-hourly		
	Oral candidiasis treatment	O	10 mg/dose (*not per kg*)	6-hourly		10 mg oral lozenge
	Intestinal candidiasis prophylaxis	O	10 mg/dose (*not per kg*)	12-hourly		
Amphotericin (liposomal) (Ambisome®) (Abelcet®)	Proven fungal infections (resistant organisms)	IV	1–5 mg/kg/day	24-hourly		*Restricted.* Indications: pre-existing renal impairment; amphotericin B associated nephrotoxicity or infusion-related toxicity.

Name	Indication	Route	Dose	Interval	Dose limit	Notes
Ampicillin	Usual dose	IV/IM	25 mg/kg/dose	6-hourly	12 g/day	Amoxycillin is used for oral administration at CHW.
	Severe infection	IV/IM	50 mg/kg/dose	4- or 6-hourly		
L-arginine	Metabolic disorder	O	Typical dose: 200–600 mg/kg/day	6- or 8-hourly		*Restricted.* Metabolic consultation required.
		IV	Load: 210 mg/kg over 90 min Maintenance: 210 mg/kg over 24 hours	Cont. infusion		
Ascorbic acid (see Vitamin C)						
Aspirin (acetylsalicylic acid)	Anti-inflammatory/ antirheumatic	O	60–120 mg/kg/day	6–12-hourly	5.2 g/day	Do not use as antipyretic. Monitor drug levels when anti-inflammatory doses are used. Low dose aspirin is used to treat Kawasaki disease when high dose IVIG is concomitantly administered.
	Antiplatelet effect and Kawasaki disease	O	2–5 mg/kg/day	daily	325 mg/day	

Drug	Indication	Route	Dose	Frequency	Max dose	Comments
Atenolol	Hypertension/arrhythmia	O	1–2 mg/kg/day	12–24-hourly (usually 24-hourly)	200 mg/day	Modify dose in renal failure. Higher doses (to 5 mg/kg/day) have been used in hypertension.
Atracurium	Neuromuscular blockade (non-depolarising)	IV bolus	Load/bolus: 0.4–0.6 mg/kg/dose	30–60 min p.r.n.		Use restricted to anaesthesia or ICU. When used as infusion, dosage titration is required to maintain neuromuscular blockade.
		IV infusion	Load as above then 5–15 micrograms/kg/min Higher doses may be required with prolonged usage.	Cont. infusion		
Atropine	Anaesthesia premedication Prevention/treatment of bradycardia	IV/IM/SC/ET	20 micrograms/kg/dose	Single dose	Child: 0.5–1 mg Adolescent: 2 mg	Refer to Poisons Information Centre for use in organophosphate/carbamate poisoning.
	Reversal of non depolarising muscle relaxants	IV	20 micrograms/kg/dose (with neostigmine 50 micrograms/kg)	Single dose		
	Organophosphate poisoning	IV	50 micrograms/kg/dose	Repeat every 2–5 min until symptoms of mild atropinisation occur	2 mg/dose	

Name	Indication	Route	Dose	Interval	Dose limit	Notes
Azathioprine	Immunosuppression	IV/O	Load: 3–5 mg/kg/day	Single dose		See specific protocols. Notify pharmacy if prescribing IV.
		IV/O	Maintenance: 1–3 mg/kg/day	24-hourly		
Aztreonam	Usual dose	IV/IM	30 mg/kg/dose	6- or 8-hourly	8 g/day	*Restricted.* Modify dose in renal failure.
	Severe infection	IV/IM	50 mg/kg/dose	6- or 8-hourly		
Baclofen	Spasticity	O	Initial 0.75 mg/kg/day, increasing every 3 days to 2.5 mg/kg/day	6- or 8-hourly	≤ 7 years: 40 mg/day > 7 years: 80 mg/day	Caution in epilepsy.
BAL (British Anti Lewisite) (see dimercaprol)						
Beclomethasone dipropionate	Inhaler or Rotacaps	Oral inhalation	Usual: 100–400 micrograms/day Range: 100–1600 micrograms/day	6–12-hourly	2000 micrograms/day	
	Nasal Spray	Nasal	50–100 micrograms/nostril/dose	12-hourly	500 micrograms/day	
Bendrofluazide	Diuretic	O	0.1–0.2 mg/kg/dose	24-hourly	10 mg/dose	
Benztropine	Drug induced dystonia	IV/IM	0.02 mg/kg/dose May be repeated after 15 min	Single dose	1 mg/dose or 6 mg/day	Use with caution in children < 3 years.

Drug		Route	Dose	Frequency	Max dose	Notes
Benzylpenicillin (Penicillin G)	Usual dose	IV/IM	30 mg/kg/dose	6-hourly	1.2 g/dose	
	Severe infection	IV/IM	60 mg/kg/dose	4- or 6-hourly	2.4 g/dose	The higher dose is recommended for meningitis. For oral dosing, use phenoxymethyl penicillin.
Bicarbonate sodium (see sodium bicarbonate)						
Biotin (Vit. H)	Metabolic disorders	O	5–20 mg/day (*not per kg*)	12-hourly	100 mg/day	*Restricted.* Metabolic consultation required.
Budesonide	Inhaler/Turbuhaler	Oral inhalation	Usual: 100–400 micrograms/day Range: 100–1600 micrograms/day	6- or 12-hourly	2400 micrograms/day	
	Croup	Neb.	2 mg/dose	Single dose		
	Nasal Spray	Nasal inhalation	100–200 micrograms/nostril/day	12- or 24-hourly		
	Inflammatory bowel disease	O	9 mg/day (*not per kg*)	24-hourly		*Restricted.* Gastroenterology
Bupivacaine	Regional anaesthesia e.g. epidural	Infusion (*not IV*)	< 6 months: not greater than 0.25 mg/kg/hour > 6 months: not greater than 0.5 mg/kg/hour		2 mg/kg or 200 mg/dose (whichever is less)	*Not for IV use.*

Name	Indication	Route	Dose	Interval	Dose limit	Notes
Calcitonin (Salmon)	Hypercalcaemia	IM/SC	Initial: 8 U/kg/day increasing to max 32 U/kg/day	6- or 12-hourly	32 U/kg/day	Ensure adequate calcium intake. Higher doses may be used in acute hypocalcaemia with endocrine consultation. For renal osteodystrophy, may be administered 3 times weekly, rather than daily.
Calcitriol (see also ergocalciferol—Vitamin D2)	Acute hypocalcaemia, hypoparathyroidism, hypophosphataemic rickets, chronic renal failure	O	15–60 nanogram/kg/day. Usual maintenance: approx. 30 nanograms/kg/day.	12–24-hourly		
Calcium carbonate (see calcium (oral) and calcium chloride)						
Calcium (oral)	Hypocalcaemia	O	20–50 mg of elemental Ca/kg/day (0.5–1.25 mmol/kg/day)	4–12-hourly		Prescribe as elemental calcium. *Calcium carbonate tablets:* 1. Caltrate® = 600 mg elemental Ca (15 mmol Ca). 2. Titralac® = 168 mg elemental Ca (4.2 mmol). 3. Cal-Sup® = 500 mg elemental Ca (12.5 mmol)
	Phosphate binder (see note)	O	600–1800 mg of elemental Ca/meal (*not per kg*)	With meals		

					Other calcium salts: 1. Sandocal® 1000 = 1000 mg elemental Ca (25 mmol) 2. Sandocal® 600 = 600 mg elemental Ca (15 mmol) For phosphate binding take immediately prior to meals. Do not use effervescent preparations for phosphate binding. Monitor Ca and phosphate levels.
Calcium chloride 10%	Hyperkalaemia (with arrhythmia), Ca channel blocker toxicity, hypermagnesaemia	IV	0.15 mmol/kg/dose (0.2 mL/kg/dose)	Single dose	27.2 mg elemental Ca/mL or 0.68 mmol Ca/mL *Caution:* Extravasation can cause tissue necrosis. Monitor Ca and phosphate levels.
	Hypocalcaemia (including tetany)	IV (slow)	0.07–0.15 mmol/kg/dose (or 0.1–0.2 mL/kg/dose)	Repeat 4–6-hourly if necessary	
	IV maintenance	IV infusion	0.5–1 mmol/kg/day Titrate to serum Ca level	Cont. infusion	

Name	Indication	Route	Dose	Interval	Dose limit	Notes
Calcium EDTA	Lead toxicity	IV infusion	1500 mg/m²/day	Continuous infusion		Consult Poisons Information Centre prior to administration. Often used with dimercaprol (BAL). Give the first dose of Ca EDTA 4 hours after the first dose of dimercaprol. Monitor hepatic and renal function.
		IM	50–75 mg/kg/day	6–12-hourly		
Calcium gluconate 10% (see also calcium chloride)	Hypocalcaemia (including tetany)	IV (slow)	0.07–0.15 mmol/kg/dose (or 0.3–0.6 mL/kg/dose)	Repeat 4–6-hourly if necessary		8.9 mg elemental Ca/mL or 0.22 mmol Ca/mL. *Caution:* Extravasation can cause tissue necrosis. Calcium gluconate is not recommended for use during resuscitation.

Captopril	Cardiac failure	O	Initial dose: 0.1 mg/kg · Maintenance: 0.3–1 mg/kg/day	6-12-hourly (usually 8)	6 mg/kg/day	Commence with a small dose and increase as tolerated. Caution if administering potassium, potassium sparing agents, or in presence of renal failure. Can cause cough. Consider changing to long-acting ACE inhibitor prior to discharge.
	Antihypertensive	O	Initial: 0.3–0.9 mg/kg/day Maintenance: 0.3–4 mg/kg/day	8-hourly		
Carbamazepine	Epilepsy, bipolar disorder, adjunct to analgesia	O	Initial: 5 mg/kg/day and increase after approx. 5 days to 10 mg/kg/day Usual maintenance: 10–30 mg/kg/day	8- or 12-hourly (usually 12-hourly)	2000 mg/day	TR: 20–40 micromol/L.
Carbimazole	Thyrotoxicosis	O	Initial: 0.5–1 mg/kg/day Dose will need modification when euthyroid.	8- or 12-hourly	60 mg/day	Endocrinology consultation recommended.

Name	Indication	Route	Dose	Interval	Dose limit	Notes
L-carnitine	Metabolic disorder	O	Commence at 50 mg/kg/day, increase slowly to 50–100 mg/kg/day	6- or 8-hourly	3 g/day	*Restricted.* Metabolic consultation required. SAS
		IV	50–100 mg/kg/day			
Cefaclor	Usual dose	O	10 mg/kg/dose	8-hourly	250 mg/dose	Modify dose in renal failure
Cefotaxime	Usual dose	IV/IM	50 mg/kg/dose	8-hourly	8 g/day	*Restricted.* Modify dose in renal failure.
	Severe infection	IV/IM	50 mg/kg/dose	6-hourly		
Ceftazidime	Usual dose	IV/IM	50 mg/kg/dose	8-hourly	6 g/day	*Restricted.* Modify dose in renal failure.
	Severe infection/cystic fibrosis	IV/IM	50 mg/kg/dose	8-hourly		
Ceftriaxone	Usual dose	IV/IM	50 mg/kg/dose	24-hourly	2 g/dose	*Restricted.* May displace bilirubin. Not recommended for neonates.
	Severe infection	IV	50 mg/kg/dose or 100 mg/kg/dose	12-hourly 24-hourly	4 g/day	
	N. meningitidis prophylaxis	IM	< 12 years: 125 mg/dose (*not per kg*) ≥ 12 years: 250 mg/dose (*not per kg*)	Single dose		
	H. influenzae type b prophylaxis	IM	50 mg/kg/dose	24-hourly × 2 days	2 g/dose	

Drug	Indication	Route	Dose	Frequency	Maximum	Notes
Cephalexin	Usual dose	O	12.5–25 mg/kg/dose	6-hourly	1 g/dose	
Cephalothin	Usual dose	IV/IM	25 mg/kg/dose	6-hourly	8 g/day	Modify dose in renal failure.
	Severe infection	IV/IM	50 mg/kg/dose	6-hourly		
Charcoal (activated)		NG/O	Initial dose: 1 g/kg/dose	Single dose	50 g/dose	Consult Poisons Information Centre.
		NG/O	Subsequent doses: 0.25 g/kg/dose	Hourly		
Chloral hydrate	Sedation	O/rectal	6–10 mg/kg/dose	6- or 8-hourly	500 mg/dose	Prolonged usage may result in accumulation in patients with renal or hepatic impairment.
	Hypnotic or premedication	O/rectal	50 mg/kg/dose Higher doses (75 mg/kg/dose) can be used.	Single dose	1 g/dose	
Chloramphenicol	Usual dose	O/IV	12.5 mg/kg/dose	6-hourly	750 mg/dose	Restricted. Only administer if less toxic antibiotics unsuitable.
	Severe infection	IV	25 mg/kg/dose	6- or 8-hourly		
Chloroquine	Malaria treatment	O	Initial: 10 mg/kg/dose Subsequent: 5 mg/kg/dose 6 hours after initial dose and on days 2 and 3	Single dose	600 mg/dose	Dose is chloroquine base.
				24-hourly		
	Malaria prophylaxis	O	5 mg/kg/dose	Weekly	300 mg/dose	
	Immune suppression	O	Initial: 12 mg/kg/dose Maintenance: 4–8 mg/kg/dose	24-hourly	600 mg/dose	

Name	Indication	Route	Dose	Interval	Dose limit	Notes
Chlorpromazine	Psychosis	O	2–6 mg/kg/day	4–6-hourly	< 5 years: 40 mg/day	Hypotension can occur with intravenous administration.
		IM	0.5–1 mg/kg/dose	6–8-hourly	5–12 years:	IV administration for psychiatric reasons is inappropriate. Intramuscular injection requires co-administration of hyalase-like compounds. Benztropine is antidote for extrapyramidal side-effects.
		Rectal	3–4 mg/kg/day	6–8-hourly	75 mg/day	
	Antiemetic, pyrexia	O/IV/IM	0.5–1 mg/kg/dose	6–8-hourly		
Chorionic gonadotropin	Cryptorchidism	IM	500–1500 U/dose	1–2/week for 5 weeks		Restricted to Endocrinology.
Cimetidine	Peptic ulcer disease, reflux > 1 month	O	20–40 mg/kg/day	6-hourly	800 mg/day	Modify dose in renal failure. Multiple drug interactions.
	Warts and molluscum contagiosum	O	20–40 mg/kg/day	24-hourly		
Ciprofloxacin	Usual dose	O	10 mg/kg/dose	12-hourly	500 mg/dose	*Restricted.* Modify dose in renal failure. Consultation with ID recommended.
	Usual dose	IV	5 mg/kg/dose	12-hourly	200 mg/dose	
	Severe infection	IV	10 mg/kg/dose	12-hourly	400 mg/dose	
	Cystic fibrosis	O	15 mg/kg/dose	12-hourly	750 mg/dose	

Drug	Indication	Route	Dose	Frequency	Maximum	Comments
Cisapride (no longer formulary)	Severe gastro oesophageal reflux	O	0.2 mg/kg/dose	6- or 8-hourly	< 36 months: 0.8 mg/kg/day Older children: 10 mg/dose	Overdose or administration with cytochrome P450 inhibitors may cause prolongation of the QT interval and ventricular arrhythmias. Multiple drug interactions.
Cisatracurium	Neuromuscular blockade (non-depolarising)	IV	Load/bolus: 0.1–0.15 mg/kg/dose	30–60 min p.r.n.		Use restricted to Anaesthesia or ICU. When used as infusion, dosage titration is required to maintain neuromuscular blockade.
		IV infusion	Load as above then 2–15 micrograms/kg/min	Cont. infusion		
Clarithromycin	Susceptible organisms including pertussis	O	7.5 mg/kg/dose	12-hourly	500 mg/dose	Restricted. Treat pertussis for 7 days
	M. avium complex, M. marinum	O	12.5 mg/kg/dose			
Clindamycin	Usual dose	O/IV/IM	10 mg/kg/dose	8-hourly	450 mg/dose	Minimum recommended oral dose is 37.5 mg every 8 hours.
	Severe infection	IV	15 mg/kg/dose	8-hourly	600 mg dose	
Clobazam	Epilepsy	O	Initial: 0.5 mg/kg/day Maintenance: 0.5–1 mg/kg/day	8- or 12-hourly	60 mg/day	

Name	Indication	Route	Dose	Interval	Dose limit	Notes
Clonazepam	Status epilepticus (neonates/infants)	IV	0.1–0.25 mg/dose (*not per kg*)	Single dose Repeat × 1		Respiratory depression can occur. Commence with the lower dose if not ventilated.
	Status epilepticus (children)	IV	0.5 mg/dose (*not per kg*)	Single dose Repeat × 1		
	Epilepsy	O	Initial: 0.01–0.03 mg/kg/day, Usual maintenance: 0.1–0.2 mg/kg/day	8- (or 12-) hourly	0.2 mg/kg/day or 2 mg/dose	
Clonidine	Antihypertensive/ autonomic dysfunction syndrome	IV	3–6 micrograms/ kg/dose Administer slowly.	6–8-hourly p.r.n.	300 micrograms/ dose	The IV preparation should be given slowly, over at least 5 minutes.
		O	3–12 micrograms/ kg/day	8-hourly	900 micrograms/ day	
	Migraine prophylaxis	O	0.5–1 micrograms/ kg/day	12-hourly		
Codeine phosphate	Analgesia	O/IM/SC	1 mg/kg/dose	4- or 6-hourly p.r.n.	60 mg/dose	Modify dose in renal failure. Antidote: naloxone.
	Antitussive	O	1 mg/kg/day	6-hourly	60 mg/day	
Cotrimoxazole (trimethoprim/ sulphamethoxazole)	Usual dose	O/IV	4 mg/kg/dose	12-hourly	Trimethoprim 320 mg/day	Dose based on trimethoprim. Modify dose in renal failure.
	Pneumocystis carinii treatment	O/IV	5 mg/kg/dose	6-hourly	Trimethoprim 1600 mg/day	
	Pneumocystis prophylaxis: children > 1 month	O	5 mg/kg/dose Alternative regimen: 5 mg/kg/dose	24-hourly 12-hourly × 3 days/week	Trimethoprim 1600 mg/day	
	UTI prophylaxis	O	2 mg/kg/dose	24-hourly		

Cromoglycate (see
sodium cromoglycate)

Cyanocobalamin
(see Vitamin B12)

Drug	Indication	Route	Dose	Frequency	Maximum	Notes
Cyclophosphamide	Immunosuppressive (nephrotic syndrome)	O	2–3 mg/kg/day	24-hourly		See specific protocols, e.g. oncology.
Cyclosporin	Autoimmune disease	O	1–4 mg/kg/day	12- or 24-hourly	12 mg/kg/day	*Restricted.* Oral dose approx. 3 × IV dose. Blood levels should guide dosage. See specific protocols.
	Nephrotic syndrome	O	5–6 mg/kg/day			
Cyproheptadine	Allergies and pruritus	O	0.25–0.4 mg/kg/day	8- or 12-hourly	16 mg/day	
Cyproterone acetate	Precocious puberty Androgen excess	O	50–150 mg/m²/day	12-hourly		Use only after consultation with Endocrinology. May cause adrenal suppression.
Desferrioxamine	Chronic iron overload	SC infusion IV infusion	500 mg/11 kg body weight/dose (rounded down to the nearest 500 mg) Infuse over at least 8 hours.	24-hourly for 6–7 nights/wk	Adults up to 6 g/day or 50 mg/kg/day	Haematology consultation recommended. Prolonged infusions are more effective. Not to be added to blood.
	Antidote (iron poisoning)	IV infusion	15 mg/kg/h up to 90 mg/kg/8 hours	Cont. infusion		

Name	Indication	Route	Dose	Interval	Dose limit	Notes
Desmopressin (DDAVP)	Central diabetes insipidus	Intranasal	Initial: 1–5 micrograms/dose Maintenance: 2–40 micrograms/day	Single dose 12–24-hourly	40 micrograms/day	Monitor electrolytes, urine output and SG. IM/IV administration has 10 × potency of nasal administration. IM/IV route should not be used for long term maintenance.
		IM/IV	Initial: 0.1–0.5 micrograms/dose Maintenance: 0.2–4 micrograms/day	Single dose 12–24-hourly	4 micrograms/day	
	Nocturnal enuresis > 6 years	Intranasal	Initial: 20 micrograms/day (nightly)	24-hourly (bedtime)	40 micrograms/day	
	Haemophilia A/Von Willebrand's type 1	IV	0.3 micrograms/kg/dose	Repeat as needed	20 micrograms/dose	
Dexamethasone	Meningitis	O/IV	0.1–1 mg/kg/day	6- or 8-hourly		Avoid rapid injection. Anti-inflammatory potency is 25–30 times greater than hydrocortisone, but has no mineralocorticoid activity. If meningitis is suspected, administer prior to antibiotics if possible.
		IV	0.6 mg/kg/day for 4 days	6-hourly		
	Croup	IV/O	0.15–0.3 mg/kg/dose	Single dose		

Drug	Indication	Route	Dose	Frequency	Max dose	Notes
Dexchlorpheniramine	Antihistamine	O	0.1–0.15 mg/kg/day	8- or 12-hourly	2 mg/dose	
Dextrose (Glucose)	Hypoglycaemia	IV	0.5 g/kg (1 mL/kg of 50% solution)			Monitor glucose level.
	Hyperkalaemia	IV	0.5g/kg (1 mL/kg of 50% solution) ± Insulin 0.1 U/kg			
Diazepam	Status epilepticus	IV	0.1–0.25 mg/kg/dose over 3–5 min	Single dose (can be repeated)	IV: 10 mg/dose	Not recommended for use in neonates. Respiratory depression can occur with IV use. Antidote: Flumanezil.
		Rectal	0.5 mg/kg/dose			
	Anxiolytic/sedative/muscle relaxant	O	0.1–0.9 mg/kg/day	6-8-hourly	40 mg/day	More frequent IV dosing may be necessary, e.g. 2nd-hourly
		IV	0.05–0.3 mg/kg/dose	4–12-hourly	0.6 mg/kg/8 hour period	
Diazoxide	Hyperinsulinism	O	5–15 mg/kg/day	6-12-hourly		Seek Endocrinology advice. Not routinely used for the treatment of hypertension.
Diclofenac	Analgesia	O, rectal	1 mg/kg/dose	8-12-hourly	3 mg/kg/day or 150 mg/day (whichever is less)	Children > 10 kg. Rectal suppositories restricted to Anaesthesia and Pain Team. Avoid in renal impairment, asthma and GI bleeding.

Name	Indication	Route	Dose	Interval	Dose limit	Notes
Dicloxacillin (see flucloxacillin)						
Digoxin (see note)	Term neonate—2 years	O/IV	Digitalisation: 10 micrograms/kg/dose × 3 Maintenance: 7 micrograms/kg/day	8-hourly 12- or 24-hourly	Maintenance: 250 micrograms/day	Monitor levels: TR = 0.5–2 ng/mL (collect at least 6 hours after last dose). Modify dose in renal failure.
	2–12 years	O/IV	Digitalisation: 10–7 micrograms/kg/dose × 3 (10 micrograms/kg at age 2 years; 7 micrograms/kg at age 12 years) Maintenance: 7–5 micrograms/kg/day (7 micrograms/kg at age 2 years, 5 micrograms/kg at age 12 years)	8-hourly 12 or 24-hourly		
	Adolescent	O/IV	Digitalisation: 5 micrograms/kg/dose × 3 Maintenance: 5 micrograms/kg/day	8-hourly 12- or 24-hourly		

Dimercaprol (BAL)	Lead toxicity	IM (deep)	4 mg/kg/dose or 750 mg/m²/day for 3–7 days	4-hourly	5 mg/kg/dose (severe)	Consult Poisons Information Centre prior to administration. Use in combination with calcium EDTA. Monitor hepatic and renal function.
Diphenhydramine	Antihistamine	O	3–6 mg/kg/day	4- or 6-hourly	300 mg/day	
		IM	5 mg/kg/day	6-hourly		
Disodium pamidronate	Hypercalcaemia	IV infusion	20–50 mg/m²/dose	Single dose over 3–4 hours	90 mg/dose	*Restricted.*
	Osteoporosis	IV infusion	See specific protocols Typical: 20–40 mg/ m²/dose slow infusion over 3–4 hours	1–2 monthly		
DMSA (see succimer)						
Dobutamine	Inotrope	IV infusion	2.5–15 micrograms/ kg/min	Cont. infusion	40 micrograms/ kg/min	Cardiovascular monitoring indicated. Titrate dose to clinical effect. Predominant β₁ adrenergic agonist.

435

Name	Indication	Route	Dose	Interval	Dose limit	Notes
Dopamine	Inotrope and vasoconstrictor	IV infusion	3–20 micrograms/kg/min	Cont. infusion	50 micrograms/kg/min	Cardiovascular monitoring indicated. Titrate dose to clinical effect. Extravasation can cause tissue necrosis.
Dornase alpha	Mucolytic enzyme for cystic fibrosis	Neb.	2.5 mg/dose (*not* per kg)	24-hourly	2.5 mg/day	*Restricted* (Respiratory Physicians). 6-monthly pulmonary function tests required.
Doxycycline	Usual dose	O	2 mg/kg/dose	24-hourly	200 mg/day	Use only in children > 8 years. Take with meals;
	Severe infection	O	4 mg/kg/dose	24-hourly		may cause oesphagitis.
	Malaria prophylaxis	O	2 mg/kg/dose	24-hourly	100 mg/dose	
Droperidol	Neuroleptic	IV/IM	0.1–0.3 mg/kg/dose	Single dose or 4–6-hourly	20 mg/dose	If using parenterally for multiple doses, concomitant use of benzodiazepine or benztropine mesylate may reduce extra-pyramidal side effects. 20 micrograms/kg/dose is usually effective for post operative/opiate-induced vomiting.
	Nausea/vomiting	IV	20–(50) micrograms/kg/dose	6–8-hourly		

Drug	Indication	Route	Dose	Frequency	Maximum	Comments
Edrophonium chloride	Diagnostic aid for myasthenia gravis	IV	0.2 mg/kg/dose Test dose: 0.02 mg/kg followed by the remainder after 30–45 s.	Single dose	10 mg/dose	
EDTA (see calcium EDTA)						
Eformoterol	Asthma	Oral inhalation	12–24 micrograms/dose	12- or 24-hourly	48 micrograms/day	1 puff = 12 micrograms Long-acting β2-adrenergic agonist.
Enalapril	Antihypertensive and cardiac failure	O	Initial: 0.1 mg/kg/day Maintenance: 0.1–1 mg/kg/day	24-hourly	40 mg/day	Commence with a small dose and increase as tolerated. Caution if coadministering potassium, potassium sparing agents, or in presence of renal failure.
Enoxaparin (low molecular weight heparin—see also Heparin)	Treatment of thromboembolism	SC	< 2 months: 1.5 mg/kg/dose ≥ 2 months: 1 mg/kg/dose	12-hourly		Seek Haematology advice. Dose should be titrated according to anti-factor-Xa levels (collect 4–6 hours after SC administration).
	Prophylaxis	SC	< 2 months: 0.75 mg/kg/dose ≥ 2 months: 0.5 mg/kg/dose			

Name	Indication	Route	Dose	Interval	Dose limit	Notes
Epoprostenol	Pulmonary hypertension and vasodilator	IV infusion	5–25 nanograms/kg/min	Cont. infusion		*Restricted.* Use in ICU only
Ergocalciferol (Vitamin D2) (see also calcitriol)	Vitamin D deficient rickets	O	Initial: 5000 IU/day (*not per kg*) for 2–3 months Maintenance: 400 IU/day (*not per kg*)	24-hourly		40 IU = 1 microgram Monitor calcium levels. Chronic ingestion of excessive doses can result in severe toxicity (hyper-calcaemia, arrested growth, renal, cardiovascular failure).
	Malabsorption states	O	Commence with 400 IU/day (*not per kg*). Higher doses (4000 IU or greater) may be required.	24-hourly		
Erythromycin	Usual dose	O	10 mg/kg/dose	6-hourly	500 mg/dose	Multiple drug interactions
	Usual dose	IV	10 mg/kg/dose	6-hourly	500 mg/dose	
Esmolol	Hypertension	IV infusion	Load: 300 micro-grams/kg over 1 min, then infuse: Usual range: 100–500 micro-grams/kg/min	Cont. infusion	1000 micrograms/kg/min	*Restricted.* Titrate by increasing/decreasing by 50 micrograms/kg/min every 5–10 min. Continuous blood pressure monitoring is advisable.

Ethambutol	Tuberculosis	O	25 mg/kg/day, then reduce to 15 mg/kg/day after 2 months	24-hourly	1.2 g/day	ID/Respiratory consult recommended. Ophthalmological monitoring required.
Ethosuximide	Anticonvulsant (petit mal seizures)	O	10–40 mg/kg/day	12-hourly	1.5 g/day or 40 mg/kg/day (whichever is less)	TR: 40–100 mg/L
Fentanyl citrate	Bolus/loading dose	IV	0.5–2 micrograms/kg	Single dose		Respiratory depression can occur—use with caution if not ventilated. Antidote: naloxone. 100+ × more potent than morphine. Higher doses may be used in ventilated patients. Withdrawal symptoms may be anticipated with prolonged use (> 5–9 days).
	Maintenance	IV infusion	Load as above followed by 1–4 micrograms/kg/hour	Cont. infusion		
Ferrous gluconate (see iron salts)						
Ferrous sulfate (see iron salts)						

Name	Indication	Route	Dose	Interval	Dose limit	Notes
Flecainide	Arrhythmia (ventricular or supraventricular)	O/slow IV	3–6 mg/kg/day Higher doses may be needed. If administered intravenously, infuse slowly over 30 min	8- or 12-hourly	100 mg/dose	This drug is not first-line therapy and should be administered only after Cardiology consultation. Modify dose in renal failure.
Flucloxacillin	Usual dose	O	12.5 mg/kg/dose	6-hourly	500 mg/dose	Modify dose in renal failure.
	Usual dose	IV/IM	25 mg/kg/dose	6-hourly	2 g/dose	
	Severe infection	IV/IM	50 mg/kg/dose	4–6-hourly		
Fluconazole	Antifungal usual dose	O/IV	3–6 mg/kg/dose	24-hourly	400 mg/dose	*Restricted.* Modify dose in renal failure. Change to oral as soon as possible. Multiple drug interactions.
	Antifungal severe infection	O/IV	12 mg/kg/dose	24-hourly	800 mg/dose	
Fludrocortisone	Chronic mineralocorticoid replacement	O	50–200 micrograms/day (*not per kg*)	24-hourly		Adjust according to BP, electrolytes and plasma renin activity. Higher doses sometimes in neonates and infants.

Drug	Indication/class	Route	Dose	Frequency	Dose	Notes
Flumazenil	Reversal of benzodiazepines	IV/IV infusion	Bolus: 5 micrograms/kg repeated every 60 sec to a total of 40 micrograms/kg then continuous infusion: 2–10 micrograms/kg/h	Minutely, then cont. infusion	Bolus: 2 mg/dose Infusion: 3 mg/h	Benzodiazepine receptor antagonist.
Fluoxetine	Depression/obsessive-compulsive disorder/self-injurious behaviour	O	Initial: 0.5 mg/kg/day Maintenance: Increase slowly to a maximum of 2 mg/kg/day	12–24-hourly (breakfast and noon)	Initial: 20 mg/day. Maintenance: 40 mg/day	*Restricted.* Consult Psychological Medicine.
Fluticasone (see also salmeterol/fluticasone)	> 4 years	Oral inhalation	100–400 micrograms/day	12-hourly	2000 micrograms/day	
Folic acid	Neonates	O/IM	100–250 micrograms/day (*not per kg*)	24-hourly	10 mg/day	
	Infants/children	O/IM	250 micrograms/kg/day	24-hourly		
Frusemide	Diuretic	O	1–4 mg/kg/day	8- or 12-hourly	6 mg/kg/dose	Infusion for use in ICU only.
		IV	0.5–2 mg/kg/dose	8- or 12-hourly		
		IV infusion	0.05–1 mg/kg/h (no loading dose)	Cont. infusion		
Fusidic acid (see sodium fusidate)						

Name	Indication	Route	Dose	Interval	Dose limit	Notes
Gabapentin	Epilepsy/Neuropathic pain (titrate more gradually)	O	day 1: 10 mg/kg/day day 2: 20 mg/kg/day day 3: 30 mg/kg/day Maintenance: up to 40 mg/kg/day	12-hourly 8-hourly 8-hourly	2400 mg/day	*Restricted to Neurology/Pain team. Review dose in renal impairment.*
Ganciclovir	CMV infection	IV	5 mg/kg/dose Infuse over 1 h	12-hourly		*Restricted.* Modify dose in renal failure. See specific protocols for transplant patients. Prophylaxis doses may differ. Use with caution in neutropenia and thrombocytopenia.
Gentamicin	Single daily dose regimen (see note)	IV/IM	< 10 years: 7.5 mg/kg/dose ≥ 10 years: 6 mg/kg/dose	24-hourly	240 mg/dose	Modify dose in renal failure. Do not use a single daily dosing regimen. for neonates, patients with renal impairment, oncological disease or streptococcal
	t.d.s. regimen	IV/IM	2.5 mg/kg/dose	8-hourly	80 mg/dose	
	Endocarditis treatment	IV	1 mg/kg/dose (synergistic dose for use in combination with other antibiotics)	8-hourly		

	Indication	Route	Dose	Frequency	Max	Notes
	Cystic fibrosis	IV	2.5–4 mg/kg/dose	8-hourly		enterococcal infection/ endocarditis. Monitor levels: Daily dosing: take a level 6–14 hours post dose and use nomogram. t.d.s. dosing: trough: < 2 mg/L, peak: 5–10 mg/L
		Neb.		8- or 12-hourly		
Glucagon	Hypoglycaemia (usually in IDDM)	IM/SC	< 5 years: 0.5 mg (*not per kg*) > 5 years: 1 mg (*not per kg*)	Every 20 min p.r.n.		1 unit = 1 mg
	Hypoglycaemia (persistent)	IV infusion	Load: 25 micro- grams/kg, then 5–20 micrograms/ kg/h	Cont. infusion	1 mg/dose	
Glucose 10% (see also dextrose)	Hypoglycaemia	IV	2 mL/kg slow IV injection. May be repeated (check glucose level).	Single dose		
Glyceryl trinitrate (nitroglycerine)	Systemic and pulmonary afterload reduction, hypertension	IV infusion	Usual: 1–4 micro- grams/kg/min (range 0.5–12 micro- grams/kg/min)	Cont. infusion	12 micrograms/ kg/min	Ensure adequate circulating blood volume. Concurrent use of an inotrope may be required.

Name	Indication	Route	Dose	Interval	Dose limit	Notes
Glycopyrrolate	Control of secretions (e.g. excessive salivation)	O	40–100 micrograms/kg/dose	6- or 8-hourly		Anticholinergic agent
		IM/IV	4–10 micrograms/kg/dose	3- or 4-hourly		
	Reversal of non-depolarising muscle relaxants	IV	0.2 mg for each 1 mg of neostigmine administered	3- or 4-hourly		
Colonlytely® (see polyethylene glycol)						
Griseofulvin	Fine particle	O	10 mg/kg/dose	24-hourly	500 mg/day	Avoid exposure to sunlight.
	Ultramicrosize particle	O	> 2 years: 5.5 mg/kg/dose	24-hourly	330 mg/day	Take with or after a meal containing a high fat content.
Growth hormone	GH deficiency/ Turner's syndrome	SC	4.5–9 mg/m²/week (= 14–28 U/m²/week)	6–7 days/week		*Restricted.* *Endocrinology only.* Cease during severe acute illness.
Haloperidol	Psychosis/Tourettes/ delirium	O	10–50 micrograms/kg/day increasing to 75–150 micrograms/kg/day if necessary	8- or 12-hourly	15 mg/day	Antidote for extrapyramidal side effects: benztropine.

Drug	Indication	Route	Dose	Frequency	Maximum	Comments
Heparin sodium (see also enoxaparin)	Anticoagulation in documented thrombosis	IV infusion	Load: 75–100 units/kg/dose Maintenance: 25 units/kg/h Titrate according to levels (usual range: 20–30 units/kg/h)	Cont. infusion		Haematology consult recommended. Monitor therapy: Heparin assay (0.1–0.2 units/mL); APTT 1.5–2.5 × pretreatment level; ACT. 1 mg = 100 units
Hydralazine	Hypertensive emergency	IV (or IM)	0.15–0.8 mg/kg/dose	4–6-hourly	25 mg/dose	
Hydrocortisone	Physiological gluco-corticoid replacement	O	12–15 mg/m²/day (Hypopituitarism: 7–10 mg/m²/day)	6- or 8-hourly		Use 3–4 × normal dose for physiological stress.
	Anti-inflammatory	O	2–8 mg/kg/day	6- or 8-hourly		
Hydrocortisone sodium succinate	Acute adrenocortical insufficiency	IV/IM	Initial: 100 mg/m²/dose Repeat if response poor.	Single dose		
		IV/IM	Continuing stress dose: 100 mg/m²/day	8–12-hourly		
	Anti-inflammatory (e.g. asthma)	IV/IM	2–8 mg/kg/day	6–12-hourly		

445

Name	Indication	Route	Dose	Interval	Dose limit	Notes
Hydromorphone	Narcotic analgesic	O	30–100 micrograms/kg/dose	4- or 6-hourly	5 mg/dose	Antidote: naloxone. 5–7 × more potent than morphine.
		IM/IV	15–30 micrograms/kg/dose	4- or 6-hourly	Usual adult dose: 2 mg/dose	
		IV infusion	1.5–6 micrograms/kg/h	Cont. infusion		
Hydroxocobalamin (see Vitamin B12)						
Hyoscine hydrobromide (Scopolamine)	Anticholinergic/ antiemetic	O/IV/IM/SC	6–10 micrograms/kg/dose	6-hourly p.r.n.	400 micrograms/dose	Avoid under 4–6 months.
	Anaesthesia premed	IM	8–10 micrograms/kg/dose 45–60 min prior to induction	Single dose		
Hyoscine N-butyl bromide (Buscopan®)	Antispasmodic	IM/IV/O	0.5 mg/kg/dose	6- or 8-hourly	20 mg/dose	
Ibuprofen	Antipyretic/analgesic and antirheumatic	O	5–10 mg/kg/dose	6- or 8-hourly	40 mg/kg/day or 2 g/day	Use paracetamol first. > 6 months only.
Imipenem and cilastatin	Usual dose	IV	15 mg/kg/dose	6-hourly	4 g/day	Restricted. Doses refer to imipenem component. Modify dose in renal failure. Seizures may occur.
	Severe infection	IV	25 mg/kg/dose	6-hourly		

Imipramine	Nocturnal enuresis (children ≥ 5 years)	O	Initially 1–1.5 mg/kg/day (increasing if necessary).	24-hourly (night)	75 mg/day or 2.5 mg/kg/day, whichever is less	Treatment period 1–3 months.
	Depression	O	Initially 0.5–1.5 mg/kg/day (increase by 1 mg/kg/day every 3–5 days)	24-hourly	5 mg/kg/day	Consult Psychological Medicine. Not effective for depression in adolescents.
Indomethacin	Anti-inflammatory/antirheumatic	O/rectal	1.5–2.5 mg/kg/day	6–8-hourly	4 mg/kg/day or 200 mg/day	Suppositories only available as 100 mg
Insulin (soluble)	Emergency management of diabetic ketoacidosis	IV infusion	0.05–0.1 Unit/kg/h	Cont. infusion		Consult Endocrinology.
	Hyperkalaemia	IV	0.1 Unit/kg/dose (with dextrose 0.5 g/kg/dose). May be repeated if clinically indicated.	Single dose		Dextrose (without insulin) may be adequate therapy.
Ipratropium bromide	Aerosol	Oral inhalation	20–40 micrograms/dose (1–2 puffs)	8-hourly	Max.: 2 puffs every 2 hours	If moderate asthma is poorly responsive to 3 doses at 20 min intervals via spacer, then use a nebuliser.
	Moderate asthma	Oral inhalation via spacer	< 6 years: 4 puffs/dose ≥ 6 years: 8 puffs/dose	Every 20 min × 3 doses or 4-hourly		

Name	Indication	Route	Dose	Interval	Dose limit	Notes
	Nebulising solution or nebules	Neb.	125–500 micrograms/dose (usual dose = 250 micrograms)	4- or 6-hourly (see note)		In the severe asthmatic nebulised ipratropium can be given every 20 min (only in the Emergency Department or ICU). See CHW asthma guidelines.
Iron salts	Prevention (Fe deficiency anaemia)	O	1–2 mg elemental Fe/kg/day	12- or 24-hourly		1 mg elemental Fe = 3 mg Ferrous sulfate (Ferro-gradumet®) or 9 mg Ferrous gluconate (Fergon®).
	Treatment (Fe deficiency anaemia)	O	6 mg elemental Fe/kg/day for 3–4 months	12- or 24-hourly		
Isoniazid	Tuberculosis treatment and prophylaxis	O	10 mg/kg/dose	24-hourly	Usual: 300 mg/dose TB meningitis: 500 mg/dose	ID consultation recommended. Treatment of TB (in combination with other anti-tuberculous drugs). Other treatment regimens also used. Consider pyridoxine supplementation.

Drug	Indication	Route	Dose	Frequency	Max dose	Notes
Isoprenaline	Bradycardia and A-V block	IV infusion	0.05–2.0 micrograms/kg/min	Cont. infusion		Hypotension may occur. Cardiovascular monitoring indicated.
Itraconazole	Antifungal	O	3–5 mg/kg/dose	24-hourly	400 mg/day	*Restricted.* Multiple drug interactions. Higher doses have been used.
	Pulmonary aspergillosis	O	Initial: 7.5 mg/kg/dose	12-hourly	300 mg/dose	
			Maintenance: 5 mg/kg/dose	12-hourly	200 mg/dose	
Ketamine	Sedation/analgesia	IV	Load: 0.2–0.75 mg/kg/dose	Single dose		For anaesthesia or intensive care use only. Note that infusion of 10–40 micrograms/kg/min will maintain anaesthesia.
		IV infusion	Load as above, then 5–20 micrograms/kg/min (titrate)	Cont. infusion		
	Anaesthetic: induction	IV	1–2 mg/kg/dose	Single dose		
		IM	5–10 mg/kg/dose	Single dose		
	Anaesthetic premedication (see note)	O	2–3 mg/kg/dose	Single dose	15 mg/dose	IV preparation is used orally. Give in conjunction with oral midazolam.
Ketoconazole	Antifungal	O	5 mg/kg/dose	24-hourly	200 mg/dose	Fluconazole preferred. Multiple drug interactions.
Labetalol	Hypertensive emergency	IV infusion	Starting dose: 1 mg/kg/h Then titrate: increase/decrease by 0.25–0.5 mg/kg/h every 30 min	Cont. infusion	3 mg/kg/h	*Restricted.* SAS. Can only be prescribed by Renal physicians.

Name	Indication	Route	Dose	Interval	Dose limit	Notes
Lactulose	Hepatic coma/ encephalopathy	O	Initial: 1 mL/kg/dose every hour until bowel cleared	1-hourly	30–45 mL/dose	Not first-line laxative.
		O	Maintenance: 1 mL/kg/dose Adjust dose to get 2–3 soft stools daily	6- or 8-hourly		
Lamotrigine	Anticonvulsant	O	Initial: 0.3–0.5 mg/kg/day Increase slowly (every 2 weeks). Usual maintenance: 10–15 mg/kg/day	12-hourly	Max. maintenance 700 mg/day	If taking sodium valproate, dose should not exceed 5 mg/kg/day without neurological consultation. Life-threatening rashes may occur.
Lignocaine	Local anaesthesia/ nerve block	Infiltrate	Up to 4.5 mg/ kg/dose	Single dose	4.5 mg/kg/dose	
	Intravenous regional anaesthesia	IV	Up to 3 mg/kg/dose	Single dose	3 mg/kg/dose	
	Antiarrhythmic	IV infusion	Load: 1 mg/kg then Maintenance: 10–50 micrograms/ kg/min	Cont. infusion		
Lisinopril	Hypertension/cardiac failure	O	0.1 mg/kg/day, increasing slowly to 0.2–0.4 mg/kg/day	12- or 24-hourly	40 mg/day	Caution if administering potassium, potassium sparing agents, or in presence of renal failure. Can cause cough.

Drug	Indication	Route	Dose	Frequency	Maximum/limits	Notes
Magnesium (oral)	Dietary supplement	O	Recommended daily intake: 0–6 months: 40 mg/day (elemental) 7–12 months: 60 mg/day 1–3 years: 80 mg/day 4–7 years: 110 mg/day 8–11 years: 160–180 mg/day Adolescents: 270–320 mg/day	8-hourly	Diarrhoea is dose limiting	Prescribe as elemental magnesium. MagMin® (magnesium aspartate) 500 mg = 1.5 mmol or 40 mg elemental magnesium. Magnesium chloride 1 mmol/mL (CHW) Note: Many different salts exist. Care should be taken when prescribing. Monitor Mg levels.
	Hypomagnesaemia	O	2.5–15 mg/ elemental Mg/kg/dose	6-hourly		
	Laxative (Magnesium sulfate as 10% solution)	O	0.25–0.5 g/kg/dose	8-hourly	2–5 years:5 g/day > 6 years:10 g/day Adults:15 g/day	
Magnesium	Hypomagnesaemia/ anticonvulsant	Slow IV	0.1–0.2 mmol/ kg/dose Dilute and repeat as necessary	Single dose	40 mmol/dose	Magnesium sulfate 50% = 2 mmol/mL or 50 mg elemental Magnesium/mL. Magnesium chloride 9.6% = 1 mmol/mL or 25 mg elemental Magnesium/mL. Monitor Mg levels. NB: MgSO$_4$ can be given IM, but is very painful.
	Antiarrhythmic (VT or VF)	IV	0.05–0.1 mmol/ kg/dose	Single dose		
	Maintenance	IV infusion	Commence: 0.15 mmol/kg/day Titrate to serum Mg level	Cont. infusion		

Name	Indication	Route	Dose	Interval	Dose limit	Notes
Mannitol	Elevated intracranial pressure	IV	0.25–1 g/kg/dose over 30–60 min	Single dose or 6-hourly	2 g/kg/dose	
	Diuretic	IV	0.25–2 g/kg/dose			
Mebendazole	Antihelminthic	O	≤ 10 kg: 50 mg/dose (not per kg) > 10 kg: 100 mg/dose (not per kg)	12-hourly or as a single dose		The number of doses varies with the infestation.
Medroxy-progesterone acetate	Dysfunctional uterine bleeding. Cyclical hormone replacement	O	2.5 to 10 mg daily for 7 to 12 days of cycle	24-hourly		Consult Endocrinology before use.
Medroxy-progesterone acetate—Depot (Depo-Provera®)	Contraception Regulation of menstrual cycle (attempted suppression)	IM	100–150 mg/dose (not per kg)	3-monthly		Consult Endocrinology before use.
Menadione (Vitamin K3)		O	0.6 mg/dose Administer daily for vitamin K supplementation in fat malabsorption.	8–24-hourly	10 mg/dose	Synthetic water soluble vitamin K. Contraindicated in infants due to hyperbilirubinaemia
Meropenem	Usual dose	IV	10–20 mg/kg/dose	8-hourly	1 g/dose	Restricted. > 3 months of age. Modify dose in renal failure.
	Severe infection	IV	40 mg/kg/dose	8-hourly	2 g/dose	

Drug	Indication	Route	Dose	Frequency	Max	Comments
Methadone	Analgesia	IV/O	0.1–0.2 mg/kg/dose	8-hourly	20 mg/dose	Equipotent with morphine. Antidote: naloxone.
Methylene blue	Drug induced methaemoglobinaemia	IV	1–2 mg/kg/dose over several min	Single dose		Repeat dose in 1 h if required.
Methyl-prednisolone (acetate/sodium succinate)	Anti-inflammatory typical dose	IV/IM	0.5–4 mg/kg/day	6- or 12-hourly		Anti-inflammatory potency is 5 times greater than hydrocortisone. Asthma protocol: 1 mg/kg/dose every 6 h on day 1, every 12 h on day 2, then oral prednisolone.
	High dose therapy	IV	See specific protocols (e.g. renal, liver transplant etc)	4–6-hourly for up to 48 h		
Metoclopramide	Antiemetic	IV/IM/O	0.15 mg/kg/dose	6- or 8-hourly	0.5 mg/kg/day or 30 mg/day	Extrapyramidal effects more likely to occur in children.
Metoprolol	Hypertension/cardiac dysrhythmias	O	Initial dose: 1 mg/kg/day, increasing every 3 days according to clinical response. Maintenance: 1–5 mg/kg/day	12-hourly	400 mg/day	Beta adrenergic blockers should be used with caution in asthmatics. IV: Monitor blood pressure and ECG.
		IV	0.1 mg/kg/dose over 5 min May be repeated twice.	Single dose	5 mg/dose	

Name	Indication	Route	Dose	Interval	Dose limit	Notes
Metronidazole	Usual dose or antibiotic-associated diarrhoea	O	10 mg/kg/dose	8- or 12-hourly	400 mg/dose	Use 8-hourly dosing for antibiotic-associated diarrhoea.
	Usual dose	IV	12.5 mg/kg/dose	12-hourly	500 mg/dose	
	Severe infection	IV	12.5 mg/kg/dose	8-hourly	500 mg/dose	
	Amoebiasis	O	15 mg/kg/dose	8-hourly	600 mg/dose	
	Giardiasis	O	30 mg/kg/dose or 6 to < 15 kg: 400 mg/dose (*not per kg*) 15 to < 20 kg: 600 mg/dose (*not per kg*) 20 to < 30 kg: 1 g/dose (*not per kg*) > 30 kg: 2 g/dose (*not per kg*)	24-hourly × 3 days	2 g/dose	
Midazolam	Sedation/seizures	IV	0.1–0.2 mg/kg/dose	Single dose (can be repeated)		Respiratory depression can occur with IV use. Antidote: flumazenil.
		IM	0.2 mg/kg/dose	Single dose		
	Sedation/status epilepticus	IV infusion	Load: 0.1–0.2 mg/kg/dose Infusion: 1–5 micrograms/kg/min	Cont. infusion		

Drug	Indication	Route	Dose	Frequency	Maximum	Notes
	Premedication	O	0.5–0.6 mg/kg/dose 0.3–0.5 mg/kg/dose (in combination with ketamine)	Single dose	15 mg/dose	
		Nasal	0.2 mg/kg/dose (Drop dose into alternate nostrils over 15 seconds)	Single dose	5 mg/dose	
Morphine	Intermittent bolus/ loading dose	IV/IM/SC	<1 month: 50–100 micrograms/kg/dose ≥1 month: 100–200 micrograms/kg/dose	2–4-hourly	15 mg/dose No dose limit for palliative care	Antidote: naloxone. Oral:IV ratio approx. 3:1. Before commencing controlled release morphine, the 24-hour requirement should first be determined using prompt release or intravenous morphine. Withdrawal symptoms may be anticipated with prolonged use (> 5 days).
		IV infusion	Load: As above, then 10–40 micrograms/ kg/h (higher doses may be required)	Cont. infusion		
	Prompt release	O	0.2–0.5 mg/kg/dose	4–6-hourly p.r.n.		
	Controlled release	O	0.2–0.8 mg/kg/dose	12-hourly		
Naloxone	Post-operative narcotic depression	IV	5–10 micrograms/ kg every 2–3 min until adequate ventilation obtained (total dose may need to be repeated at 1–2 h intervals)	Every 2–3 min p.r.n.	10 mg (cumulative dose)	Duration of action may be shorter than many narcotics, hence careful observation is needed.

Name	Indication	Route	Dose	Interval	Dose limit	Notes
	Narcotic overdose (known or suspected)	IV/SC/IM or ET	100 micrograms/kg/dose May be repeated once	Single dose	2 mg/dose	*Note:* The post-operative narcotic depression dose is 10 fold less than that for known or suspected narcotic intoxication.
	Infusion	IV infusion	5–20 micrograms/kg/h	Cont. infusion		
Naproxen	Analgesia/anti-inflammatory	O	10–20 mg/kg/day	8- or 12-hourly	1 g/day	
Nedocromil	Asthma prophylaxis	Oral inhalation	8–16 mg/day	6–12-hourly	16 mg/day or 4 actuations/day	1 actuation = 2 mg
Neostigmine	Myasthenia gravis	O IM/SC	2 mg/kg/day 0.08–0.5 mg/kg/day	3–6-hourly 2–3-hourly	10 mg/kg/day Usual adult dose: 5–20 mg/day	
	Reversal of non-depolarising muscle relaxants	IV	50 micrograms/kg/dose (with atropine 20 micrograms/kg)	Repeat as required	Total dose 5 mg	
Niacin/nicotinic acid (see Vitamin B3)						
Nifedipine	Hypertensive crisis	O	0.5–1 mg/kg/dose. Repeat if needed every 4–6 h.	Single dose	20 mg/dose 3 mg/kg/day	Capsules no longer available. If using controlled release preparation administer daily.
	Maintenance	O	Initial: 0.5 mg/kg/day Maintenance: 1–1.5 mg/kg/day	12-hourly (see note)	10–30 mg/dose	

Drug	Indication	Route	Dose	Frequency		Comments
Nitrazepam	Epilepsy	O	0.3–1 mg/kg/day	8–12-hourly	3 mg/kg/day	
Noradrenaline	Vasopressor and inotrope	IV infusion	0.05–1 microgram/kg/min	Cont. infusion		Cardiovascular monitoring indicated. α- and β_1-adrenergic agonist. Should be administered only via a central line.
Norethisterone	Dysfunctional bleeding/ cyclical hormone replacement	O	10 to 15 mg daily for 7 to 12 days of cycle (*not per kg*)	8- or 12-hourly		
Nystatin	Antifungal	O	< 2 years: 50,000–100,000 U/dose	6- or 8-hourly		Poorly absorbed from the gastrointestinal tract.
		O	≥ 2 years: 100,000–500,000 U/dose			
Octreotide	Acute variceal bleeding	IV infusion	Load: 1 microgram/kg/dose, then 1–5 micrograms/kg/h for a maximum of 48 hours (increase every 8 hours if no effect)	Cont. infusion	50 micrograms/h	*Restricted.* Gastroenterology/ Endocrinology.
	Intractable diarrhoea	SC/IV	1–10 micrograms/kg/dose	8-hourly	500 micrograms/dose	
	Refractory hypoglycaemia (neonate)	IV/IV infusion	5–10 micrograms/kg/day	8-hourly or Cont. infusion		

Name	Indication	Route	Dose	Interval	Dose limit	Notes
Oestrogen preparations	Induction and maintenance of puberty	O	2.5–30 micrograms of ethinyloestradiol or equivalent. Dose varies according to indication, age, body size and preparation used.			Consult Endocrinology before use. Multiple preparations with different potencies.
Omeprazole	Refractory oesophagitis, gastritis, duodenal ulcer, Zollinger Ellison syndrome	O	0.5–1 mg/kg/day	24-hourly	60 mg/day	H_2 antagonist should be used initially. Convert IV to oral as soon as possible.
		IV	Initial: 2 mg/kg/dose	Single dose	80 mg/dose	
			Maintenance: 1–2 mg/kg/day	12- or 24-hourly	80 mg/day	
Ondansetron	Chemotherapy/ radiotherapy induced nausea and vomiting	IV/O	5 mg/m²/dose	8- or 12-hourly	8 mg/dose	
	Postoperative nausea and vomiting		0.1–0.15 mg/kg/ dose	8- or 12-hourly p.r.n.	4 mg/dose	*Restricted to 3 doses. Use metoclopramide first for other causes of vomiting (wait 20 min before considering ondansetron).*
Oxandrolone	Maturational delay	O	0.075–0.1 mg/kg/ day	24-hourly	20 mg/day	
	Turner's Syndrome	O	0.05 mg/kg/day	24-hourly		Sometimes used as an adjunct to growth hormone therapy.

Oxybutynin hydrochloride (Ditropan®)	Neurogenic bladder/ incontinence	O	0.4–0.8 mg/kg/day	6–12-hourly	5 mg/dose	Restricted to Urology if < 5 years.
Pancreatic extract (lipase microspheric preparation)	Pancreatic insufficiency	O	Infants: Starting dose: ½ capsule per breast feed or ½ capsule per 120 mL of infant formula. Children: 1–30 capsules/day.	With meals and snacks	5000 IU/kg/day	Lipase: 5000 IU/ capsule Capsules can be opened and offered in an infant fruit gel. Use a small amount of gel and offer to the infant on a feeding spoon. If patients have ongoing oily stools despite optimal compliance, consider the use of ranitidine or omeprazole concomitantly to increase intestinal pH.
Pancuronium	Neuromuscular blockade (non-depolarising)	IV	0.1–0.15 mg/kg/ dose	30–60 min p.r.n.		Use restricted to anaesthesia or ICU. Duration of action prolonged in renal failure. Decrease dose in hepatic insufficiency.

Name	Indication	Route	Dose	Interval	Dose limit	Notes
Paracetamol	Analgesic	O/rectal	15–20 mg/kg/dose (maximum 1 g/dose)	4-6-hourly	90 mg/kg/day up to 4 g/day	Hepatotoxicity is recognised in children with a prodromal illness and prolonged fasting taking frequent regular doses. If charted regularly, review after 48 hours. For prolonged use and at risk patients, reduce to 10 mg/kg/dose.
	Antipyretic	O/rectal	10–15 mg/kg/dose (maximum 1 g/dose)	4-6-hourly	60 mg/kg/day up to 3 g/day	
Paraffin liquid (mineral oil)	Disimpaction	O	15–30 mL/year of age/dose Repeat daily if necessary	Single dose	240 mL/dose	Do not use if < 1 year.
	Laxative and lubricant	O	1–3 mL/kg/day	Daily	50 mL/day	Do not use if < 1 year. If dose exceeds 30 mL, can be given as divided doses.
Paraldehyde	Status epilepticus	Rectal	0.15–0.3 mL/kg/dose	Single dose or 4-6-hourly	10 mL/dose	IM route should be avoided. Dilute 2–10-fold with olive oil or normal saline. Use a glass syringe.

Drug	Indication	Route	Dose	Frequency	Max	Notes
Penicillamine	Heavy metal chelator/ Cystinuria and Wilson's Disease.	O	30–40 mg/kg/day	6- or 8-hourly	2 g/day	Should be administered only on expert advice. Administer on an empty stomach. May require pyridoxine supplements for prolonged use.
Penicillin (see benzyl penicillin and phenoxymethyl penicillin)						
Pentamidine	Pneumocystis carinii	IV/IM	4 mg/kg/dose	24-hourly		*Restricted.* Modify dose in renal failure.
Pethidine	Analgesia	IV	0.5–1 mg/kg/dose	3–4-hourly	50 mg/dose	Antidote: naloxone. 8 × less potent than morphine
		IM/SC	1–2 mg/kg/dose	3–4-hourly	100 mg/dose	
Phenobarbitone	Status epilepticus	IV/IM	Load: 10–20 mg/kg/dose	Single dose	500 mg/dose	Monitor levels. TR: 80–120 micromol/L.
	Epilepsy	O/IV/IM	Maintenance: 3–5 mg/kg/day	12–24-hourly	600 mg/day	
Phenoxybenzamine	Cardiac surgery	Slow IV	0.5–1 mg/kg/dose	8–12-hourly		IV form: *restricted SAS*
	Phaeochromocytoma (preoperative)	O	Initial: 0.2 mg/kg/day Gradually increase over 7–10 days to 1 mg/kg/day	8–12-hourly		

Name	Indication	Route	Dose	Interval	Dose limit	Notes
Phenoxymethyl penicillin (penicillin V)		O	10–12.5 mg/kg/dose	6–12-hourly	2 g/day	
	Post splenectomy and rheumatic fever prophylaxis	O	< 2 years: 125 mg/dose ≥ 2 years: 250 mg/dose	12-hourly		
Phenytoin	Status epilepticus	IV	Load: 15–20 mg/kg/dose	Single dose	Loading dose: 1.5 g	Younger children and infants require higher maintenance doses than older children. Monitor drug levels. TR: 40–80 micromol/L
	Epilepsy	IV/O	Maintenance: 4–10 mg/kg/day	8–12-hourly (usually 12-hourly)		
Phosphate salts (oral)	Hypophosphataemic rickets	O	30–100 mg/kg/day	8-hourly		Phosphate Sandoz® (effervescent tablet). Contains: 500 mg phosphorus (16.1 mmol), 469 mg sodium (20.4 mmol), 123 mg potassium (3.1 mmol) per tablet. Monitor electrolytes and renal function.
	Hypophosphataemia	O	250–2000 mg/day	6-, 8-, 12- or 24-hourly		

Drug	Indication	Route	Dose	Frequency	Max	Notes
Phosphate salts (IV)	Hypophosphataemia	IV infusion	Initially 0.15–0.3 mmol/kg/dose over 4–6 h repeated until adequate blood levels.	Cont. infusion		Potassium dihydrogen phosphate = 1 mmol phosphate/mL and 1 mmol K/mL. Sodium dihydrogen phosphate (156 mg/mL) = 1 mmol phosphate/mL and 1 mmol K/mL
	Maintenance	IV infusion	0.5–1.5 mmol/kg/day	Cont. infusion		
Physostigmine	Anticholinergic drug overdose/anticholinergic psychosis	IV	Initially 0.02 mg/kg over at least 1 min. May be repeated at 5–10 min intervals, if necessary.	Every 5–10 min p.r.n.	2 mg/dose	Use in life-threatening situations only after discussion with Poisons Information Centre. Atropine should be available to reverse effects.
Phytomenadione (Vitamin K1) (see also menadione)	Prevention of haemorrhagic disease of the newborn	IM	1 mg immediately post-partum	Single dose	1 mg/dose	Give slowly if administered intravenously.
		O	2 mg/dose at birth, 3–5 days and 4 weeks of age			
	Vitamin K deficiency	IV/IM/O	0.3 mg/kg/dose	24-hourly or according to coagulation studies	10 mg/dose	

Name	Indication	Route	Dose	Interval	Dose limit	Notes
Piperacillin	Usual dose	IV/IM	50 mg/kg/dose	6-hourly	24 g/day or 6 g/dose	*Restricted.* Modify dose in renal failure.
	Severe infection	IV/IM	50 mg/kg/dose	4-hourly		
	Cystic fibrosis	IV	225–450 mg/kg/day	8-hourly		
Piperacillin/ tazobactam (Tazocin®)	Usual dose	IV/IM	100 mg/kg/dose	8-hourly	4 g/dose	*Restricted.* Doses refer to piperacillin component.
Polyethylene glycol (+ electrolytes) (Colonlytely®)	Colonic lavage, bowel washout, meconium ileus equivalent	O/NG	25 mL/kg/h until rectal effluent is clear (usually 4–8 hours). If administering orally, give no more than 250 mL every 10 minutes.		1.5 L/h, 4 L total	Consult Poisons Information Centre if used for poisoning. Use with caution if < 2 years. Chilled solution more palatable and nasogastric route may be preferable.
Potassium chloride	Maintenance	IV	1–3 mmol K⁺/kg/day administered with maintenance IV fluids.	Cont. infusion		ECG monitoring and frequent K⁺ levels required if infusion rate > 0.4 mmol/kg/h. See also phosphate salts (potassium dihydrogen phosphate).
	Hypokalaemia	IV infusion	0.1–0.4 mmol K⁺/ kg/h Concentrated K⁺ infusion is potentially dangerous and should be avoided if possible.	Cont. infusion	0.5 mmol/kg/h	

Potassium salts (oral)	Maintenance	O	1–3 mmol/K⁺/kg/day		5–10 mmol/kg/day may be needed if on concurrent diuretic therapy or other losses. Chlorvescent® = 14 mmol K⁺/ tablet Span K® tablet = 8 mmol K⁺/ tablet KCl suspension = 10 mmol K⁺/15 mL
Prednisolone, Prednisone	Typical anti-inflammatory dose	O	2 mg/kg/day	6–12-hourly	Anti-inflammatory potency is 4 times greater than hydrocortisone.
	Croup	O	1 mg/kg/dose for 48 hours	8- or 12-hourly	
Probenecid	Antibiotic therapy adjunct	O	Load: 25 mg/kg/ dose then 10 mg/ kg/dose	6-hourly	500 mg/dose
Procainamide	Arrhythmia	O	15–50 mg/kg/day	4-hourly	4 g/day
		IV infusion	Load: 3–6 mg/kg/ dose over 15 min. Load may be repeated if arrhythmia not controlled.	May be repeated	100 mg/dose and total load of 15 mg/kg
		IV infusion	Maintenance: 20–80 micrograms/ kg/min	Cont. infusion	2 g/day
Prochlorperazine		O/IM	0.2 mg/kg/dose	8–12-hourly	15 mg/dose

Name	Indication	Route	Dose	Interval	Dose limit	Notes
Promethazine	Antihistamine/antiemetic	IM/IV	0.125–0.5 mg/kg/dose	6-hourly	150 mg/day	Not recommended for children < 2 years.
	Sedative	IM/IV	0.5–1 mg/kg/dose	6-hourly or single night time dose		
Propranolol	Hypertension/cardiac dysrhythmias	O	Initially: 0.5–1 mg/kg/day	6–12-hourly	160 mg/day	Beta adrenergic blockers should be used with caution in asthmatics.
		O	Maintenance: 2–4 mg/kg/day	12-hourly		
	Migraine prophylaxis	O	Initially: 10 mg/dose and increase up to 2 mg/kg/day if necessary	12–24-hourly	See above	
Propylthiouracil	Thyrotoxicosis	O	5–10 mg/kg/day	8-hourly		Endocrinology consultation recommended. Modify dose in renal failure.
Prostaglandin E1 (see alprostadil)						
Protamine sulfate	Heparin reversal	Slow IV	1 mg/100 units of heparin (administered < 30 min previously)	Single dose	50 mg/10 min period *or* 100 mg/2 h period	Specific antidote to heparin. *Note:* A smaller dose is indicated if heparin to be reversed was administered > 30 min previously.

Drug	Indication	Route	Dose	Frequency	Maximum	Notes
Pyrantel embonate	Pinworm, threadworm	O	10 mg/kg/dose	Single dose		Dose refers to pyrantel base/kg.
	Roundworm, hookworm	O	20 mg/kg/dose	Single dose	750 mg /dose	
Pyrazinamide	Tuberculosis	O	25–35 mg/kg/day	8-, 12- or 24-hourly	1.5 g/day	In combination with other anti-tubercular drugs.
Pyridoxine (see Vitamin B6)						
Ranitidine	Ulcer treatment and prophylaxis	O	4–12 mg/kg/day	8–12-hourly	150 mg/dose	Dosage reduction may be necessary in severe renal impairment.
		Slow IV	2–4 mg/kg/day	8-hourly	50 mg/dose	
Resonium (see sodium polystyrene sulfonate)						
Riboflavine (see Vitamin B2)						
Rifampicin	Usual dose	O/IV	10 mg/kg/dose	24-hourly	600 mg/dose	*Restricted* (except for pruritis). Colours body fluids orange–red (urine, faeces, saliva, sweat, tears). Ceftriaxone may be used for *Neisseria* prophylaxis.
	Severe infection	O/IV	10 mg/kg/dose	12-hourly		
	Neisseria meningitidis prophylaxis	O	Neonates: 5 mg/kg/dose Children: 10 mg/kg/dose	12-hourly for 2 days		
	Haemophilus influenzae type b prophylaxis	O	Neonates: 5 mg/kg/dose Children: 10 mg/kg/dose	24-hourly for 4 days		
	Pruritis secondary to liver disease	O	10 mg/kg/dose	24-hourly	300 mg/day	

Name	Indication	Route	Dose	Interval	Dose limit	Notes
Risperidone	Psychosis (adolescents)/ Tourettes/severe aggression	O	Initial: 0.5 mg/day (*not* per kg) increasing by 0.25 mg/day every 5–7 days Maintenance: 0.75–1.5 mg/day	12-hourly	6 mg/day	*Restricted.* Psychological Medicine. Not generally recommended for use in children. Modify dose in renal failure.
Rocuronium	Neuromuscular blockade (non-depolarising)	IV	Load/bolus: 0.6–0.9 mg/kg/dose	Every 30–60 min p.r.n.		Use restricted to Anaesthesia or ICU. When used as infusion, dosage titration is required to maintain neuromuscular blockade.
		IV infusion	Load as above, then 5–15 micrograms/kg/min	Cont. infusion		
Roxithromycin	Usual dose	O	4 mg/kg/dose	12-hourly	150 mg/dose	
Salbutamol	Bronchopulmonary dysplasia	Neb.	0.1 mg (0.02 mL of 0.5% sol.)/kg/dose	6-hourly		If mild to moderate asthma is poorly responsive to 3 doses at 20 min intervals via spacer, then use a nebuliser. See CHW asthma guidelines.
	Asthma	Oral inhalation	100–400 micrograms/dose (1–2 puffs)	4–6-hourly		
	Mild–moderate asthma	Oral inhalation via spacer	< 6 years: 6 puffs ≥ 6 years: 12 puffs	Every 20 min × 3 doses or 1–4-hourly		

	Asthma	Neb.	< 5 years: 2.5 mg/dose (0.5 mL of 0.5% sol.) > 5 years: 5 mg/dose (1 mL of 0.5% sol.)	1–4-hourly, every 20 min or continuous depending on severity		An IV loading dose may be considered (15 micrograms/kg) in the patient not responding to nebulisers. 20 min or continuous nebulisation should only be used in ICU or Emergency Dept.
	Severe asthma	IV infusion	1–5 micrograms/kg/min	Cont. infusion	15 micrograms/kg/min	
	Hyperkalaemia	Neb.	< 5 years: 2.5 mg/dose (0.5 mL of 0.5% sol.) > 5 years: 5 mg/dose (1 mL of 0.5% sol.)	Single dose (may be repeated in 2 hours).		
Salmeterol	Bronchodilator/asthma	Oral inhalation	50 micrograms/dose (2 puffs)	12-hourly	100 micrograms/dose	Long-acting β2 adrenergic agonist. Should not be used for relief of acute symptoms. > 4 years.
Salmeterol/fluticasone (Seretide®)	Long-acting bronchodilator/steroid	Oral inhalation	50–100 micrograms/dose Strengths: Sal 25 with Flu 50, 125, 250; Sal 50 with Flu 100, 250, 500.	12-hourly	100 micrograms/dose	Dose based on Salmeterol. Back titrate steroid component to minimum effective dose. Prolonged higher dose associated with adrenal suppression.
Scopolamine (see hyoscine hydrobromide and also papaveretum)						
Sennoside (Senokot®)	Laxative	O	2–6 years: 3.75–7.5 mg/day (not per kg)	24-hourly	30 mg/day	

Name	Indication	Route	Dose	Interval	Dose limit	Notes
		O	6–12 years: 7.5–15 mg/day (*not per kg*)	24-hourly		
	Bowel evacuation	O	1 mg/kg/dose on the day before examination	Single dose	72 mg/dose	
Sertraline	Depression	O	Initially 12.5–25 mg (*not per kg*) increasing slowly as required over several weeks until desired response	24-hourly	200 mg/day	*Restricted.* Consult Psychological Medicine.
Sodium benzoate	Disorders of urea cycle metabolism	O	Typical dose: 250 mg/kg/day	6-hourly	500 mg/kg/day	*Restricted.* Metabolic consultation required.
		IV	Load: 250 mg/kg over 90 min Maintenance: 250 mg/kg over 24 hours	Cont. infusion		
Sodium bicarbonate	Urinary alkalinisation/ chronic acidosis (renal failure or renal tubular acidosis)	O	1–3 mmol/kg/day	4–8-hourly		Correction of base deficit = ⅓ [base deficit (mmol) × body weight (kg)]
	Resuscitation (cardiac arrest)	IV	Initial dose: 1 mmol/kg Subsequent doses: 0.5 mmol/kg	Every 10 min		

Drug	Indication/form	Route	Dose	Frequency	Max dose	Notes
Sodium cromoglycate	Inhaler	Oral inhalation	10 mg/dose (2 puffs)	8-hourly		1 puff of Forte = 5 mg 2 puffs twice daily (20 mg/day) sometimes effective once control achieved.
	Nebuliser	Neb.	60 mg/day	8-hourly	120 mg/day	
Sodium fusidate		IV/O	20–30 mg/kg/day	8-hourly	1500 mg/day	580 mg Diethanolamine fusidate is equivalent to 500 mg sodium fusidate.
Sodium nitroprusside	Hypertension and afterload reduction in CCF	IV infusion	Usual: 0.5–4 micrograms/kg/min. Higher doses can be used for short periods (see note).	Cont. infusion	10 micrograms/kg/min	Cover syringe with foil to protect from light and use black opaque infusion tubing. Prolonged infusion, particularly in the presence of renal impairment, may be associated with cyanide toxicity.
Sodium phenylbutyrate	Disorders of urea cycle metabolism	O	250 mg/kg/day	4- or 6-hourly	600 mg/kg/day	Restricted. Metabolic consultation required.
Sodium polystyrene sulphonate (resonium A)	Hyperkalaemia	O/rectal	0.5–1 g/kg/dose	6-hourly or as needed to correct hyperkalaemia	30 g/dose	Contains approx. 100 mg of sodium per gram (= 4.1 mmol/g). 4 level tsp = 15 g

Name	Indication	Route	Dose	Interval	Dose limit	Notes
Sodium valproate (valproic acid)	Epilepsy	O	Initial: 10 mg/kg/day Increase after approx. 5 days to 20 mg/kg/day Usual maintenance: 20–60 mg/kg/day	8- or 12-hourly (usually 12-hourly)	60 mg/kg/day	Modify dose in renal failure. Monitor renal function.
Sorbitol 70%	Constipation	O	1–3 mL/kg/day	6-, 8-, 12- or 24-hourly	30 mL/dose	
Sotalol	Acute arrhythmia	IV	0.5–1.5 mg/kg/dose over 10 min	6-hourly	100 mg/dose	Consult cardiology before use.
	Prevention/maintenance	O	Initially 1–2 mg/kg/dose increasing to 4 mg/kg/dose	8- or 12-hourly	200 mg/dose	Modify dose in renal failure.
Spironolactone	Potassium sparing diuretic	O	Initially 1–4 mg/kg/day	8-, 12- or 24-hourly	200 mg/day or 9 mg/kg/day	Monitor serum electrolytes, especially potassium, sodium.
	Ascites secondary to cirrhosis	O	5 mg/kg/day			
Succimer (meso 2,3-dimercapto-succinic acid, DMSA)	Lead toxicity	O	30 mg/kg/day for 5 days, then: 20 mg/kg/day for 14 days	8-hourly 12-hourly		*Restricted* (SAS). Consult Poisons Information Centre before administering.

Drug	Indication	Route	Dose	Frequency	Max	Comments
Sucralfate	Ulcer prophylaxis	O O O	6 months–2 years: 1 g/day (*not* per kg) 3–12 years: 2 g/day (*not* per kg) > 12 years: 4 g/day (*not* per kg)	6-hourly	4 g/day	Do not administer to children < 6 months of age, and use with caution in patients with renal impairment (contains aluminium). Avoid in renal failure.
Sulfasalazine	Inflammatory bowel disease	O	25–50 mg/kg/day	4- to 8-hourly	8 g/day	Enteric coated preparation available.
	Remission	O	30 mg/kg/day	6-hourly	2 g/day	
Suxamethonium	Neuromuscular blockade (depolarising)	IV IM	1–2 mg/kg/dose 2–4 mg/kg/dose	Single dose Single dose	150 mg/dose	Depolarising agent. Avoid in patients with known muscle disorders. Use with caution for weeks after trauma, including burns. Preadministration of atropine is generally advised.
Tacrolimus	Immunosuppression for organ transplantation	O	0.05–0.3 mg/kg/day. *Note:* Dose varies according to type of transplantation.	12-hourly		*Restricted.* See specific protocols. Blood levels should guide dosage. Modify dose in renal failure.

Name	Indication	Route	Dose	Interval	Dose limit	Notes
Tazocin® (see piperacillin/tazobactam)						
Teicoplanin	Septicaemia/ osteomyelitis, septic arthritis	IV/IM	Load: 10 mg/kg/ dose for 3 doses. Maintenance: 6–10 mg/kg/dose	12-hourly 24-hourly	400 mg/dose	*Restricted* Modify dose in renal failure.
Temazepam	Premedication/ hypnotic	O	0.3 mg/kg/dose	Single dose or nocte	20 mg/dose	Round dose to nearest 5 mg.
Terbutaline	Turbuhaler	Oral inhalation	One actuation/dose	4–6-hourly	2000 micrograms/ day	Turbuhaler: 500 micrograms/ metered dose. Aerosol: 250 micrograms/ metered dose. Salbutamol is used via nebuliser, or intravenously at CHW.
	Metered aerosol	Oral inhalation	250–500 micro- grams/dose (1–2 puffs)	4–6-hourly		
Theophylline (sustained release)	Bronchodilator	O	10–20 mg/kg/day	12-hourly	600 mg/day	Different slow release preparations are not interchangeable. Therapeutic monitoring advised. TR: 55–110 micro- mol/L (4 hours post dose)

Drug	Indication	Route	Dose	Frequency	Max dose	Notes
Thiabendazole	Antihelminthic	O	25 mg/kg/dose	12-hourly	1.5 g/dose	Duration of treatment varies according to the helminth. Caution in patients with renal and/or hepatic impairment.
Thiopentone sodium	Induction of anaesthesia, anticonvulsant	IV	2–5 mg/kg/dose Note: An infusion may be used for status epilepticus (see ICU protocols).	Single dose. Can be repeated.	5 mg/kg/dose	Causes hypotension and decreased cardiac output. Use with extreme caution in patients with shock, cardiac disease. May also be used to treat raised intracranial pressure (see ICU protocols).
Thioridazine	Psychosis (second line antipsychotic)	O	1–4 mg/kg/day	6–12-hourly	600 mg/day	Restricted Psychological Medicine. Modify dose in hepatic or renal failure. Considerably higher doses have been given (individualise according to condition and response).

Name	Indication	Route	Dose	Interval	Dose limit	Notes
Thyroxine (see also triiodothyronine)	Congenital hypothyroidism (neonatal)	O	Initial: 10 micrograms/kg/day	24-hourly	Usual adult dose: 100–150 micrograms/day	Adjust on basis of 2–4 weekly thyroid function tests.
	Hypothyroidisn	O	Maintenance: 80–100 micrograms/m²/day	24-hourly	Usual adult dose: 100–150 micrograms/day	Regular thyroid function tests required.
Ticarcillin and clavulanic acid	Usual dose	IV	50 mg/kg/dose	6-hourly	3 g/dose	*Restricted.* Dose refers to Ticarcillin.
	Severe infection	IV	50 mg/kg/dose	4-hourly		
(Timentin®)	Cystic Fibrosis	IV	300–450 mg/kg/day	8-hourly	18 g/day	Modify dose in renal failure.
Timentin® (see ticarcillin and clavulanic acid)						
Tinidazole	Giardiasis	O	50 mg/kg/dose	Single dose	2 g/dose	
	Acute Amoebic Dysentery	O	50 mg/kg/dose for 3 days	24-hourly		
Tobramycin	t.d.s. regimen	IV/IM	2.5 mg/kg/dose	8-hourly	2.5 mg/kg/dose	Modify dose in renal failure.
	Single daily dosing regimen (see note)	IV/IM	< 10 years: 7.5 mg/kg/dose ≥ 10 years: 6 mg/kg/dose	24-hourly		Do not use a single daily dosing regimen for neonates, patients with renal impairment, oncological disease
	Cystic Fibrosis	IV/IM	7.5–12 mg/kg/day	8-hourly		
		Neb.	< 9 years: 80 mg/dose (*not* per kg)	8–12-hourly		

					≥ 9 years: 120 mg/dose (not per kg)	or streptococcal/enterococcal infection/endocarditis. Monitor levels: Daily dosing: take a level 6–14 hours post dose and use nomogram. t.d.s. dosing: trough: < 2 mg/L, peak 5–10 mg/L
Topirimate	Epilepsy	O	Initial: 1 mg/kg/day Maintenance: 3 mg/kg/day	8- or 12-hourly	18 mg/kg/day	
Triiodothyronine	Hypothyroidism when oral thyroxine cannot be taken	IV	0.2–1.2 micrograms/kg/day	6–24-hourly		*Restricted.* Neurology. Titrate by pulse rate and free T3 measurement. May be given as a continuous infusion.
Trimeprazine	Antihistamine/allergy	O	0.5–1.5 mg/kg/day	6-hourly	100 mg/day	
	Premedication	O	2–4 mg/kg/dose	Single dose		
Trimethoprim	Usual dose	O	6 mg/kg/day	12- or 24-hourly	300 mg/day	
	Prophylaxis	O	2 mg/kg/dose	24-hourly (at night)	100 mg/dose	
Trimethoprim/ sulfamethoxazole (see cotrimoxazole)						

Name	Indication	Route	Dose	Interval	Dose limit	Notes
Ursodeoxycholic acid	Cholestasis/biliary atresia	O	10–30 mg/kg/day	12-hourly		*Restricted.* SAS.
Valproic acid (see sodium valproate)						
Vancomycin	Usual dose	IV	10 mg/kg/dose	6-hourly	500 mg/dose	*Restricted.* Modify dose in renal failure. Monitor levels. Trough: 5–10 mg/L Peak: 25–40 mg/L
			20 mg/kg/dose	12-hourly	1 g/dose	
	Severe infection	IV	15 mg/kg/dose	6-hourly	1 g/dose	
	Pseudomembranous colitis (see note)	O	10 mg/kg/dose	6-hourly	500 mg/day (125 mg/dose)	Metronidazole is first-line therapy for pseudomembranous colitis.
Vecuronium	Loading dose or intermittent bolus	IV	0.1–0.2 mg/kg/dose	May be repeated every 30–60 min		Use restricted to anaesthesia or ICU. Patients with severe renal or hepatic failure may experience prolonged neuromuscular blockade.
	Continuous infusion	IV infusion	50–200 micrograms/kg/h	Cont. infusion		
Verapamil	Arrhythmia	IV	0.1–0.3 mg/kg/dose. Administer slowly, over 2 min.	A repeat dose may be given 30 min after initial dose	Initial: 5 mg/dose. Subsequent: 10 mg/dose	Adenosine is the drug of choice for SVT. Relatively contraindicated in

		Route	Dose	Interval	Max dose	Comments
		O	Maintenance: 3–9 mg/kg/day	8-hourly	360 mg/day	acute SVT for children < 12 months (only administer on Cardiology advice). Caution with β-adrenergic blockers.
Vigabatrin	Epilepsy	O	Initial: 50 mg/kg/day.	24-hourly	2 g/day	May cause permanent peripheral visual field defects.
		O	Usual maintenance: 50–150 mg/kg/day	12- or 24-hourly	4 g/day	
Vitamin A (retinol)	Severe measles	O	100 000 IU/dose for 3 doses	Repeat next day and on day 28	200 000 IU/dose	Severe measles: 200 000 IU (single dose) is recommended by some. Doses > 25 000 IU/day may be associated with hypervitaminosis A. Micelle A Plus E® = Vitamin A 2210 IU/mL and Vitamin E 102 IU/mL. Capsules = 5000 IU Vitaplex® capsules = Vitamin A 2500 IU and Vitamin D 100 IU 1 IU = 0.3 micrograms of retinol
	Malabsorption states (chronic cholestasis, cystic fibrosis)	O	5,000–15,000 IU/day (*not* per kg)	24-hourly		
	Dietary supplement	O	< 6 months: 1500 IU; 6 months–3 years: 1000 IU; 4–7 years: 1200 IU; 8–11 years: 1700 IU	24-hourly	5000 IU/day	

Name	Indication	Route	Dose	Interval	Dose limit	Notes
Vitamin B1 (thiamine) (see note)	Treatment of deficiency (Beriberi)	O/IM/(IV)	1–2 mg/kg/day	24-hourly	IM/IV: 25 mg/day O: 50 mg/day	Consult Metabolic Service before use in metabolic disorders. Dose may vary considerably depending upon the defect. Anaphylaxis can occur. Administer slowly IV.
	Dietary supplement	O	6–12 months: 0.4 mg/day 1–7 years: 0.5–0.7 mg/day > 8 years: 0.8–1.2 mg/day	24-hourly		
Vitamin B2 (riboflavine)	Treatment of deficiency	O	5–10 mg/day (*not per kg*)	24-hourly		Consult Metabolic Service for dose in metabolic disorders.
	Dietary supplement	O	< 6 months: 0.4 mg/day 6–12 months: 0.6 mg/day 1–3 years: 0.8 mg/day 4–7 years: 1.1 mg/day 8–11 years: 1.3–1.4 mg/day			

Vitamin B3 (niacin, niacinamide, nicotinic acid)	Treatment of deficiency	O	100–300 mg/day (*not* per kg)	8-hourly	Dosages of niacin and niacinamide as vitamin supplements are equal.
	Dietary supplement	O	< 6 months: 4 mg/day 6–12 months: 7 mg/day 1–3 years: 9–10 mg/day 4–7 years: 11–13 mg/day 8–11 years: 14–16 mg/day	24-hourly	
Vitamin B6 (pyridoxine)	Hereditary pyridoxine dependency syndrome including seizures.	IV/IM	Neonates: Initially 50–100 mg/dose (*not* per kg)	Single dose	CPR facilities needed if given IV. Consult Metabolic Service if metabolic disorder suspected (higher maintenance doses may be needed).
		O	Maintenance Infants: 2–200 mg/day	24-hourly	
		O	Maintenance Children: 10–250 mg/day	24-hourly	
	Deficiency	O	5–25 mg/day (*not* per kg)	24-hourly	
	Prophylaxis (peripheral neuritis in patients on isoniazid therapy).	O	5–10 mg/day (*not* per kg)	24-hourly	

Name	Indication	Route	Dose	Interval	Dose limit	Notes
Vitamin B12 (cyanocobalamin, hydroxocobalamin)	Pernicious anaemia or vitamin B12 malabsorption	IM	Initial: 30–50 micrograms/day (*not per kg*) for 2 or more wks (total of 1–5 mg)	24-hourly		IM route (or deep SC for cyanocobalamin) is recommended for initial therapy. Hydroxocobalamin and cyanocobalamin have equivalent B12 activity. Seek Haematology advice.
			Maintenance: 100 micrograms/dose (*not per kg*)	monthly		
		O (see note)	5 mg/dose (*not per kg*)	24-hourly		
	Metabolic disorders	O (see note)	5–10 mg/day	24-hourly		Metabolic consultation advisable for metabolic disorders Oral preparation: cyanocobalamin 5 mg/mL (CHW formula)
	Dietary supplement	O	< 6 months: 0.3 micrograms/day 7 months–1 year: 0.6 micrograms/day 1–3 years: 1 micrograms/day 4–7 years: 1.5 micrograms/day 8–11 years: 1.5 micrograms/day > 11 years: 2 micrograms/day	24-hourly		

		O/IV/IM			
Vitamin C (ascorbic acid)	Treatment of deficiency		100–300 mg/day (*not per kg*)	8- or 12-hourly	100 mg/kg/day up to 6 g/day (if given IV)
	Dietary supplement	O	< 6 months: 25 mg/day (*not per kg*) ≥ 7 months: 30 mg/day		
Vitamin D (see calcitriol and ergocalciferol—Vitamin D2)					
Vitamin E (alpha tocopherol acetate)	Cystic fibrosis	O	50–400 IU/day (*not per kg*)	24-hourly	1 IU = 1 mg all racemic (RRR) alpha tocopherol acetate = 0.67 mg alpha tocopherol equivalents. Micelle A Plus E® = Vitamin A 2210 IU/mL and Vitamin E 102 IU/mL. Micelle E® = 156 IU/mL Vitaplex® capsules = 500 IU
	Cholestasis and malabsorption	O	20–300 IU/kg/day	12- or 24-hourly	
Vitamin K1 (see phytomenadione)					

Name	Indication	Route	Dose	Interval	Dose limit	Notes
Warfarin	Loading: (days 1 and 2 of therapy)	O	0.2 mg/kg/dose 0.1 mg/kg/dose if patient has prolonged baseline INR or liver dysfunction	24-hourly	10 mg/dose	Consult Haematology. Target INR is usually 2.0–3.5. Dosage should be adjusted by increasing or decreasing in 20% increments. Round dose to nearest 0.5 mg where possible. Multiple drug interactions. Antidote: vitamin K
	Maintenance (adjust according to INR)	O	0.05–0.3 mg/kg/dose	24-hourly		
Zinc sulfate	Deficiency	O	1 mg (elemental Zn)/kg/day	8-, 12- or 24-hourly	100–200 mg/dose	Prescribe as elemental zinc. 220 mg zinc sulfate = 50 mg elemental zinc
		IV	100 micrograms (elemental Zn)/kg/day	24-hourly	5 mg/day	

References

Advanced Life Support Committee of the Australian Resuscitation Council. Paediatric advanced life support. Australian Resuscitation Council Guidelines. *Med J Aust*, 1996; 165: 199–201

Allen J and Fisher R. *The Feeding Guide* (4th edn). James Fairfax Institute of Paediatric Clinical Nutrition, Children's Hospital at Westmead, 2001: 34

Asthma Management Handbook 2002 (6th edn). Melbourne: National Asthma Council of Australia, 2002: 159–60

Australasian College of Sexual Health Physicians. *National Management Guidelines for Sexually Transmissible Infections*. 2002: 272

Children's Hospital at Westmead. *Acute pain manual*. Sydney: The Children's Hospital at Westmead, <www.chw.edu.au>

Children's Hospital at Westmead. *Trauma manual*. Sydney: The Children's Hospital at Westmead, <www.chw.edu.au>

Daniel Jr WA. *Adolescents in Health and Disease*, Saint Louis: CV Mosby Co., 1977: 261

Diem, K, (ed.). *Documenta Geigy Scientific Tables* (6th edn). Basle: JR Geigy SA., 1962: 348

Hamill PVV, Drizd TA, Johnson CL, et al. Physical growth: National Center for Health Statistics percentiles. *Am J Clin Nutr*, 1979; **32**: 609

Hicks CL, von Baeyer CL, Spafford P, et al. The faces pain scale-revised: toward a common metric in pediatric pain measurement. *Pain*, 2001; **93**: 173–83

NHMRC. *The Australian Immunisation Handbook* (8th edn). Canberra: Australian Government Publishing Service, 2003: 138, 355

MIMS Australia. eMIMS Sydney: IMS Publishing, 1998: 36

NSW Department of Health. *Acute management of young children and infants with gastroenteritis. Clinical Practice Guidelines.* Sydney: New South Wales Department of Health, 2002: 206

Tanner JM. *Growth and Adolescence* (2nd edn). Oxford: Blackwell Scientific Publications, 1962: 261

Therapeutic Guidelines: Antibiotic (12th edn). Melbourne: Therapeutic Guidelines Ltd, 2003: 110, 125, 239

Todd J, Fishnaut M, Kapral F and Welch T. Toxic shock syndrome associated with phage group 1 staphylococci. *Lancet*, 1978; **2**: 1116–8

Turrell G. Compliance with the Australian Dietary Guidelines in the early 1990s: have population-based health programs been effective? *Nutrition and Health*, 1997; **11**: 271–88

Many of these publications are available through Kidshealth, The Children's Hospital at Westmead: tel (612) 9845 3585; fax (612) 9845 3562; email <kidsh@chw.edu.au>; website <www.chw.edu.au>

Index

Page numbers in *italics* refer to figures and tables.

abbreviations in drug documentation, 410–11, *411*
ABC; E (CPR steps), 13–14
ABCC (head injury priorities), 241
ABCDE (primary trauma survey), 375–6
abdomen, 103, 184–5, 368–70
Abelcet ®, *417*
absence seizures, 230–1
abuse, *see* child abuse
accidents, *see* trauma
ACE inhibitors, *263–4*
acetazolamide, *412*
N-acetylcysteine, *412*
acetylsalicylic acid (aspirin), 60, *418*
aciclovir, 120–1, *121–2*, *413*
acid burns to the eye, 320
acidosis, 75, 109, 219, *see also* diabetic ketoacidosis
activated charcoal, 338–9, *427*
acute adrenal insufficiency, 186–9
acute asthma, 170–4, *171*, *172*
acute decompensation in chronic anaemia, 53
acute pain, defined, 58
acute renal failure (ARF), 256–8
adenosine, *413*
ADH (antidiuretic hormone), 191
adolescents, 276–91, *see also* children
chronic illness, 285–6
development, 276–7, *278*, 280–2
sexual health, 288–90, *290*
suicidality, 266–8, 273, 287
symptomatic (undiagnosable), 291
adrenal hyperplasia, congenital, 189–90
adrenal insufficiency, acute, 186–9
adrenaline, 20, 24, *414*
age-related reference ranges, *see* laboratory reference ranges
airway obstruction, 164–70, *165*, 375

albumin, in hypervolaemia, 254
allergies, 41, 345
allopurinol, *414*
alprostadil, *414*
ambiguous genitalia, 189–90, 366
Ambisome ®, *417*
amenorrhoea, 281
amethocaine, 65
amikacin, *415*
amiloride, *415*
aminoglycosides, *114*, 114–15
aminophylline, *415*
amiodarone, *416*
amitriptyline, *416*
amlodipine, *416*
amoxycillin, *416*
amphotericin, *417*
ampicillin, *418*
anaemia, 52–3
blood transfusion, 43–4
leukaemia, 293
anaesthesia, 343–5, 347
in diabetes, 208–10
local, 65
analgesia, 59–60, *see also* pain
burns, 357
cancer pain, 296
lacerations, 380
anaphylaxis, 23–4, 342
ankles, fractures of, 379
anorexia nervosa, 283
antagonist drugs, 339–40, 351–2
anti-haemophilic factor (AHF), 49
anti-infective drugs, *see* antibiotic therapy
antibiotic therapy, 112–15, *114*, *116–20*
burns, 357
cardiac lesion prophylaxis, 159–60
cystic fibrosis, 183
gastroenteritis, 221

487

meningitis, 129–30, *130*
neonatal sepsis, 92
osteomyelitis, 133
pneumonia, 178
septic arthritis, 134
septicaemia, 132
toxic shock syndrome, 136
UTI prophylaxis, 250–1
antidiuretic hormone (ADH), 191
antiepileptic drugs, 232–7
antihistamines, in anaphylaxis, 24
antihypertensives, 261, *262–4*
antimicrobials, *see* antibiotic therapy
antisepsis, lacerations, 379
antivenom, 341–2
L-arginine, *418*
arms, fractures of, 378
arrhythmias, 162–3
arterial blood gas analysis, 88
arterial oxygen, 85–9
arterial PCO$_2$, 88
ascites, 228
ascorbic acid (vitamin C), *483*
aspirin (acetylsalicylic acid), 60, *418*
asplenic patients, prophylaxis in, 150,
    151
asthma, acute, 170–4, *171, 172*
atenolol, *419*
atonic seizures, 230
atopic dermatitis, 312–13
atracurium, *419*
atresia, 370–1
atropine, *419*
Atrovent, 173, *447–8*
Augmentin Duo®, *416*
autoimmune haemolytic anaemia, 43, 52
autopsies, 386
azathioprine, *420*
aztreonam, *420*

babies, *see* infants; neonates
baclofen, *420*
bacteraemia, *see* septicaemia
bacterial endocarditis, *119*, 159
bacterial infections, *see* infections
bacterial meningitis, 125–30

BAL (dimercaprol), *435*
balanitis, 364–5
beclomethasone dipropionate, *420*
bed availability information, Newborn
    ICU, 83
bendrofluazide, *420*
benign focal epilepsy of childhood,
    230–1
benzodiazepines, 235
benztropine, 352, *420*
benzylpenicillin, *421*
bereavement care, 387
beta-blockers, *264*
bicarbonate, 204, *470*
bilious vomiting, 371–2
biochemical genetic emergencies,
    104–11
biochemistry reference ranges, 8–11,
    9–11
biopsy, renal, 253, 255
biotin, *421*
'black eyes' (blowout fractures), 322–3
blast cells, 294–5
bleeding, 335
    disorders, 46–53, 294
blood gas analysis, 88
blood pressure measurement, 259–60,
    see also hypertension
blood products, 46–50
blood specimen collection, 5–6, 8, 11
blood transfusion, 42–6, 360
blowout fractures of the orbit, 322–3
blunt ocular trauma, 321–3
body surface area nomograms, *391*
body weight, *see* anorexia nervosa;
    bulimia nervosa; obesity
boils, *118*
botulism, 241
brain abscesses, *117*
breast milk jaundice, 93, 96
breastfeeding, 30–2
    gastroenteritis, 221
    preoperative, 345
breasts, *278*, 280–1
breath-holding attacks, 231–2
breathing, 375, *see also* respiratory
    distress
    noisy, 164–6, *165*
British Anti Lewisite (dimercaprol), *435*

bronchii, inhaled foreign bodies, 327
bronchiolitis, 174–6
budesonide, *421*
bulimia nervosa, 283–4
bullous impetigo, 309
bupivacaine (Marcain), 65, *421*
burns, 320, 355–62
Buscopan®, *446*

calcitonin, *422*
calcitriol, *422, see also* ergocalciferol
calcium, *422–3, see also* hypercalcaemia;
    hypocalcaemia
calcium carbonate, *423*
calcium-channel blockers, *263*
calcium chloride, *423*
calcium EDTA, *424*
calcium gluconate, *424*
calculations
    drug dosage, 410–11
    fluid therapy, *68–71, 69–70, 74,* 219,
        358–9
cancer, 292–6
capillary collection techniques, 5
captopril, *425*
carbamazepine, 233, *425*
carbimazole, *425*
carbohydrate malabsorption, 37
carbon monoxide poisoning, 356
cardiac disease, 154–63, *see also*
    congenital heart disease
    catheterisation, 162
    dysrhythmia, 87
    heart failure, 155–7
    infections, *119*
    murmurs, 158–9
    neonatal examination, 102
    schedule of surveillance, *409*
    surgery, 160–1
cardiopulmonary resuscitation (CPR),
    13–14, 17, 385–6
cardiorespiratory arrest, 12–18, *15*
cardiovascular risk factors, 161
L-carnitine, *426*
catecholamines, urinary collection for,
    41
catheter intervention, 162
cefaclor, *426*
cefotaxime, *426*

ceftazidime, *426*
ceftriaxone, *426*
cellulitis, *117–18*, 324–5
central lines, fever and, 226–7
central nervous system infections, *117*
cephalexin, *427*
cephalothin, *427*
cerebral infarction, 54–5
cerebral oedema, 205–6
cerebrospinal fluid, *11*, 107, *see also*
    shunt problems
cervical spine control, 375
CFRDM, 185
charcoal, activated, 338–9, *427*
chelating agents, 339–40
chemicals
    accidental ingestion of, 337–8
    burns to the eye, 320
chemotherapy, 295
chest X-rays, neonates, 83, 87
chickenpox, 141, *142*, 146
    aciclovir for, 121
child abuse, 297–306
    head injury, 245
    reporting, 297–9
child health surveillance, *see*
    developmental assessment
Child Protection Unit (CPU), 297–9,
    301–2, 304–6
children, 2–4, *see also* adolescents
    disruptive, 270–2
    recommended food intake, 31–2
    types of pain in, 57–8
chloral hydrate, *353, 427*
chloramphenicol, *427*
chloroquine, *427*
chlorpromazine, *428*
cholangitis, *119*
cholestasis, 94
chorionic gonadotropin, *428*
chronic anaemia, 43–4, 53
chronic illness and disability, 285–6
chronic persistent pain, defined, 58
cimetidine, *428*
ciprofloxacin, *428*
circulatory failure (shock), 18–20, *19*
    blood transfusion, 43
    burns, 356–60
    gastrointestinal bleeding and, 225

inotropic drugs, 20
trauma, 375
circumcision, 363
cisapride, *429*
cisatracurium, *429*
clarithromycin, *429*
clavicle fracture, 378
clavulanic acid, *416, 476*
cleft palate, 103
clindamycin, *429*
clobazam, 235, *429*
clonazepam, 235, *430*
clonidine, *430*
closure methods (lacerations), 380–1
CMV negative blood, 45–6
coagulation factors, 48–50
treatment with, 51–3
coagulation studies, *6*
coarctation of the aorta, 102
codeine, 60, *430*
coeliac disease, diets in, 38
cold agglutinin titre, 8
Colonlytely®, *464*
colostomy, 221
coma, 20–3, *21*
combined oral contraceptive pill
(COCP), 288
communication with parents, 4
complex partial seizures, 229–30
condoms, 288
congenital adrenal hyperplasia, 189–90
congenital coagulation disorders, 51–3
congenital errors of metabolism, *see*
metabolic disorders, inherited
congenital gut evisceration, 372–3
congenital heart disease, 154–5
cyanosis and, 87
foetal diagnosis, 161–2
long-term outcome, 158
neonatal examination, 102
schedule of surveillance, *409*
congenital hip dislocation, *409*
congenital hypothyroidism, 197–8
congenital sucrase-isomaltase deficiency,
37
conjunctival damage, 318–19, 321
conjunctivitis, 323–4
conscious sedation, 347
consent to procedures, 343, 350

constipation, 65, 384
contraception, 288–9
convulsions, *see* epilepsy; febrile
convulsions
corneal damage, 319–21
coroner's cases, 386
corticosteroids, in asthma, 173
cotrimoxazole, *430, 477*
cow's milk protein intolerance, 37
CPR, *see* cardiopulmonary resuscitation
CPU, *see* Child Protection Unit
critical care, *see* emergencies; medical
retrieval
critical incident debriefings, 387–8
croup, 25, 166–9
crusted impetigo, 308–9
cry, neonatal examination, 101
cryoprecipitate, 48
CSF, *see* cerebrospinal fluid
CT scans after head injury, 242
cyanocobalamin (vitamin B12), *482*
cyanosis, 85–9, 156
cyanotic breath-holding attacks, 231–2
cyclophosphamide, 255, *431*
cyclosporin, 255, *431*
cyproheptadine, *431*
cyproterone acetate, *431*
cystic fibrosis, 179–85
therapeutic diets, 38
cystourethrograms, 250
cytomegalovirus negative blood, 45–6

DDAVP, *432*
death, 383–8, *see also* perimortem
evaluation
debriefings (after deaths), 387–8
decimal prescribing guidelines, 410
decompensation in chronic anaemia, 53
deep sedation, 347
deficit therapy, 67, 71–5, *see also* fluid
therapy
dehydration, 72–3, *see also* fluid therapy
gastroenteritis, *217*, 217–20
metabolic disorders, 109
neonates, 99
delayed puberty, 280
dental emergencies, 331–6
dental procedures, antibiotic prophylaxis,
160

dentition, *see* teeth
Department of Community Services (DoCS), 298, 301–2, 304
Depo-Provera®, *452*
depression, 272–3, 287
dermatitis, 312–13
dermatological conditions, *see* skin conditions
desferrioxamine, *431*
desmopressin, *432*
developmental assessment, 404–9, *406–7, 409*
dexamethasone, *432*
dexchlorpheniramine, *433*
dextrose, *see* glucose (dextrose)
diabetes insipidus, 190–1
diabetes mellitus, 200–15
  cystic fibrosis-related, 185
  fasting and surgery in, 207–10
  therapeutic diets, 38
diabetic ketoacidosis (DKA), 74–5, 201–7
diagnosis, 1–2
dialysis, 109, 257–8
diaphragmatic hernia, 373
diarrhoea, *145*
diarrhoea-associated HUS, 258–9
diazepam, 236, *433*
diazoxide, *433*
diclofenac, *433*
dicloxacillin, *434*
diet and nutrition, 30–41, *see also* infant feeding
  adolescent patients, 282–4
  burns, 361
  food allergies, 41
  gastroenteritis, 221
  recommended intake, 31–2
  therapeutic diets, 37–41, 110
  total parenteral nutrition, 78–9
digoxin, 410, *434*
dimercaprol (BAL), *435*
dimercaptosuccinic acid (DMSA), 250, *435*
diphenhydramine, *435*
diphtheria, *144*
  diphtheric croup, 167
disodium pamidronate, *435*
disruptive children, 270–2

Ditropan, *459*
diuretics in head injury, 243–4
DKA, *see* diabetic ketoacidosis
DMSA (succimer), 250, *435*
dobutamine, *435*
DoCS, *see* Department of Community Services
DoCS Helpline, 298–9
doctors
  critical incident debriefings, 387–8
  infectious disease notifications, *152–3*
dopamine, 20, *436*
dornase alpha, *436*
dosage, *see* drug dosage
doxycycline, *436*
droperidol, *436*
drug dosage, 410–11, *411–84*
drugs, *see also* antibiotic therapy; prescriptions
  accidental ingestion of, 337–8
  cardiac arrest, 16–17
  disruptive children, 271–2
  epilepsy, 232–7
  gastroenteritis, 220–1
  hypertension, 261, *262, 263–4*
  hypoglycaemia in neonates, 98
  neonatal stabilisation, 82–3
  sedation, *353–4*
  surgery and, 345
dying, 383–8
dysmenorrhoea, 281–2
dyspnoea, palliative care, 385

ears, discharge from, 329
ECGs, 87
echocardiography, 88, 162–3
eczema, 312–14
edema, cerebral, 205–6
edrophonium chloride, *437*
EDTA, *424*
EEGs, 232, 238–9
eformoterol, *437*
electrocardiograms (ECG), neonates, 87
electroencephalograms (EEG), 232, 238–9
electrolytes, *9*, 67–79
  acute renal failure, 257
  burns, 360
  content of antibiotics, 115

diabetic ketoacidosis, 203–4
gastroenteritis, 218–19
metabolic disorders, 109
replacement after burns, 357–9
emergencies, 12–29
haematological, 52–6
head injury, 241–5
inherited metabolic disorders, 109–10
oncological emergencies, 293–5
emergency patient transport, 25–9, 80–3
emergency team, 13–14
EMLA (lignocaine and prilocaine), 65
emotional abuse and neglect, 305–6
empiric antibiotic therapy guidelines, 115, *116–20*
Employee Assistance Program, 388
enalapril, *437*
encephalitis, 120
endocarditis, 159
endocrinology, 186–200, *see also* diabetes mellitus
endotracheal intubation (ET), 24–5, *25*, *see also* tube feeds
cardiac arrest, 14, 16
tube size and length, 25, *25*, 170
energy intake, 31–2
enoxaparin, *437*, *see also* heparin
ENT conditions, 327–30
envenomations, 340–2, *see also* poisoning
epidemic haemolytic uraemic syndrome, 258–9
epidural abscesses, *117*
epiglottitis, 168–70
epilepsy, 229–37
epistaxis, 329–30
epoprostenol, *438*
ergocalciferol, *438*, *see also* calcitriol
eruption times (teeth), *336*
erythromycin, *438*
esmolol, *438*
esophageal atresia, 370–1
ethambutol, *439*
ethosuximide, 235, *439*
euthyroidism, sick, 199–200
exchange transfusion in jaundice, 95, 95–6
eyeball lacerations, 321
eyelid lacerations, 321
eyes, *see also* ocular emergencies

acute red eye, 323–4
equipment for examining, 318
neonatal examination, 101–2
vision, 101, *406–7*, *409*

facial emergencies, 331–6
Factor Eight Bypassing Activity (FEIBA), 50
factor VIII concentrates, 48–9, 51–2
factor IX concentrates, 49–52
fasting
in diabetes, 207–10
before sedation, 345, 349–50
febrile convulsions, 237–9
febrile neutropenia, 295
feet, neonatal examination, 103
FEIBA, 50
femoral epiphysis, 285
femur fracture, 378
fentanyl citrate, *439*
ferrous gluconate, *see* iron salts
ferrous sulfate, *see* iron salts
fever, 123–5, *126*
antibiotic therapy, *115*
cancer and, 294–5
in chronic liver disease, 226
febrile convulsions, 237–9
heart disease and, 159
liver transplant patients, 227
in patients with a central line, 226–7
postoperative, 373
severe infections and, 125–38
UTIs and, 250
fibula, fracture, 378
fine motor skills, *406–7*
fingers, fractures of, 379
first aid, 341, 355–62
flecainide, *440*
flucloxacillin, *440*
fluconazole, *440*
fludrocortisone, *440*
fluid therapy, 67–79, *69*, *70*
burns, 357–9
calculations, *68–71*, 69–70, 74, 219, 358–9
cardiac arrest, 17
diabetes and, 203, 206, 213
gastroenteritis, 219–20
hyperbilirubinaemia, 95

intravenous lines, 98–100
liver transplant patients, 228
neonates, 95, 98–100
surgical conditions, 75–8
flumazenil, 352, *441*
fluoride, 32
fluoxetine, *441*
fluticasone, *441*, *469*
foetal cardiac diagnosis, 161–2
folic acid, *441*
food, *see* diet and nutrition
foreign bodies, 327–8
in eyes, 318–19
foreskin, 363–4
formulae, *see* infant formulae
fractures, 332–3, 377–9
fresh frozen plasma (FFP), 48
frusemide, *441*
fungal infections, *see* infections; tinea
furunculosis, *118*
fusidic acid, *471*

G6PD deficiency, 52
gabapentin, *442*
galactosemia, 40
ganciclovir, *442*
gastric lavage, 339
gastro-oesophageal reflux, 222–3
gastroenteritis, *118–19*, 216, 216–21
dehydration, 74, *217*, 217–18
gastroenterology, 216–28
gastrointestinal bleeding, acute, 223–5
gastrointestinal disease, septicaemia and,
131
gastrointestinal symptoms in palliative
care, 384
gastrostomy, 221
generalised tonic-clonic seizures
('grand mal'), 230–1
genetic autopsy, 110–11
genetic metabolic disorders, *see*
metabolic disorders, inherited
genital maturity, *see* puberty
genitalia, 103
ambiguous, 189–90, 366
gentamicin, *442–3*
German measles (rubella), *143*
gingivostomatitis, 121, 314
Glasgow Coma Scale, 22–3, *23*, 241

glaucoma, 323
glomerulonephritis, 252
glucagon, 194, *443*
glucose (dextrose), 192, *433*, *443*, *see also*
hyperglycaemia; hypoglycaemia
neonates, 97–8
glue ear, 329
gluten-free diets, 38
glyceryl trinitrate, *443*
glycopyrrolate, *444*
grafting skin after burns, 362
'grand mal' seizures, 230–1
griseofulvin, *444*
gross motor skills, *406–7*
growth charts, 389–90, *391–403*, *see also*
adolescents, development
growth hormone, *444*
Guillain-Barré syndrome (GBS), 240
gut evisceration, congenital, 372–3
gynaecomastia, 281

haemangiomas, 315–16
haematology, 42–56
laboratory reference ranges, 5–8, *6*, *7*
haemodialysis, 109, 257–8
haemoglobin, 6, 8
GIT bleeding and, 225
haemolysis, 52, 93
haemolytic anaemia, 43, 52
haemolytic uraemic syndrome, 221,
258–9
haemophilias, 51–3
blood factor concentrates, 48–50
Haemophilus influenzae type b, 144
haemoptysis, 184
haloperidol, *444*
head circumference, 389, *396–7*, *402–3*,
409
head injury, 241–5
health professionals, critical incident
debriefings, 387–8
health screening, 408
hearing, *406–7*, *409*
neonatal examination, 101
heart, *see* cardiac
height measurement, 389, *398*, *400*, *409*
heparin, 5–6, *445*, *see also* enoxaparin
hepatitis, 140–1, *143–4*
hernias, 367–8, 373

herpes simplex infection, 314
heterophile antibody agglutination test, 8
high blood pressure, *see* hypertension
hip examinations, 103, *409*
Hirschsprung's disease, 371–2
HIV prophylaxis after needlestick injury, 141
hormonal contraception, 288–9
hospitalisation, 2–3
HSV infection, neonatal, 120
humerus fracture, 378
hydralazine, *445*
hydration, *see* fluid therapy
hydroceles, 366
hydrocephalus, 245–7
hydrocortisone, *445*
    in acute adrenal insufficiency, 188–9
    in hypoglycaemia, 194
hydromorphone, *446*
hydroxocobalamin, *482*
hyoscine hydrobromide, *446*
hyoscine N-butyl bromide, *446*
hyperbilirubinaemia, 94–5
hypercalcaemia, 196–7
hypercyanotic spells, 157
hyperglycaemia, 214–15
hyperinsulinism, 194
hyperkalaemia, *258*
hypernatraemia, 74, 100, 219
hyperoxia test, 88
hypersensitivity reactions, 345, *see also* anaphylaxis
hypertension, 259–61, *262*, *263–4*
    centrally acting drugs in, *264*
    measurement, 259–60, *260*
hyphaema, 321–2
hypocalcaemia, 194–6
hypoglycaemia, 192–4, 214
    in diabetes, 210–12
    epilepsy diagnosis and, 232
    metabolic disorders, 109
    neonates, 96–8
    neurogenic, 193, 211
    neuroglycopenic, 193, 211
hypokalaemia, 218
hyponatraemia, 74, 99
    gastroenteritis, 218
hypothyroidism, congenital, 197–8

hypovolaemia, 254
hypoxaemia, 85–9

ibuprofen, *446*
IDDM (diabetes Type 1), 200
IgA nephritis, 252
ileostomy, 221
imaging, 239
    epilepsy, 232
    head and neck, 170, 242
    neonates, 83, 87, 94
imipenem and cilastatin, *446*
imipramine, *447*
immediate hypersensitivity reactions, *see* anaphylaxis
immobilisation of fractures, 379
immunisation, 147–50, *148*
    cancer treatment and, 296
immunocompromised patients, 121, 131
immunoglobulins in IgA nephritis, 252
immunosuppression, 254–5, 295
impetigo, *118*, *145*, 308–9
in utero transfer bed status, 83
inborn errors of metabolism, *see* metabolic disorders, inherited
incubation periods for infectious diseases, 141, *142–5*
indomethacin, *447*
infant feeding, 30–1, *see also* diet and nutrition
infant formulae, 30–3, *33*
    in gastroenteritis, 221
    special, 33, *34–7*
infantile botulism, 241
infantile eczema, *see* atopic dermatitis
infantile spasms, 30
infants, *see also* neonates
    vomiting, 371–2
infections
    blood diseases and, 55–6
    burns, 360–1
    facial, 334
    fever and, 125–38
    glomerulonephritis and, 252
    haemolytic uraemic syndrome, 258–9
    neonatal, 89–92
    preoperative assessment, 344
    presenting as napkin rash, 316
    shunt problems, *117*, 246–7

sickle cell disease, 55
urinary tract, *118*, 131, 248–51
infectious diseases, 139–53
'infectious' periods, 141, *142–5*
oncological emergencies, 295
prophylaxis in asplenic patients, 150, *151*
informed consent, 343, 350
ingested foreign bodies, 328
inguinal hernia, 367–8
inhaled foreign bodies, 327
injections, dissolving antibiotics for, 113
injury, *see* trauma
innocent murmurs, 158–9
inotropic drugs, 20
insulin, 204–10, *see also* diabetes
hyperinsulinism, 194
during intercurrent illness, 213–15
soluble, *447*
Internet, *see* web addresses
intersex, *see* ambiguous genitalia
intestinal obstructions, 76–7
intracardiac access, 16
intracranial infections, *see* meningitis
intracranial pressure, raised, 127–8
intramuscular opioids, 61
intraocular foreign bodies, 319
intraosseous access (IO), 14
intravascular haemolysis, 52
intravenous lines
analgesia, 59, 61–2
blood transfusion, 45
calcium, 195
cardiac arrest, 14
fever and, 226–7
gastroenteritis, 220
glucose, 97–8, 193–4
neonates, 97–100
septicaemia, 131
intussusception, 78, 369
ipratropium bromide, 173, *447–8*
iritis, 323
iron-loaded patients, 55–6
iron salts, *448*
irradiated blood, 45
ischaemia in burns, 360
isoimmunisation, 95–6
isoniazid, *448*
isoprenaline, *449*

itch from opioid analgesics, 64
itraconazole, *449*
IV, *see* intravenous lines

jaundice, 92–6, *95*
jaws, trauma, 331–2
juvenile myoclonic epilepsy, 230–1

Kawasaki syndrome, 136–8, *137*
keratitis, 324
ketamine, *353*, *449*
ketoacidosis, *see* diabetic ketoacidosis
ketoconazole, *449*
ketogenic diet, 40–1
kidneys, *see* renal disease
kyphosis, 284

labetalol, *449*
laboratory investigations
burns, 359
dehydration, 73
diabetic ketoacidosis, 202
infectious disease notifications, *152–3*
poisoning, 340
laboratory reference ranges, 5–11, *6*, *7*, *9–11*
lacerations, 379–81
oro-facial, 330, 332
lactase deficiency, 37
lactulose, *450*
lamotrigine, 234, *450*
laryngotracheitis, 166
lateral airways (neck) X-rays, 170
lavage, 339
legs, fractures of, 378
length measurement, 390, *392*, *394*
Lennox-Gastaut syndrome, 230
lens damage (eye trauma), 322
leukaemia, 292–3
leukocoria (white pupil), 325
lichen sclerosus et atrophicus, 365
life-sustaining treatment, limiting, 385–6
lignocaine (Xylocaine), 65, *450*
limb fractures, 377–9
limb ischaemia in burns, 360
limb weakness, 240–1, 294
limp, 381, *382*
lines, *see* intravenous lines

lipase microspheric pancreatic preparation, 459
liquid medications, guidelines, 410
lisinopril, 450
liver disease, 225–6
liver function tests, 9–10
liver transplant patients, 227–8
local anaesthetics, 65
lower airway obstruction, 165–6
  bronchiolitis, 174–6
lumbar puncture, 128–9, 238
Lyclear, 307–8
lysate studies, 6

magnesium, 451
magnesium sulfate in poison removal, 339
maintenance fluids, see fluid therapy
malrotation, 372
mannitol, 243–4, 452
Marcain (bupivacaine), 65, 421
measles, 141, 142, 146–7
measurement of children, 389–90, 391–403
mebendazole, 452
mechanical ventilation, 84–5
meconium, delayed passage of, 372
medical care, principles of, 3–4
medical retrieval, 25–9
  neonates, 80–3
medications, see drugs
medroxyprogesterone acetate, 452
menadione, 452, see also phytomenadione
menarche, 281
meningitis, 125–31, 130
meningococcal infection, 145
menstrual disorders, 281–2
mental state examination, 270, see also psychiatric conditions
meropenem, 452
metabolic acidosis, see acidosis; diabetic ketoacidosis
metabolic disorders, inherited, 104–10
  screening tests, 106–7, 108
  therapeutic diets, 40, 106
metacarpal fractures, 378
metatarsal fractures, 379
methadone, 61, 453

methyl-prednisolone, 453
methylene blue, 453
metoclopramide, 453
metoprolol, 453
metronidazole, 454
micturating cystourethrograms, 250
midazolam, 353, 454–5
milk, 33, 371–2, see also breastfeeding; infant formulae
  cow's milk intolerance, 37
mineral intake, 32
mineral oil, 460
molluscum contagiosum, 313–14
Monofix, 49
mononucleosis antibodies, 8
Moro test, 101
morphine, 60–2, 455
mouth conditions, see oral conditions
mumps, 142
myoclonic seizures, 230–1
myositis, 241

NAI, see non-accidental injury
naloxone, 351, 455–6
napkin rash, 316–17
naproxen, 456
nasal discharge, 327
nausea, palliative care and, 384
nebuliser therapy in asthma, 171–2
neck X-rays, 170
nedocromil, 456
needlestick injury, 140–1
neglect, see emotional abuse and neglect
neonates, 80–103, see also infants
  blood transfusion, 42–3
  cholestasis, 94
  HSV infection, 120
  hypercalcaemia, 196
  hypocalcaemia, 194
  ICU availability, 83
  jaundice, 92–6, 95
  sepsis, 89–92
  surgery, 76
  thyrotoxicosis, 199
  transport, 80–3
  undescended testes, 366
  vomiting, 370–2
neostigmine, 456
nephritis, 251–3

nephrotic syndrome, 253–5
neurobehaviour, neonatal, 100–1
neurology, 229–47, 376
neutropenia, 53–4, 294–5
newborns, *see* neonates
niacin (nicotinic acid), *see* vitamin B3
NIDDM (Type 2 diabetes), 200
nifedipine, *456*
nitrazepam, 235, *457*
nitroglycerine, *443*
nitrous oxide, 65–6, *354*
noisy breathing, 164–6, *165*
nomogram for body surface area, *391*
non-accidental injury, 245, 323
    self-harm, 266–8, *see also* suicide
nonsteroidal anti-inflammatory drugs, 60
noradrenaline, 20, *457*
norethisterone, *457*
normal ranges, 5–11, *6*, *7*, *9–11*
notifiable infectious diseases, 152, *152–3*
Novoseven (Activated Factor VIIa), 50
NSAIDs, 60
nystatin, *457*

obesity, 282–3
    drug dosage and, 411
    therapeutic diets, 39–40
obstructive jaundice, 94
occupational therapy for burns, 361
octreotide, *457*
ocular emergencies, 318–26, *see also* eyes
oedema, cerebral, 205–6
oesophageal atresia, 370–1
oestrogen preparations, *458*
omeprazole, *458*
oncological emergencies, 292–6
ondansetron, *458*
opioid analgesics, 59–65
oral analgesia, 59–61
oral bleeding, 335
oral conditions in palliative care, 384
oral lacerations, 330
oral progestogen-only pill, 289
oral rehydration therapy (ORT), 220
orbital cellulitis, 324–5
oro-facial emergencies, 331–6
orthopaedic problems, 284–5
    trauma, 374–82
Osgood-Schlatter disease, 284

osteomyelitis, *120*, 132–3
otitis media, *116*, 328–9
overhydration, 99
oxandrolone, *458*
oxybutynin hydrochloride, *459*
oxygen tension (hypoxaemia), 85–9
oxygen therapy, 89, 171

paediatric doses, *see* drug dosage
paediatrics, 1–4
pain, 57–66, 296, *see also* analgesia
    dental, 335–6
        pain faces scale, 58, *58*
        palliative care, 384
palate, neonatal examination, 102–3
palliative medicine, 383–5
pallid breath-holding attacks, 232
pancreatic extract, *459*
pancuronium, *459*
paracetamol, 59–60, *460*
paraffin liquid, *460*
paraldehyde, 237, *460*
paraphimosis, 365
parenteral opioids, 61
paroxysmal disorders, 231–2, *see also*
        epilepsy
partial seizures, 229–30
pathogens, *see* infections
patient-controlled analgesia (PCA),
        63–4
pelvic examination, 280
penetrating injury, avoidance of, 139–40
penicillamine, *461*
penicillin G, *421*
penicillin V, *462*
penis development, *278*
penis surgery, 363–5
pentamidine, *461*
percentile charts, 390, *391–403*
perimortem evaluation of metabolic
        disorders, 110–11
peritoneal dialysis, 109
peritonitis, acute, *119*
permethrin, 307–8
pertussis, *142*
pethidine, *461*
'petit mal' seizures, 230–1
pharmacological antagonists, 339–40
    sedation and, 351–2

pheniramine, *433*
phenobarbitone, 235–7, *461*
phenoxybenzamine, *461*
phenoxymethyl penicillin, *462*
phenylketonuria (PKU), 40
phenytoin, 235–6, *462*
phimosis, 363–4
phosphate salts, *462, 463*
phototherapy in jaundice, *95,* 95–6
physical abuse, *see* child abuse
physiotherapy for burns, 361–2
physostigmine, *463*
phytomenadione, *463, see also* menadione
piperacillin, *464*
pituitary emergencies, 190–1
PKU (phenylketonuria), 40
plantar warts, 312
plasma studies, 6
platelet concentrates, 47–8
play, 4
pleural effusion, 178
pneumatoceles, 178–9
pneumonia, *116,* 177–9
    septicaemia and, 131
pneumothorax, 183–4
poisoning, 337–40
    carbon monoxide, 356
    envenomations, 240, 340–2
Poisons Information Centre, 337–41
poliomyelitis, 241
polycystic ovary syndrome, 282
polyethylene glycol, *464*
post-traumatic seizures, 244
postinfectious glomerulonephritis, 252
postoperative period
    acute adrenal insufficiency, 188
    fever, 373
    fluid therapy, 76
    ocular problems, 326
potassium, 71, 74–5, *see also*
        hyperkalaemia; hypokalaemia
    diabetic ketoacidosis, 204
potassium chloride, *465*
potassium salts (oral), *464*
preanaesthetic preparations, 343–5
precipitated sulfur, 307–8
precocious puberty, 280
prednisolone, *453, 465*
    in nephrotic syndrome, 254–5

prednisone, *465*
premature babies, formula for, *35*
premedication, 344
preoperative period, 75, 343–5
prescriptions, *see also* drug dosage
    abbreviations in, 410–11, *411*
preseptal cellulitis, 324–5
pressure ulcers, 385
probenecid, *465*
procainamide, *465*
procedures, sedation for, 346–54
prochlorperazine, *465*
progestogen, 289
promethazine, *466*
prophylaxis
    asplenic patients, 150, *151*
    cardiac lesions, 159–60
    contacts of infectious diseases, 141,
        142–5
    needlestick injury, 141
    tetanus, 380–1
    UTIs, 250–1
propranolol, *466*
proptosis, unilateral, 325–6
propylthiouracil, *466*
prostaglandin E1, *414*
protamine sulfate, *466*
protein
    intake, 31–2, 41
    proteinuria, 255–6
    replacement after burns, 357–9
prothrombinex, 50
pseudomembranous croup, 166
psychiatric conditions, 265–75
    assessment by non-psychiatrists,
        268–70
    medical presentation of, 273–4,
        274–5
psychogenic abdominal pain, 370
puberty, 277, *278,* 280
pubic hair development, *278*
pull-to-sit manoeuvre, 101
pulmonary hypertension, 102
pupils (of eyes), 20–1, 325
pyelonephritis, antibiotic therapy, *118*
pyloric stenosis, 77, 371
pyrantel embonate, *467*
pyrazinamide, *467*
pyridoxine, *481*

radius fracture, 378
ranitidine, *467*
rape, 304–5
rash in septicaemia, 131
recombinant coagulation factors, 48–50
red eye, acute, 323–4
reflux, 222–3
rehydration, *see* fluid therapy
renal disease, 248–64
  indicatons for biopsy, 253, 255
  therapeutic diets, 39
rescue retrieval services, 26
resonium, *471*
respiratory diseases, 164–85
respiratory distress, *see also* breathing
  dyspnoea in palliative care, 385
  neonates, 83–7, *85*
  oncological emergencies, 294
  trauma survey, 375
respiratory examination of neonates, 102
respiratory foreign bodies, 164
respiratory tract infections, *116*
respiratory tract injury from burns, 356
resuscitation
  dehydration, 73
  diabetic ketoacidosis, 202
  gastroenteritis, 218
  metabolic disorders, 109
  sedation and, 348
  trauma, 376
retinal detachment, 322
retinol (vitamin A), *479*
Rhesus isoimmunisation, 95–6
riboflavine, *480*
rifampicin, *467*
risperidone, *468*
rocuronium, *468*
route of administration guidelines, 410
roxithromycin, *468*
RSV, infectious disease
  recommendations, *145*
rubella, *143*

salbutamol, 171–3, *468–9*
salmeterol, *469*
salmon calcitonin, *422*
scabies, 307–8
scalded skin syndrome, 309–10
scalp, tinea, 310

scar problems from burns, 362
school exclusion for infectious diseases,
  141, *142–5*
schoolwork in hospital, 4
sclera, lacerations of, 321
scoliosis, 284, *409*
Scopolamine, *446*
screening tests, 408
  cystic fibrosis, 179–80
  metabolic disorders, 106–7
scrotum, *278*, 365–7, *see also* testes
seborrhoeic dermatitis, 313
sedation, 346–54, *353–4*
  in diabetes, 208–10
  lacerations, 380
seizures, 229–30, 244, *see also* febrile
  convulsions
self-harm, 266–8, *see also* suicide
sennoside laxative (Senokot®), *469–70*
sepsis, neonatal, 89–92
septic arthritis, *120*, 133–4
septicaemia (bacteraemia), 124–5, 130–2
Seretide®, *422*
sertraline, *470*
serum drug levels, *10*
serum ferritin, 6
sexual abuse, 302–5
sexual ambiguity, *see* ambiguous genitalia
sexual assault, 304–5
sexual development, *see* puberty
sexual health, 288–90, *290*
sexually transmitted diseases, 289–90,
  290
sharps, disposal of, 139–40
shock, *see* circulatory failure (shock)
short gut syndrome, 221
short stature, 280
shunt problems, *117*, 245–7
sick euthyroidism, 199–200
sickle cell disease, 54–5, 150
simple partial seizures, 229
skin conditions, 307–17
  dermatitis, 312–13
  grafting for burns, 362
  infections, *117–18*, 120
  lacerations, 379–81
  in palliative care, 385
skull fractures, 244–5
skull X-rays, 242

sleep disturbance in palliative care, 385
slipped capital femoral epiphysis, 285
snake bite, 240, 340–2
snoring, 164, 166
social skills, normal milestones, *406–7*
social workers, 361–2
sodium, 71, *see also* hypernatraemia;
    hyponatraemia
  deficit therapy, 74, 100
  diabetic ketoacidosis, 203–4
sodium benzoate, *470*
sodium bicarbonate, *470*
  diabetic ketoacidosis, 204
sodium cromoglycate, *471*
sodium fusidate, *471*
sodium nitroprusside, *471*
sodium phenylbutyrate, *471*
sodium polystyrene sulphonate, *471*
sodium valproate, 234, *472*
soft tissue lacerations, oro-facial, 332
solid food, introduction of, 31
somatisation, 291
sorbitol 70%, *472*
sotalol, *472*
spasmodic croup, 166
special formulae, *see* infant formulae
specimen collection, blood, 5–6
speech, normal milestones, *406–7*
spider bite, 340–2
spine
  control during trauma surveys, 375
  neonatal examination, 102
  spinal cord lesions, 240
spironolactone, *472*
spleen, 54–5, 150, *151*
stabilisation of neonates, 80–3
standing height measurement, 389
staphylococcal scalded skin syndrome,
    309–10
staphylococcal tracheitis, 166
Staphylococcus aureus TSS, 134–6
status epilepticus, 236–7
STDs, 289–90, *290*
steroids, preoperative assessment, 345
strabismus, 325
streptococcal TSS, 135–6
stridor, 165–6
stroke, *see* cerebral infarction
subcutaneous insulin, 206–7

subcutaneous opioids, 61
subdural empyema, *117*
succimer (DMSA), 250, *472*
suck, neonatal examination, 101
sucralfate, *473*
sucrase-isomaltase deficiency, 37
suicide
  depression and, 273
  high-risk groups, 287
  non-accidental self-harm, 266–8
sulfasalazine, *473*
sulfur, precipitated, 307–8
sulphamethoxazole/trimethoprim, *430*,
    477
superglue in eyes, 320–1
supine length measurement, 390
supplementary feeds, 41
supraglottitis, 168–9
supraventricular tachycardia (SVT), 14,
    162–3
surface area nomograms, *391*
surgery, 363–73, *see also* anaesthesia;
    postoperative period; preoperative
    period
  acute adrenal insufficiency and, 188
  diabetes and, 207–10
  fluid therapy, 75–8
  neonates, 76
  sedation for, 346–54
surveillance, child health, *see*
    developmental assessment
suxamethonium, *473*
sweat tests, for cystic fibrosis, 180
symptom control in cancer, 296
symptomatic adolescents, 291
syncope, 231
syrup of ipecac, outmoded, 339

tacrolimus, *473*
tazobactam/piperacillin, *464*
Tazocin®, *464*
teenagers, *see* adolescents
teeth
  eruption times, *336*
  trauma, 331–5
teicoplanin, *474*
telephone numbers
  child protection social worker, 297
  DoCS Helpline, 298

Employee Assistance Program, 388
infectious disease notifications, 152
medical retrieval, 28–9
Newborn ICU availability, 83
Poisons Information Centre, 337
temazepam, *474*
terbutaline, *474*
terminal dyspnoea, 385
testes, 365–7, *409, see also* scrotum
tetanus prophylaxis, 380–1
thalassaemia, 55–6
theophylline, 173, *474*
therapeutic diets, *see* diet and nutrition
thiabendazole, *475*
thiamine (vitamin B1), *480*
thiopentone sodium, *475*
thioridazine, *475*
thrombocytopenia, 47–8, 53
leukaemia and, 294
thyroid disorders, 197–200
thyroid function tests, *11*, 198
thyroidectomy, 200
thyrotoxicosis, 198–9
thyroxine, *476, see also* triiodothyronine
tibia, fracture, 378
ticarcillin and clavulanic acid
(Timentin®), *476*
tick bite, 240
tinea, 310–11
tinidazole, *476*
tobramycin, *476–7*
tocopherol, *483*
toes, fractures of, 379
tonsillitis, *116*, 328
tooth, *see* teeth
topirimate, *477*
tortion of the testis, 365
total parenteral nutrition, 78–9
toxic shock syndrome (TSS), 134–6,
136
TPN, 78–9
tracheal intubation, *see* endotracheal
intubation
transfusion reactions, 46
transplants, liver, 227–8
transport, *see* emergency patient
transport
trauma, *see also* head injury
eyes, 318–23

oro-facial, 331–4
orthopaedic, 374–82
post-traumatic seizures, 244
triiodothyronine, *477, see also* thyroxine
trimeprazine, *477*
trimethoprim, *477*
trimethoprim/sulphamethoxazole, *430,
477*
TSS, *see* toxic shock syndrome
tube feeds, *36*, 41, *see also* endotracheal
intubation (ET)

ulna fracture, 378
umbilical hernia, 368
undescended testes, 366–7
unilateral proptosis, 325–6
urine
collection and analysis, 41, 249
output in burns, 359
tests for metabolic disorders, 107
urinary tract infections (UTIs), *118*,
131, 248–51
ursodeoxycholic acid, *478*
UTIs, *118*, 131, 248–51

vaccination, *see* immunisation
valproic acid, *see* sodium valproate
vancomycin, *478*
varicella zoster infections, 121, 146
vascular disease risk factors, 161
vasculitis, 136–8, *137*
vecuronium, *478*
venereal diseases, *see* sexually transmitted
diseases
venom identification, 340–1
venous access, *see* intravenous lines
ventral suspension, 101
verapamil, *478–9*
vigabatrin, 234, *479*
viral infections
bronchiolitis, 174–6
febrile illness and, 124
IgA nephritis and, 252
laryngotracheitis, 166
myositis, 241
neonatal sepsis, 92
universal precautions against, 139–40
vision, *406–7, 409*
neonatal examination, 101

visual analogue scale (of pain), 58
vitamin A (retinol), *479*
vitamin B1 (thiamine), *480*
vitamin B2 (riboflavine), *480*
vitamin B3 (niacin), *481*
vitamin B6 (pyridoxine), *481*
vitamin B12 (hyroxocobalamin), *482*
vitamin C (ascorbic acid), *483*
vitamin D2 (ergocalciferol), *438, see also*
    calcitriol
vitamin E (tocopherol), *483*
vitamin H, *421*
vitamin K1 (phytomenadione), *463*
vitamin K3 (menadione), *452*
vitamins, 32, 71
vitreous haemorrhage, 322
vomiting, 370–2
    gastro-oesophageal reflux and, 222
    opioid analgesics, 64
    palliative care, 384

walking movements, neonatal
    examination, 101
warfarin, *484*

warts, 311–12
water requirements, 67, *69,* 69–70, *70,*
    see also fluid therapy
    neonates, 98–9
web addresses
    gastroenteritis management, 221
    genetic autopsy protocol, 111
    medical retrieval, 29
weight, 390, *409*
    charts, *393, 395, 399, 401*
wheeze, 165–6
whole bowel lavage, 339
whooping cough (pertussis), *142*
Wilson's disease, 225–6
wound healing in burns, 360–1

X-rays
    chest, 83, 87
    neck, 170
Xylocaine, *see* lignocaine

Yersinia septicaemia, 55–6

zinc sulfate, *484*